COMMERCE
AND THE SPREAD OF
PESTS AND DISEASE VECTORS

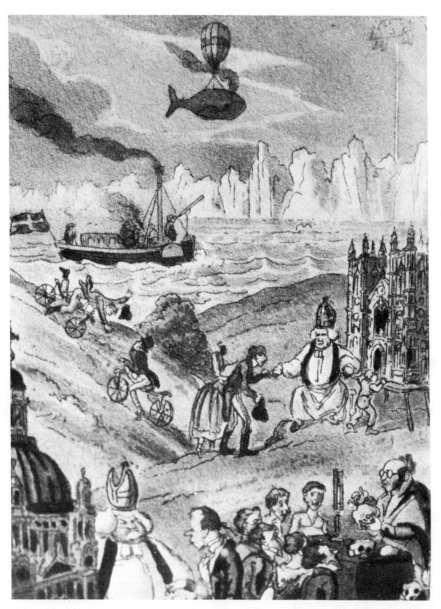

Hand-colored in the original, the George Cruikshank frontispiece was first published in the same role in Francis Moore's "The Age of Intellect: or Clerical Showfolk, and Wonderful Layfolk" (London: William Hone, 1819). The reader is referred to this amusing though tedious poem for the clerical allusions; those concerning transportation are mentioned in the Preface.

COMMERCE
AND THE SPREAD OF
PESTS AND DISEASE VECTORS

Edited by

Marshall Laird

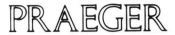

PRAEGER SPECIAL STUDIES • PRAEGER SCIENTIFIC

New York • Philadelphia • Eastbourne, UK
Toronto • Hong Kong • Tokyo • Sydney

Library of Congress Cataloging in Publication Data

Main entry under title:

Commerce and the spread of pests and disease vectors.

Based on a symposium held at the XV Pacific Science
Congress in Dunedin, New Zealand, Feb. 1–11, 1983.
Bibliography: p.
Includes index.
1. Pest introduction—Congresses.   2. Aeronautics,
Commercial—Congresses.   3. Pest control—Congresses.
4. Vector control—Congresses.   5. Insects as carriers
of diseases—Congresses.   6. Insect control—Congresses.
I. Laird, Marshall.   II. Pacific Science Congress (15th :
1983 : Dunedin, N.Z.)
SB990.C65   363.7'8   83–16627
ISBN 0–03–062137–2

Published in 1984 by Praeger Publishers
CBS Educational and Professional Publishing
a Division of CBS Inc.
521 Fifth Avenue, New York, New York 10175 U.S.A.

© 1984 by Praeger Publishers

456789   052   987654321

Printed in the United States of America
on acid-free paper

Dedication

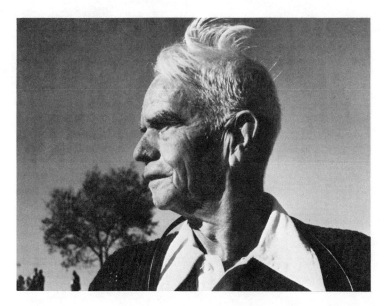

Bill Sullivan (1908-1979) at Simpson's Gap
Northern Territory, Australia
17 August 1972

Photo Credit:
Lynnaire Clark Hawker

A modest and kindly gentleman with an endearing sense of
humor, the late Dr. William Nicholas Sullivan, Jr., served
his country and humanity well. He was a distinguished
researcher whose innovative investigations took him around
the world and to out-of-the-way assignments and places,
including radiological monitoring in the nuclear clouds
during the July 1946 atomic bomb tests held at Bikini Atoll,
and a visit to Australia's Red Center on his way to participate in the 14th International Congress of Entomology
(Canberra, August 1972). His coinvention (with Dr. Lyle
D. Goodhue) of the aerosol "bomb" (World War II's "bug
bomb") materially reduced allied mosquito-vectored disease
casualties in the Pacific theater and elsewhere, opened the
way to practical aircraft disinsection on the scale demanded

by the postwar flourishing of aviation, and was fundamental to the development of today's aerosol industry. Among his many honors and awards, one that came late in life and that meant a great deal to him had rarely been granted to a Westerner. This was his (1977) doctorate from the Tokyo University of Agriculture.

This book is dedicated to Bill for his vision, qualities of friendship, and unflagging eagerness to cooperate with others in working towards a happier and healthier world.

Acknowledgments

It was a pleasure collaborating with Dr. J. S. ("Mani") Pillai of the Department of Microbiology, University of Otago, in his capacity as Convener of Section J, Entomology, 15th Pacific Science Congress. His speedy handling of preliminary correspondence and communications generally allowed us to keep in close contact despite the distance separating our institutions. In fact, all participants in Symposium 7—the presentations from which form the basis of this book—are to be complimented for providing their contributions rapidly enough to allow of publication towards the end of the same year in which our session took place (February 9 and 10, 1983) in Dunedin, New Zealand. A special word of thanks is due to the Coorganizer of Symposium 7, Dr. Pat S. Dale (Ministry of Agriculture and Fisheries, Auckland) for his friendly assistance in chairing the meeting. Appreciation is expressed to the authorities of the Memorial University of Newfoundland (MUN) for supporting the editorial burden in various ways. Finally, thanks are due to Mr. Roy Ficken (photographer, Biology Department, MUN) for processing a number of illustrations, and especially to Ms. Ruby Strang for invaluable secretarial assistance.

Preface

This book had its genesis at the joint slide presentation on "Aircraft Disinsection—its history, status, and future" presented by the editor and the late Dr. W. N. Sullivan, Jr., during the 14th International Congress of Entomology (Canberra, Australia, August 22-30, 1972). The 11th Session of WHO's Expert Committee on Insecticides, "Aircraft Disinsection," in Geneva (September, 19-24, 1960) had envisaged an early transition from hand-held single-use aerosol insecticide dispensers to built-in semiautomatic spraying systems for in-flight treatment of all enclosed spaces of aircraft with suitable vapor pressure pesticides. Having chaired that Session and soon afterwards joined the WHO Secretariat for a 6-year term, I enjoyed associations with Dr. Sullivan while he was undertaking a task on WHO's behalf, that was intended to be the final research and development phase preceding the general adoption of such built-in systems. Unhappily, this task was set aside in the early 1970s because it was demonstrated that some harm to certain materials of aircraft construction might result from the routine use of vapor pressure insecticides in aircraft. By this time I had returned to academic life; I shared with Dr. Sullivan growing misgivings that failure to achieve a standard semiautomatic solution to aircraft disinsection was now associated with a combination of rapid increase in global aviation (inevitably favoring insect dispersal hazards) and steady decrease in the conscientiousness with which airport insect control and disinsection were being regarded by many countries.

Appreciating that the public relations aspects of disinsection were involved too, at a time when the DDT controversy and speculation about possible adverse effects of aerosols on the ozone layer were occasioning widespread concern, we decided to write a joint book objectively presenting all the facts of the case. Dr. Sullivan's death came at a time when we were well advanced in assembling the relevant background information. Moreover, during the 1970s there were worrying new developments involving additional establishments of medically and economically important insects, through transportation, particularly in the Pacific. The transportation in question included not only larger and faster aircraft but also shipping containers, which were now beginning to dominate the carriage of cargo by sea—and to a growing extent by jumbo jets, too.

On being invited to organize one of the symposia in Section J (Entomology) of the XV Pacific Science Congress (Dunedin, New Zealand, February 1-10, 1983), I thus felt it appropriate to suggest *Accidental Introductions of Insects Through Human Agency* as the topic. So titled, Symposium 7 of the Congress brought together a number of scientists to consider all aspects of this subject on February 9 and 10, 1983. This book's chapters were expanded from papers then presented (these were duly abstracted in Programme Volumes 1 and 2, distributed to participants). While the titles of Symposium 7 and the present work were deliberately made comprehensive in recognition of the essentially global nature of the problem discussed, the Pacific is always at the center of the stage. This both reflects our topic's relevance to the Congress theme of *Conservation, Development and Utilization of the Resources of the Pacific* (all of which goals necessarily suffer when new insect pests and disease vectors arrive), and the fact that so many Pacific lands (particularly isolated islands) have proved especially vulnerable to imported fauna able to thrive in previously underutilized ecological niches—often in the absence or near-absence of natural predators, parasites, and pathogens.

Our frontispiece was originally published in 1819. Its artist, George Cruikshank, was clearly comfortable abreast of profound contemporary changes that must have made his era as intellectually stimulating as ours. Thus, in the aftermath of the Napoleonic Wars, sea transportation was about to be revolutionized by the steam engine. With two more years remaining before little ships of the type he sketched first came into service on the Dover-Calais channel crossing, Cruikshank nicely captured the birth of a new means of locomotion that was destined to accelerate the long-distance spread of insect stowaways and eventually to augment beyond all imagining the volume of cargo carried aboard individual vessels.

Balloons were much in the news at the time. Already there had been notable balloon voyages and even pertinent high-altitude experimentation with insects (see Chapter 15) foreshadowing the Apollo IV research mentioned in Chapter 2. Cruikshank's balloon-whale whimsy (a Mr. Egg having made a rival case for steam-propelled balloon-packets between London and Paris) anticipated the commercial resumption of animal transport—intentional and unintentional—by international aviation a little more than a century afterwards. The practical history of aircraft disinsection commenced at the conclusion of the first trans-Atlantic passenger flights to the USA made by the German dirigible *Graf Zeppelin* in 1928 (see Chapters 2 and 15). Since then, not only has an extensive literature accumulated concerning the inadvertent transportation of pests and vectors by heavier-than-air planes, but also the carriage of the largest mammals (including whales!) aboard jumbo jets has become a reality.

Recognizing that of late years there has been widely diminishing concern with enforcement of the national and international recommendations and regulations that emerged from over half-a-century's experience of accidental importations—and sometimes establishments—of insect pests and vectors through ever-expanding aviation and changing shipping practices, the coauthors of this book have attempted to provide a status report in hopes of its being of some service in redirecting attention to relevant problems intimately concerned with human health and welfare.

It is regretted that one aspect of commerce has not been adequately covered in this book through failure to locate a scientist from Latin America in a position to discuss the role of road transportation in the spread of insect pests and vectors. Reverting to the frontispiece, Cruikshank's illustration of two velocipedes (the ancestral bicycle, only just invented in that same year of 1819) presaged the giant leap forward in land transportation that was to come later in his century and to be so greatly amplified in ours. The Pan-American Highway might have served as an outstanding example of a route along which serious truck-borne insect dispersal hazards exist, in a phase of political instability and at a time, moreover, when containerization is increasingly involving the transshipment of unopened cargo modules from both ships and aircraft to ground haulage vehicles.

It should be observed in closing that a modest amount of overlap has been countenanced between individual chapters so that these can better stand alone.

Marshall Laird
St. John's, Newfoundland, Canada
June 15, 1983

List of Contributors

I. D. Carter: WHO, Geneva, Switzerland

P. S. Dale: Ministry of Agriculture and Fisheries, Auckland, New Zealand

E. Dharmaraju: University of the South Pacific, Alafua Campus, Apia, Western Samoa

L. M. Forster: Otago Museum, Dunedin, New Zealand

J. M. Goldsmid: University of Tasmania, Hobart, Tasmania, Australia

G. Grodhaus: California Department of Health Services, Berkeley, CA, USA

D. K. Hayes: USDA, Beltsville, MD, USA

D. Jewell: San Mateo County Mosquito Abatement District, Burlingame, CA, USA

H. Kurahashi: National Institute of Health, Tokyo, Japan

Marshall Laird: Research Professor, Memorial University of Newfoundland, St. John's, Newfoundland, Canada

W. A. Langsford: Commonwealth Department of Health, Woden, ACT, Australia.

P. A. Maddison: Entomology Division, DSIR, Auckland, New Zealand

J. A. R. Miles: University of Otago, Dunedin, New Zealand

J. S. Pillai: University of Otago, Dunedin, New Zealand

N. Rajapaksa: Commonwealth Department of Health, Woden, ACT, Australia

S. Ramalingan: University of Malaya, Kuala Lumpur, Malaysia

R. C. Russell: Commonwealth Institute of Health, University of Sydney, Sydney, NSW, Australia

L. S. Self: World Health Organization, WPRO, Manila, Philippines

A. Smith: WHO, Geneva, Switzerland

S. Takahashi: Narita Airport Quarantine Station, Narita, Japan

R. A. Ward: Walter Reed Army Institute of Research, Washington, D.C., USA

P. I. Whelan: Northern Territory Health Department, Darwin, NT, Australia

Glossary of Abbreviations

ACT	Australian Commonwealth Territory
APHIS	Animal and Plant Health Inspection Service (USDA)
ARS	Agricultural Research Service (USDA)
BOAC	British Overseas Airways Corporation (present successor, British Airways)
CER	Closer Economic Relations (a trade agreement between Australia and New Zealand signed in November 1982)
CPA	Canadian Pacific Airlines
CSIRO	(Australian) Commonwealth Scientific and Industrial Research Organization
DDT	1,1,1-Trichloro-2,2-di(4-chlorophenyl) ethane
DDVP	dichlorvos
DHF	Dengue haemorrhagic fever
DSIR	(New Zealand) Department of Scientific and Industrial Research
FAO	Food and Agriculture Organization (U.N.)
FIFRA	(United States) Federal Insecticide, Fungicide and Rodenticide Act
HMSO	Her Majesty's Stationery Office
IATA	International Air Transport Association
ICAO	International Civil Aviation Organization
IHR	International Health Regulations (WHO)
ISR	International Sanitary Regulations
JE	Japanese B encephalitis
NASA	National Aeronautics and Space Administration (USA)
NSW	New South Wales, Australia
NT	Northern Territory, Australia
PNG	Papua New Guinea
QIMR	Queensland Institute of Medical Research
RRV	Ross River virus
ULV	ultra-low volume
UNDP	United Nations Development Programme
USDA	United States Department of Agriculture
USPHS	United States Public Health Service
WHO	World Health Organization

Contents

Chapter 1

International Transportation of Mosquitoes of Public Health Importance

A. Smith and I. D. Carter

> *It ain't the things we don't know that hurt us.*
> *It's the things we do know that ain't so.*
> —Artemus Ward

INTRODUCTION

There are many published records of mosquitoes found in aircraft operating on international flights and a smaller number of such records of these insects found in international shipping, examples of which are given in the Appendix. There are also some published reports of mosquitoes established through international transport in receptive areas where they were previously absent (see Appendix), and presumably other unobserved or unrecorded incidents have occurred. For the entomologist these records may provide very interesting data for a variety of reasons, but for the epidemiologist they are of no consequence unless they clearly show that the insects in question present a threat of introduction or spread of disease. It is therefore constructive to identify situations in which mosquitoes have been introduced into new areas, established themselves as a significant part of the local fauna, and taken an active role in transmission of disease. It is also relevant to be informed of incidents in which people have become infected in the vicinity of international airports—located in nonendemic areas—through the bite of an infective mosquito introduced

1

from an endemic area by an international aircraft. The significance of these findings can then be considered in terms of the risk of establishment of exotic diseases into new areas and in relation to planning and implementing appropriate cost-effective control measures.

REPORTS OF MOSQUITO-BORNE DISEASES
TRANSMITTED BY THE INTRODUCTION AND
ESTABLISHMENT OF SPECIES NOT KNOWN
TO HAVE BEEN ESTABLISHED PREVIOUSLY

Mauritius

Malaria was unknown in Mauritius until the second half of the nineteenth century when between 1867 and 1868 there was an epidemic of malaria that caused 32,000 deaths. This catastrophe has been attributed to the introduction of *Anopheles gambiae s.1.* by shipping from Madagascar or the mainland of Africa and its establishment on Mauritius (Bruce-Chwatt 1969).

Brazil

Anopheles gambiae s.1., which was unknown in Brazil until 1930, established itself in great numbers and was the principal vector of an epidemic of malaria involving 300,000 cases and 16,000 deaths before it was eradicated in 1940. Subsequently five living *A.* gambiae s.1.* were discovered in 1943 at Natal, Brazil, where there is an international airport. It was considered that *A. gambiae s.1.* was first introduced into Brazil by fast shipping operating between Brazil and West Africa, or perhaps by aircraft (Soper and Wilson 1943; WHO 1955).

---

*Throughout this book generic names of mosquitoes have been abbreviated to the initial letter only. While the convenient practice of abbreviating to the second letter to avoid confusing e.g. *Anopheles* with *Aedes* is currently much used by mosquito workers, it is not customary in broader zoological usage, and is held inappropriate to a work in which organisms of various other taxa besides Culicidae are under discussion–Ed.

Egypt

In Egypt there was an epidemic of malaria between 1942-44 with about 170,000 cases and 12,000 deaths. The epidemic followed the introduction of *A. gambiae s.1.* possibly by shipping coming down the Nile from the Sudan. This vector was eradicated by 1945 following "a costly and stubborn campaign" (WHO 1955).

Guam

In Guam, Marianas, an outbreak of dengue fever, involving some cases of dengue haemorrhagic fever (DHF) occurred in 1975, transmitted by *Aedes albopictus,* which was first detected on the island between 1944-45 (see Chapter 8). Control was effective and carried out in an emergency program by the combined military forces on the island.

Prior to World War II Guam was well within that part of the Pacific known as the "malaria-free zone" because of the absence of anopheline mosquitoes. In 1966 six cases of malaria were reported in Guam, there being good evidence that introduced autochthonous malaria was responsible for two of them. Similarly in 1969, when six malaria cases were diagnosed, one of the victims had not previously left the continental United States and would appear to have been infected either by a mosquito recently introduced by aircraft from a malarious area or by a vector breeding in Guam. *Anopheles indefinitus,* established in Guam about 1948, could have acquired an infection locally from military personnel who contracted malaria in Southeast Asia and were evacuated to Guam for hospitalization (Nowell 1977; see Chapter 8).

RECORDS OF MALARIA CASES IN THE VICINITY OF EUROPEAN INTERNATIONAL AIRPORTS ARISING FROM IMPORTED INFECTIVE VECTORS

Switzerland

In August 1970 two military recruits, who had never visited malaria-endemic areas and who were stationed close to Zurich International Airport, became infected with *Plasmodium falciparum*. A third autochthonous case due to *P. falciparum* was reported in August 1972 and one involving *P. malariae* infection occurred in an old woman who lived close to Zurich International Airport and had never visited endemic areas. The most probable explanation of the occurrence of these malaria cases is the transport by air of malaria-infected anophelines from endemic areas, and their subsequently transmitting the infection to people in the immediate surroundings of the airport.

France

Nine cases of autochthonous "airborne malaria" were detected between 1974 and 1978 (eight with *P. falciparum* and one with *P. vivax*). The infections occurred in the vicinity of Paris airports and were considered to have been transmitted by anophelines carried by aircraft arriving from tropical areas (Gentilini and Danis 1981).

Netherlands

The last autochthonous malaria case in the Netherlands was recorded in 1958. On August 27, 1978 an infection with *P. falciparum* was reported in a 24-year-old woman who had never left the Netherlands. She lived in Hoofddorp, a village about 1.5 km distance from Schiphol Airport, where her home was next to one of the landing and take-off strips of the airport. In the past the local vector *Anopheles labranchiae* ssp. *atroparvus* had only transmitted *P. vivax* malaria when this disease was endemic in the Netherlands. Local transmission of *P. falciparum* had not been recored before. It is most likely that the first autochthonous *P. falciparum* infection in this country was transmitted by an imported infective *Anopheles* transported to Schiphol by an aircraft (Anonymous 1979b). In 1981 another autochthonous case (*P. falciparum*) was detected in a 10-year-old child who had never been in a malarious country. The girl, living in Amsterdam, sailed on the Nieuve Meer (New Lake) situated at about 1,500 m distance from Schiphol Airport. She passed the night on board the boat in a side canal of the lake where she was badly bitten by mosquitoes. It is most likely that this second autochthonous case of *falciparum* malaria was transmitted by an infected *Anopheles* mosquito imported by an aircraft (Anonymous 1981).

Belgium

Two cases of autochthonous malaria (*P. falciparum*) occurred in August 1982 in a community situated about 2 km from the International Airport of Zaventern. Two brothers aged 18 and 24 years, respectively, who had never been abroad, fell ill a week apart. They had probably been bitten by infected mosquitoes that had been imported by aircraft from a tropical country (Anonymous 1982).

FACTORS AFFECTING THE ESTABLISHMENT OF
MOSQUITO VECTORS AND THE INTRODUCTION
OF MOSQUITO-BORNE DISEASES INTO NEW AREAS

When considering the factors that affect the establishment of mosquito vectors and the introduction of mosquito-borne diseases into new areas, it is interesting and important to consider why the number of newly established mosquito vectors, and the introduction of mosquito-borne diseases, has not increased in relation to the enormous increase in volume, speed, and varied nature of international transportation, particularly air traffic, over the last 20 years (Figure 1-1).

Some factors mitigating against the establishment of mosquito vectors and the introduction of mosquito-borne diseases into new areas, are:

1. The greatest volume of international air traffic operates between temperate countries, for instance, those of Europe and North America where the risk of mosquito vectors and of mosquito-borne diseases being introduced is low.
2. A considerable volume of air traffic operates between countries with a similar mosquito fauna and mosquito-borne diseases, for example, African countries south of the Sahara.
3. An important group of vectors, that is, certain aedines of the subgenus *Stegomyia,* are relatively uncommon in mosquito collections from aircraft. The risk of their introduction into new areas by this means may thus be low (WHO 1955). Nevertheless, *Aedes albopictus* may have been introduced into Guam aboard insufficiently disinsected aircraft (Morrill et al. 1952). Chapters 5, 6, 8, 12 and 15 of this book cite further examples of recent range extensions for this mosquito and *Aedes (Stegomyia) aegypti.* The prospect that females of the latter already harboring yellow fever virus might enter aircraft departing from a country where this disease is endemic, subsequently transmitting the infection to humans either during the journey or following escape in a receptive zone, has

Figure 1-1. Passengers, freight, and mail.

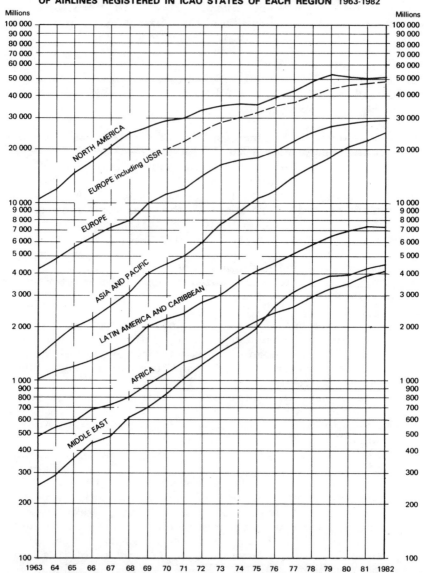

LONG-TERM REGIONAL TRENDS

**TOTAL TONNE-KILOMETRES PERFORMED BY SCHEDULED SERVICES
OF AIRLINES REGISTERED IN ICAO STATES OF EACH REGION** 1963-1982

Note. — The figures shown for each region include all operations of airlines registered in the region. The regions are divided on a geographical basis as used in ICAO statistical publications. (North America comprises Canada and the United States only).

Source: Annual Report of the Council 1982, published as Doc 9382 by the International Civil Aviation Organization, Montreal, 1983. Reproduced by permission of ICAO.

in the past been a major factor according high priority to aircraft disinsection and airport mosquito control specifically aimed at *A. aegypti,* in such receptive areas. Vigilance in these connections should certainly continue.

4. Some countries, even if vulnerable to the introduction of new vector species, are not receptive—or have a low receptivity—to them, for instance, *Anopheles farauti* might have difficulty in establishing itself in New Zealand due to the cool winter there.

5. In some tropical countries most international aircraft arrive and depart in daytime, thus reducing the risk of *Anopheles* entering them, even in heavily anopheline-infested airport areas.

6. Many mosquitoes found in aircraft are dead when collected, and living mosquitoes have a number of hazardous steps in their life-cycle to overcome before breeding can be established in a new area, for example, leaving the aircraft, obtaining a blood-meal, surviving to lay eggs, and locating a suitable breeding site.

7. Although, in the past, shipping has been implicated in the transportation of *Anopheles gambiae s.1.* into Mauritius, Brazil, and Egypt, marine shipping does not, in general, appear to be an important means of international transportation of *Anopheles,* since it is slow and largely ocean-going. Coastal craft do, however, present *Aedes* and *Anopheles* problems in some areas, for instance, the Torres Straits between Australia and Papua New Guinea (PNG). Coastal shipping has been claimed to be a cause of reinfestation by *Aedes aegypti* in South America.

8. Varying levels of vector surveillance and control are maintained in international airports and seaports as provided for in the International Health Regulations (WHO 1983). In some areas, such as the South Pacific with its "malaria-free zone," particular attention is also given to aircraft disinsection.

9. As can be seen from the above incidents of airport-associated malaria in Europe where nearly all cases were *Plasmodium falciparum* infections, the risk of an outbreak of malignant tertian malaria is negligible since the parasite will not infect the local European vector *Anopheles maculipennis* and the climate is too cold to support breeding of imported tropical vectors.

FACTORS CONTRIBUTING TO THE ESTABLISHMENT OF MOSQUITO VECTORS AND THE INTRODUCTION OF MOSQUITO-BORNE DISEASES INTO NEW AREAS

1. Lack of the necessary technical information to enable value judgements to be made by health administrations on the level of risk of the introduction of mosquito vectors, on their becoming established, and on the transmission of disease.

In particular,

a) *Insufficient identification of those specific air routes and international airports to which particular attention should be given to surveillance in and around the airports.* While on a global and even interregional scale the majority of air routes and international airports present a negligible risk of exotic mosquitoes being transported from one country to another, there may be certain routes, for example, Denpasar (Indonesia) to Darwin (NT, Australia), which present a relatively high risk.

b) *Insufficient identification of the specific flights or aircraft and the relative risk of their introducing disease vectors.* The relatively few incidents of airport-associated malaria in Europe referred to above suggest that some unusual set of factors occurs from time to time, such as the involvement of particular cargo flights or special cargoes. Were the cause associated with routine flights, one could expect there to have been many more such events. Documented evidence of individuals contracting malaria as a result of being bitten on a plane has not been seen.

c) *Insufficiency in terms of detail and timeliness of much of the available information.* Many records of mosquitoes found in aircraft do not make it clear as to whether specimens were found alive or dead or whether the aircraft were disinsected or not. Even when there are records as indicated below showing that mosquitoes may be found alive in disinsected aircraft, very few of them relate to findings within the last five years:

(1) Of 12,825 mosquitoes found in disinsected aircraft arriving at seven American airports, that is, Brownsville, Fort Worth, Honolulu,

Miami, New Orleans, San Juan, and Terminal Island between 1937 and 1947, 817 (6%) were alive (WHO 1955).

(2) Of 20,692 mosquitoes found in disinsected aircraft arriving at Brownsville, Houston, Honolulu, Miami, New Orleans, New York, and San Juan between 1947 and 1960, 2,468 (12%) were alive. Four of the nonindigenous species (*Anopheles grabhamii, A. neomaculipalpus, A. vestitipennis* and *Culex tarsalis* were alive when found (Hughes 1961).

(3) Of 6,115 aircraft arriving at Bombay Airport between January 1955 and June 1959, 35 aircraft (0.6%) were found live *Culex* mosquitoes that had survived routine aircraft disinsection. The number of mosquitoes varied from one to six per aircraft.

(4) A live engorged female *Aedes aegypti* and female *Anopheles subpictus,* both vector species absent from Japan, were captured in aircraft arriving at Haneda (then Tokyo's International Airport) on flights routinely subject to disinsection prior to arrival (Ogata et al. 1974).

d) *Insufficiency in terms of technique and resources.* The presently used techniques for collecting mosquitoes in aircraft are inadequate. The financial and human resources allocated to vector surveillance and control are frequently either insufficient or inappropriately distributed.

e) *Insufficient identification of shipping routes and nature of vessels with respect to the risk of importing vector species.* As suggested above shipping does not, in general, appear to constitute a major problem. Nevertheless, there are situations—such as those between Australia and PNG, and between South American countries—where there is a risk of importing vector species, for example, *Aedes aegypti* and *A. albopictus.* The eggs and larvae of these species are readily transported in water barrels in coastal craft.

2. Lack of implementation of control measures.

a) *Insufficient application of IHR pertaining to mosquito surveillance and control in and around international airports and seaports.* In many tropical areas insufficient priority is given to this aspect of public health so that the necessary level of funding and trained staff is not available for effective surveillance (Msangi et al. 1973). In other situations staff are not employed in the most cost-effective manner. Actual routine surveillance and prompt control of vectors in and around an airport may well achieve more than the routine spraying of aircraft on the presumption that vectors are being introduced.

b) *Inappropriate methods of aircraft disinsection.* While aircraft disinsection using an aerosol formulation and method found suitable by WHO is effective if carried out properly, the method has a number of operational deficiencies:

(1) In-flight disinsection is difficult to supervise, and cabin staff are presented with a conflict between carrying out aerosol spraying thoroughly, on the one hand, and causing as little disturbance as possible to passengers, on the other.

(2) Aircrew in particular, and also some passengers, dislike inhaling the aerosol insecticide formulations; crew and passenger resentment to aircraft disinsection is consequently expressed.

(3) On-arrival spraying by airport personnel can lead to more effective aircraft disinsection, but it increases aircraft "turnaround" time that is sometimes critical on short routes.

REQUIREMENTS FOR IMPROVING VECTOR CONTROL AND SURVEILLANCE IN INTERNATIONAL TRANSPORTATION OF MOSQUITOES OF PUBLIC HEALTH IMPORTANCE

In the foregoing pages we have attempted to place in perspective, against the background of past incidents, the risks that new mosquito vectors and mosquito-borne diseases might become established in areas from which they are presently absent. Reference has been made to transportation by aircraft and shipping. There is also an unquantified risk through international land transport and construction of international highways. Relevant documentation is scarce, but the rapid spread of *Aedes aegypti* through the jungles of South America and Thailand, where this species is becoming established in villages close to international highways, is well known. Thus, when the construction of the fully surfaced trans-Sahara highway is complete, there will be an enhanced risk that *Anopheles arabiensis* may move into Algeria from Niger (Stafford Smith 1981).

One of the difficulties is to obtain a perspective of the overall change in a mosquito population resulting from increased communication on a gradual basis. This has inevitably occurred with time just as has the more obvious change resulting from a sudden direct linkage, for instance, that provided by a major highway. From available records it would appear that the risk of mosquitoes of public health importance establishing in areas where they are presently absent, and then proceding to take a significant part in disease transmission, is extremely low when considered on a global basis. Clearly, though, there are areas at relatively high risk. The first prerequisite to cost-effective prevention and control measures, is therefore to obtain the necessary detailed information by means of which sound judgements can be made. The type of information includes:

1. Accurate records of which indigenous vector species occur within international airports (or ports), in the vicinity of such airports (or ports), and along transcontinental highways.
2. Records of any exotic vectors that have become established in international airports (or ports), or in their vicinity, or along transcontinental highways.
3. Detailed records of vectors found in international transport, that is, species, whether living or dead, sex and, if female, whether unfed, blood-fed or gravid. If large numbers of living specimens are found, it may be possible to carry out insecticide susceptibility tests as has already been done with houseflies (Ogata et al. 1974).
4. The bionomics of exotic vectors found in international transport should be studied through scientific literature and consultations to determine: (a) whether these vectors could establish themselves within presumptive receptive areas, and (b) what the limiting factors are.
5. The sources of exotic vectors found in international transport should be identified as far as possible through study of flight and shipping schedules. All findings of vectors should be recorded, together with

registration details of the relevant international aircraft or shipping.

In the case of the yellow fever vector, *Aedes aegypti,* assessment of risk not only concerns its possible establishment in a potentially receptive area from which it is presently absent (for example, New Zealand), but also the introduction of the virus into a yellow fever-free country where *Aedes aegypti* is established, for instance, India, Pakistan, or Australia. Introduction of the virus could theoretically occur through the bite of an infective mosquito accidentally imported aboard an aircraft, or possibly through transovarian transmission following the vector mosquito's escape from the aircraft to lay eggs in the receptive area. Receptive countries have not been able to quantify this risk. Consequently, the finding of even a single live adult female *Aedes aegypti* in international transport that has originated from or previously visited a yellow fever-infected area should be treated as a matter of great concern.

APPROPRIATE PREVENTATIVE AND CONTROL MEASURES MAY BE CONSIDERED UNDER TWO BROAD CATEGORIES

A. *Surveillance within the receptive areas.*

Surveillance involves a country's maintenance of effective detection and control measures, to prevent establishment within it of exotic vectors of disease. The WHO Expert Committee on Malaria, 1952 (WHO 1952), considered that "the most effective means of avoiding transference of anophelines is through the rigid sanitation of airfields and their vicinity in order to remove the risks of anopheline invasion of aircraft, or of the multiplication of imported anophelines. No measures of disinfestation of aircraft can lessen the importance of these precautions." This view has been repeatedly emphasized by successive WHO Expert Committee meetings. The first national priority is therefore maintenance of effective antimosquito measures within and around international airports (and ports).

These measures should include:

1. Appropriate sanitary engineering in the design and maintenance of international airports to minimize vector breeding and vector entry into buildings.
2. Regular entomological surveys and application of larvicides to breeding places. Residual and ultralow

volume (ULV) formulations of insecticides may also be necessary for treatment of buildings within and around airports (and ports). Adequate insecticides and techniques are available and, providing that insecticides to which the vectors are susceptible are used, limitations to vector control will be budgetary rather than technological.

Surveillance procedures also include detection and control of exotic vectors in international aircraft and shipping. This aspect of surveillance needs more precise study than at present with the objective of pinpointing the sources of infestation of aircraft and ships. The risk of vector infestation of aircraft is much greater on some routes than on others. When the vulnerable routes have been identified, it may be possible to redirect this aspect of surveillance to only those international aircraft plying those routes. The method of disinsecting passenger cabins immediately *after* disembarkation, as practiced in the US, merits wide trial. Other methods of aircraft disinsection that are acceptable to crew and passengers require development.

B. *International cooperation to control the mosquito vectors at source.*

Governments with international airports in areas infested with mosquito vectors should be encouraged to undertake the following:

1. Make in-depth entomological (and other vector) studies in and around their international airports (and ports).
2. Assess the international implications of the findings.
3. Describe the vector control activities currently being conducted and indicate the degree of control achieved.
4. Indicate the constraints that exist where there is failure to maintain vector control in and around airports (and ports).
5. Publish the results; WHO would be pleased to assist in this respect wherever possible.
6. Consult with other countries concerned, and with WHO, as to how these constraints, including technical, personnel and financial, may be reduced.

The intention of this approach is to encourage the problem to be better defined, brought into the open, and resolved through international cooperation rather than "enforcement," which is impracticable. WHO contributes by

3. In 1933 *Anopheles gambiae s.1.* adults were found in aircraft arriving at Kisumu, Kenya, from Juba, Sudan, and Entebbe, Uganda (Anonymous 1935).

4. In 1935 a survey of sailing vessels, lighters, dhows, and other country craft entering Bombay, India, for local trade revealed that the drinking-water barrels or tanks of 458 out of 898 harbored larval *A. aegypti* (Bana 1936).

5. During 1936–41 81 dead and 7 living mosquitoes were found in 321 aircraft arriving at Honolulu, Hawaii, from California. The living specimens comprised five *Culex quinquefasciatus* and two species not found breeding in Hawaii, a female *Anopheles pseudopunctipennis* and *Culiseta incidens* (Pemberton 1944).

6. In 1937–38 live insects were found in 28 of 84 flying boats arriving at Durban, South Africa, from abroad. Among mosquitoes collected, *Anopheles* and *Aedes* were detected twice (Park Ross 1938)

7. In 1941–42 seven *Anopheles gambiae s.1.* were recovered from planes arriving in Brazil from Africa (Highton and van Someren 1970).

8. During 1942–45 352 *Anopheles gambiae s.1.* were found on board flying boats and aircraft from Africa arriving at the airports of Belem, Fortazala, Natal, and Recife in Brazil (Mendonça and Cerqueira 1947).

9. During 1946–60 2,468 live and 16,475 dead mosquitoes were found in international aircraft arriving in Brownsville, Honolulu, Houston, Miami, New York, and San Juan, Puerto Rico. Four of the nonindigenous species *Anopheles grabhamii, A. neomaculipalpis, A. vestitipennis* and *Culex tarsalis* were alive when found (Hughes 1961).

10. In 1950 three *Anopheles superpictus* were discovered in Cyprus in passenger cabins of a ship coming directly from Portugal at a time when this mosquito no longer existed on the island (WHO 1955).

11. In April 1950 a living female of *Aedes aegypti* (which is not established in New Zealand) was discovered in the passenger compartment of a DC3 aircraft arriving at Whenuapai Airport (Auckland) from Nausori, Fiji. In the same month, one live and five dead females and two dead males of *Culex annulirostris* were collected in aircraft arriving at Whenuapai. The living female was found in the forward luggage compartment of a DC4 aircraft on arrival from Sydney, Australia (Laird 1951).

12. During 1951 insects were collected from 111 of 343

aircraft arriving at Whenuapai. Among them was a live female *Culex annulirostris* found in the passenger compartment of a DC3 from Fiji (Laird 1952)

13. In 1960-61 the baggage compartments of 210 aircraft arriving at New Orleans, 89 arriving at Honolulu, and 1,831 arriving at Miami yielded 42 mosquitoes (all dead or moribund following spraying). The cabins of these aircraft yielded 178 mosquitoes (some of which were alive). All of five identified species taken from aircraft arriving at Miami were indigenous to Louisiana, but of nine identified from aircraft arriving at Honolulu only *Culex quinquefasciatus* was indigenous. The exotic ones were: *Aedes nigripes, Aedes sollicitans, Anopheles annularis, Anopheles nigerrimus, Culex annulirostris, C. sitiens, C. tritaeniorhynchus,* and *Mansonia uniformis* (Evans et al. 1963).

14. During 1964-68 14,264 aircraft were searched at Manila, Philippines; 52 living and 482 dead mosquitoes were recovered. The live examples include three disease vectors: *Anopheles subpictus, Culex tritaeniorhynchus,* and *Culex quinquefasciatus* (Basio et al. 1970).

15. In 1968 living larvae of *Aedes aegypti* and *Culex cinerellus* were detected in an aircraft arriving in Kansas directly from abroad. The larvae were present in water that had accumulated on a tarpaulin used as a cover for cargo that had been stored in an open area in Liberia prior to loading on the aircraft (Pippin et al. 1968).

16. In March and April 1968 the following mosquitoes were found in 27 aircraft arriving at Nairobi, Kenya, mainly from other African countries (Highton and van Someren 1970):

> *Anopheles gambiae s.1.* (1 ♂, 2 ♀♀)
> *Mansonia uniformis* (1 ♂, 2 ♀♀)
> *Aedes cumminsii* (1 ♂, 1 ♀)
> *Aedes dentatus* (1 ♂, 1 ♀)
> *Aedes hirsutus* (1 ♀)
> *Aedes lineatopennis* (1 ♂, 1 ♀)
> *Culex antennatus* (1 ♂, 1 ♀)
> *Culex pipiens* (7 ♂♂, 1 ♀)
> *Culex quinquefasciatus* (33 ♂♂, 95 ♀♀)
> *Culex theileri* (1 ♂, 1 ♀)

17. Between November 1968 and July 1969 the following mosquitoes were found in 65 aircraft of nine airlines arriving at Nairobi, Kenya, mainly from other African

countries (Highton and van Someren 1970):

> *Anopheles gambiae s.1.* (1 ♂, 3 ♀♀)
> *Mansonia uniformis* (1 ♂, 1 ♀)
> *Aedes lineatopennis* (1 ♂, 1 ♀)
> *Culex antennatus* (1 ♂, 1 ♀)
> *Culex pipiens* (5 ♂♂, 7 ♀♀)
> *Culex quinquefasciatus* (44 ♂♂, 265 ♀♀)
> *Culex univittatus* (2 ♂♂, 1 ♀)

In addition, two non-African species were recorded, *Aedes sollicitans* (1 ♂, 1 ♀) and *Culiseta annulata* (1 ♂, 1 ♀).

18. During 1972-73 living mosquitoes were captured in 42 aircraft arriving at Haneda, then Tokyo's International Airport (Ogata et al. 1974). Species exotic to Japan were: *Anopheles subpictus* (1 ♀), *Aedes aegypti* (1 ♀), *Culex gelidus* (2 ♀♀), and *C. sitiens* group (1 ♀). Other species captured in the aircraft and present in other parts of Japan but not in the Tokyo area were: *Culex quinquefasciatus* (9 ♂♂, 15 ♀♀), *C. pseudovishnui* (1 ♀), and *Mansonia uniformis* (1 ♀) (Ogata et al. 1974; see also Chapter 4).

19. Between 1974-79 *Anopheles sundaicus* and *A. subpictus*, malaria vectors that do not occur in Australia, were found in aircraft arriving at Darwin, NT, from Bali, Indonesia (Anonymous 1979a; see Chapter 7).

B. *Likely and proven reports of vectors becoming established through international transportation in receptive areas where they were previously absent.*

1. It has been conjectured that in or about 1860 *Anopheles gambiae s.1.* was brought to Mauritius from Madagascar or the African mainland by sailing vessel (Bruce-Chwatt 1969).

2. In 1930 *Anopheles gambiae s.1.* became established in Brazil probably by a rapid sea voyage from West Africa. Following a protracted and intensive campaign, it was eradicated by 1940 (Soper and Wilson 1943; WHO 1955).

3. In 1942 *Anopheles gambiae s.1.* became established in Egypt, possibly through river traffic from the Sudan. It was eradicated by 1945 following "a costly and stubborn campaign" (WHO 1955).

4. *Aedes aegypti,* absent from Wake Island up to 1941, was established there by 1947, presumably due to

importation during or immediately after World War II (Rosen et al. 1948).

5. The first record of *Anopheles stephensi* in Egypt was of larvae found in 1966 about one mile from the Gulf of Suez in an area of newly discovered oil fields. It was thought likely that the species had been introduced by air transport from Saudi Arabia (Bruce-Chwatt 1969).

6. At least 18 species of mosquitoes have become established on the island of Guam, 15 of them through international (primarily aerial) transportation, mostly since World War II (Nowell 1977; Ward et al. 1976; see Chapter 8). A full listing and discussion are presented in Chapter 8, but the extent of the problem is evident from the fact that on this previously anopheline-free island of the Marianas the establishment of the five hereunder has now been confirmed—with the exception of *Anopheles indefinitus* (first collected on Guam in 1948), all of them were first reported from 1970-76:

> *Anopheles barbirostris*
> *Anopheles indefinitus*
> *Anopheles litoralis*
> *Anopheles subpictus*
> *Anopheles vagus*

7. In 1979 *Aedes aegypti* reinfested Grand Cayman in the Caribbean, probably via small private aircraft not subjected to quarantine inspection (Anonymous 1980).

8. The reappearance of *Aedes aegypti* in areas of the South American continent where eradication had been claimed, and the invasion of other areas from which it was previously unknown, have been attributed to transportation services, possibly including aviation (Anonymous 1980).

9. In 1944 a live late-instar larva of *Anopheles albimanus* was found in a canal near the military airfield of Boca Raton, Florida. An investigation proved that 15 days earlier an aircraft had arrived from Puerto Rico and had not been disinsected. It was surmised that a female *A. albimanus* might have escaped from this aircraft and oviposited in the canal (Mulrennan et al. 1945).

REFERENCES

Anonymous. 1935. *Rec. Med. Res. Lab. Nairobi*, No. 6.
————. 1978. Weekly Epidemiological Record No.

47:338.

————. 1979a. Arthropod-borne vectors of human disease discovered on aircraft. *Aust. Comm. Dis. Intell. Bull.* 79:20.

————. 1979b. Weekly Epidemiological Record No. 10:79.

————. 1980. *Aedes aegypti* campaign. *Pan American Hlth Org. Epidem. Bull.* 2:5-7.

————. 1981. Weekly Epidemiological Record No. 22:174.

————. 1982. Relève epidemiologique hebdomadaire 35ème semaine, 29/8 to 4/9/1982. Belgium: Ministry of Public and Family Health.

Bana, F. D. 1936. A practical way of dealing with *Aedes aegypti (Stegomyia fasciata)* mosquito breeding in country craft. *Indian med. Gaz.* 71:79-80.

Basio, R. G., M. J. Prudencio, and I. E. Chanco. 1970. Notes on the aerial transportation of mosquitoes and other insects at the Miami International Airport. *Philipp. Ent.* 1:407-8.

Bruce-Chwatt, L. J. 1969. Global review of malaria control and eradication by attack on the vector. *Misc. Publ. ent. Soc. Amer.* 7:7-27.

Datta, S. K. 1960. Need for disinsectisation of aircrafts on international flights. *Bull. Nat. Soc. Ind. Mal. Mosq. Dis.* 8:153-57.

Evans, B. R., C. R. Joyce, and J. E. Porter. 1963. Mosquitoes and other arthropods found in baggage compartments of international aircraft. *Mosquito News,* 23:9-12.

Gentilini, M., and M. Danis. 1981. Le paludisme autochtone. Médecine et Maladies Infectieuses, 11:356-62.

Graham, D. H. 1939. Mosquito Life in the Auckland District. *Trans roy. Soc. N.Z.* 69:210-24.

Griffitts, T. D. H., and J. J. Griffitts. 1931. Mosquitoes transported by airplanes. *Publ. Hlth Rpts.* (Wash.) 46:2775-2782.

Highton, R. B., and E. C. C. van Someren. 1970. The transportation of mosquitoes between international airports. *Bull. Wld Hlth Org.* 42:334-35.

Hughes, J. H. 1961. Mosquito interceptions and related problems in aerial traffic arriving in the United States. *Mosquito News* 21:93-100.

Laird, M. 1951. Insects collected from aircraft arriving in New Zealand from abroad. Wellington: *Zool. Publs Victoria Univ. Coll.* No. 11.

————. 1952. Insects collected from aircraft arriving in

New Zealand during 1951. *J. Aviation Med.* 23:280-85.

Mendonça, F. C. de, and N. Cerqueira. 1947. Insects and other arthropods captured by the Brazilian Sanitary Service on landplanes or seaplanes arriving in Brazil between January 1942 and December 1945. *Bol. Ofic. Sanit. Panamer.* 26:22-30.

Morrill, A. W., Jr., A. N. Dandoy, M. S. Johnson, J. F. Poole, and R. H. Vincent. 1952. Mosquito control on army posts in the Far East. *Mosquito News,* 12:110-15.

Msangi, A. N., R. J. Tonn, and Y. H. Bang. 1973. Mosquito control and evaluation at Dar-es-Salaam International Airport. WHO/VBC/73.450. Mimeographed.

Mulrennan, J. A., M. Goodwin, and R. C. Shannon. 1945. The importation of exotic anophelines into the United States. *J. nat. Malar. Soc.* 4:56-58.

Nowell, W. R. 1977. International quarantine for control of mosquito-borne diseases on Guam. *Aviation, Space envi. Med.* January 1977:53-60.

Ogata, K., I. Tanaka, Y. Ito, and S. Morii. 1974. Survey of the medically important insects carried by international aircraft to Tokyo International Airport. *Jap. J. sanit. Zool.* 25:177-84.

Park Ross, G. A. 1938. Le destruction automatique des moustiques dans les aeronefs et le vecteur de la fièvre jaune dans les traversées aeriènnes en Afrique. *Bull. Off. Int. Hyg. Pub.* 30:2002-2031.

Pemberton, C. E. 1944. Insects carried in transpacific airplanes. *Hawaii. Plant Rec.* 48:183-86.

Pippin, W. F., S. Thompson, and R. Wilson. 1968. The interception of living larvae of *Aedes aegypti* (L.) and *Culex cinerellus* Edw. in aircraft. *Mosquito News* 28:646.

Rosen, L., W. C. Reeves, and T. Aarons. 1948. *Aedes aegypti* in Wake Island. *Proc. Hawaii. ent. Soc.* 13:255-56.

Soper, F. L., and D. B. Wilson. 1943. *Anopheles gambiae* in Brazil 1930 to 1940. New York: The Rockefeller Foundation.

Stafford Smith, D. M. 1981. Mosquito records from the Republic of Niger with reference to the construction of the new "Trans-Sahara Highway." *J. trop. Med. Hyg.* 84:95-100.

Ward, R. W., B. Jordan, A. R. Gillogly, and F. J. Harrison. 1976. *Anopheles litoralis* King and *An. barbirostris* group on the island of Guam. *Mosquito News* 36:99-100.

WHO. 1952. Expert Committee on Malaria (1951). Geneva: *WHO Techn. Rep. Ser.,* No. 39.

————. 1955. The control of insect vectors in international air traffic: A survey of existing legislation. Geneva: WHO.

————. 1983. International Health Regulations (1969). Third annotated ed. Geneva: WHO.

Chapter 2

The History and Present Status of Aircraft Disinsection

D. K. Hayes

At present aircraft disinsection research in USDA is conducted by the Livestock Insects Laboratory, Agricultural Environmental Quality Institute, Agricultural Research Service, USDA, located at Beltsville, Maryland. The name of the Laboratory has changed several times over the years since aircraft disinsection research began and as the study of aircraft disinsection has continued.

In the present chapter* aircraft disinsection studies are reviewed from the U.S. perspective. Related investigations arising from these studies and our [USDA] present approaches are presented.

Aircraft disinsection is the intransit control of hitch-hiking insects in aircraft from a country or within a country where they are indigenous to a destination where they are exotic. The need for this was recognized by Sasser (1928), Griffitts and Griffitts (1931), Cummings (1938), and others.

In the United States, the leader in aircraft disinsection research was Dr. W. N. Sullivan, Jr. In his doctoral thesis

---

*This chapter reports the results of research only. Mention of a commercial product or a pesticide in this paper does not constitute a recommendation for use by the USDA nor does it imply registration under the U.S. Federal Insecticides Fungicide and Rodenticide Act (FIFRA) as amended.

Sullivan (1976) wrote, "The development of great intercontinental transportation systems has often proceeded
without an awareness of the need or the will for quarantine
action to prevent the pollution of man's environment to his
disadvantage by the introduction of foreign insect vectors
of disease and agricultural pests harmful to man, his crops,
fibers, and animals. Unless rectified, this problem will
become acute as more and more food is needed to feed the
ever growing world population; many of them huddled and
poorly fed in city slums will become prime targets for
malaria, yellow fever, typhus, plague, and other insect-
borne diseases."

The results of research done in our laboratory on the
optimal techniques for aircraft disinsection are utilized in
USDA by the Animal and Plant Health Inspection Service
(APHIS), the transportation industry, and other private
sector concerns. We also cooperate with the Department of
Defense, the Public Health Service, and the World Health
Organization, and we interact appropriately with the private
sector.

The first interception of insects in aircraft in the United
States occurred in 1928 when Max Kisluik (1929) boarded
the large, lighter-than-air craft *Graf Zeppelin* and found
ten species of hitchhiking insect pests. Interest in in-
tercepting insects hitchhiking on aircraft continued through
the 1930s and early 1940s. In the 1930s there were essentially no synthetic insecticides of the type we know today,
but L. D. Goodhue and W. N. Sullivan, among others,
began to work on methodology for disseminating materials in
airplanes to kill insects. There are several historical
accounts of the development of gas-propelled aerosols; in
the 1960s and early 1970s at least five authors in addition
to Sullivan wrote accounts to keep the record straight
(Shepherd 1961; Evens 1955; Goodhue 1965; Fales 1973;
Sanders 1970).

Eric Roheim (1933) received a U.S. patent for a method
of spraying coating compositions by dissolving the coatings
in dimethyl ether, confining the solution under pressure,
and discharging the solutions through a valve. Carl
Iddings (1937) made an especially valuable contribution by
making liquids such as insecticides self-propelled by using
Freon. Sullivan, Goodhue, and Fales (1941) tried both
burning and dropping insecticide onto a hot plate for
dispersal; however, this method was cumbersome and was
also an obvious fire hazard aboard aircraft. In the spring
of 1941, according to Sullivan (1976), Lyle Goodhue
(Goodhue and Sullivan 1943a; Goodhue 1942; Sullivan et al.
1942) "mixed pyrethrum oleoresin and sesame oil (a syner-

gist) with chloroform and filtered the mixture into an evacuated 5 lb ICC9 cylinder. . . . The chloroform was evaporated and the tank was connected to another tank containing liquid Freon 12 (CF_2Cl_2). The Freon tank was inverted, the insecticide tank to be filled placed in ice water, the valves opened, and the liquid Freon flowed rapidly into the cold tank. An oil burner nozzle was attached to a 45° angle valve on the tank containing the insecticide. When the valve was opened, the solution sprayed out under the pressure of the Freon (82 lb/sq inch at 20° C) (14.6kg/sq cm at 20°C). The Freon immediately evaporated and left the insecticide dispersed as an aerosol (fog or mist). . . . [this] was logistically attractive (1 lb [454 g] aerosol formulation was equivalent to 1 gallon [3.8 l] of pyrethrum-kerosene fly spray then in use). The U.S. Patent Office granted Goodhue and Sullivan (1943b) Patent No. 2,321,023 for this method of applying parasiticides and assigned it to the Secretary of Agriculture and his successors in office . . ." Figure 2-1 shows the young Sullivan operating one of these early aerosol dispensers.

In 1942, Sullivan was commissioned in the U.S. Army and assigned to the Aeromedical Laboratory, Army Service Command, Wright Patterson Army Air Force Base where advanced work was underway on gases. At this base Sullivan's "duty was . . . to obtain an insecticidal aerosol package suitable for use in the tropics where malaria and other insect-borne diseases were a serious drain on U.S. manpower. In cooperation with the Westinghouse Electrical Company, the tank of about 454 g capacity that was being used to hold Freon in household refrigeration systems was modified into an aerosol dispenser. A screw cap was developed to seal the package between uses. This was the prototype (see Figure 2-1) of 30,000,000 insecticidal aerosol "bombs" used to protect personnel against disease, and since 1947, liquified gas-propelled aerosols have been the standard method for preventing the spread of insects on common carriers" (Sullivan 1971).

Later the ingredients were changed and DDT plus pyrethrum in kerosene (Fales et al. 1951) became the standard aerosol formulation until the late 1960s when newer formulations were promulgated.

When Sullivan returned to Beltsville after the war, he worked with the Beltsville Pesticide Chemicals Research Branch and developed the aerosols used in disinfection. He was responsible for the U.S. protocol in which aircraft were sprayed at "blocks-away" with a formulation of Freons 11 and 12 (Propellents 11 and 12), pyrethrins (0.4%), DDT, (3%) and kerosene (Sullivan et al. 1964). Fulton et al.

Figure 2-1. The late Dr. W. N. Sullivan using prototype aerosol "bomb" as for aircraft disinsection, 1942.

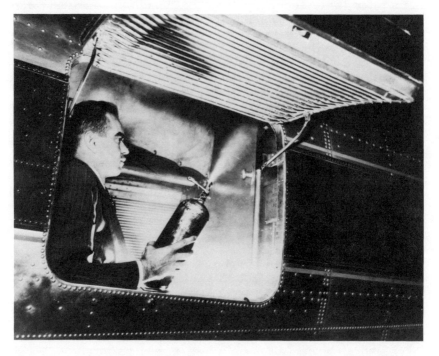

(1949) and McBride et al. (1950) working with Sullivan evaluated residual deposits in aircraft and concluded that these were not practical for control of insects.

Park Ross (1938) and later Schechter and Sullivan (1972) described the selection of candidate insecticide as follows:

1. It should be toxic to a reasonably wide spectrum of insects.
2. It should have some residual activity on the order of a day or two. (Sullivan and Schechter believed a residue lasting longer could become a problem.)
3. It should have low toxicity to mammals.
4. It should be stable in aerosol or dust formulations, and the formulations should be readily dispersible.
5. It should have little or no odor, be nonirritating and should leave no stains.
6. It should have no deleterious effects on the electronic components, metal parts, fabrics, or plastics (especially plastic windows) used in

aircraft.
7. If it is to be used in an aerosol, it should be possible to formulate it in a high concentration (at least 7.5%); 20% may be needed and usable.
8. If used in the presence of passengers, it should be dischargable within a minute or two, even in the largest aircraft, before any food or drink is served.

During this time Sullivan (Sullivan et al. 1958; Knipling and Sullivan 1957, 1958; Sullivan and Thompson 1959; Senior-White and Kirkpatrick 1949; Porter and Hughes 1950) also evaluated temperature extremes, atmospheric composition and high g-forces on insects. He found some eggs such as those of the tent caterpillar resistant to cold at high altitudes on airplanes and in balloons. It was at this time that Dr. Sullivan became interested in survival of insects in outer space. The ultimate aircraft for disinsection is a space vehicle—and Sullivan became interested in determining what would happen to insects in those vehicles. He probably believed that when a more or less permanent satellite is put up to mine the moon and the asteroids, cockroaches and other insects will become established on this new man-made heavenly body.

After some unsuccessful attempts to arrange an experiment with National Aeronautics and Space Administration (NASA) in which effects of space on rhythms of the Madeira roach were to be determined, Sullivan, Hayes, Schechter, and Morrison (1977) finally succeeded in putting 700 gypsy moth (*Porthetria dispar*) eggs onto Skylab IV to determine if diapause would be broken early. Many of them became desiccated in the lower atmospheric pressure in the space vehicle but about one percent of the eggs broke diapause early and one female hatched on return to earth. She was reared to adulthood (see Figure 2-2) and mated. She laid about 400 eggs; these eggs did not hatch and the experiment was terminated (Sullivan et al. 1977). Subsequent experiments by Leppla et al. (1983) demonstrated that the velvetbean caterpillar (*Anticarsia gemmatalis* Hübner) behaved and reproduced normally when returned from space.

During the Skylab IV study, we learned that apparently two mosquitoes had stowed away on one of the earlier flights in the space capsule. Attempts to confirm this after 8 years are still in progress.

During the 1960s and 1970s other work related to rhythms and diapause grew out of the work in space as exemplified by reports on wavelength of light required to prevent diapause in the laboratory (Norris et al. 1969), on

Figure 2-2. Female gypsy moth (*Porthetria dispar*) hatched on return to earth from eggs put into space aboard "Skylab IV" for diapause experimentation.

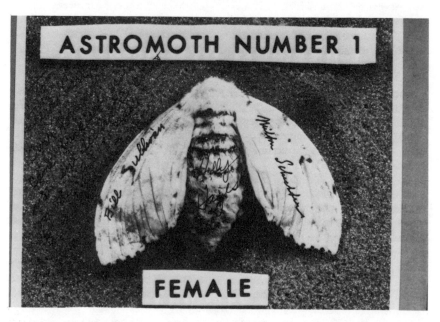

prevention of diapause in the field (Hayes et al. 1970), and on insect survival in photoperiodic shifts (Hayes 1976).

In 1968 Sullivan and Schechter, becoming increasingly concerned by the need for newer technology for disinsection of aircraft, initiated investigations that have continued to this day (Sullivan et al. 1972; Schechter and Sullivan 1972; Schechter et al. 1976). Plane cabins were simulated with tractor trailers for semitrucks and test insecticides were applied as aerosols or as dusts propelled with CO_2 gas. Initially insects were released into the trailer; however, problems of quantitative recapture led to the subsequent use of caged insects. Extensive tests were conducted in commercial training flights and even, at one point, in the Presidential aircraft, Air Force ONE.

During these developments, synthetic pyrethroids such as resmethrin showed promise. Eventually this compound was rejected because it decomposes in sunlight (UV light) with one by-product being phenylacetic acid, which has a pronounced urinelike odor (Sullivan et al. 1975). Other synthetic pyrethroids were also tested. Schechter and Sullivan finally recommended 2% d-phenothrin made up in Freons 11 and 12 (propellents 11 and 12) (Schechter et al.

1974). Kerosene (euphemistically referred to as petroleum distillate) has been left out of our current recommendation after Sullivan showed in cooperation with Colonel Marshall Steinberg (M. S. Schechter, personal communication) that when kerosene aerosols were inhaled by rabbits lung damage was observed.

In the early 1970s Sullivan embarked on a round-the-world trip for the World Health Organization to test his formulations. Sullivan and his coworkers (Sullivan et al. 1972) endorsed the WHO (1961) recommendation for disinsection of the cabins at "blocks-away"—that is, as the blocks are pulled away from the wheels of the airplane and it taxis to the take-off point. In South Africa and New Zealand, aircraft disinsection treatments are carried out just before or immediately upon landing—before passengers disembark (Hayes, unpublished).

Dusts have been tested (Hill et al. 1970; Schechter and Whittam 1973; Whittam and Schechter 1974; Sullivan et al. 1972); although effective, these are not generally favored by pilots.

During the 1970s new concerns have arisen. These include:

1. Concern for the effects on passengers of disinsection.
2. Concern for the ozone layer.
3. Continuing problems in resistance to insecticides.
4. Some concerns on our part for areas in the world which have new airlines, especially after civil disturbances have permitted build up of undesirable pests.
5. Desire to develop techniques that can be used in the absence of passengers.
6. Efficient handling of a growing body of data on aircraft disinsection trials.

In addition a new, effective, although costly, method for particle size determination has been developed in which a forward scattering laser has revealed that more small particles are present than had earlier been reported (Cawley et al. 1977).

Our approach at present is the following: We receive samples of insecticides from industrial laboratories that have desirable properties for aircraft disinsection previously mentioned. We check these against several species in a commercially available wind tunnel (Morgan and Retzer 1981); and if we find them promising we formulate them in Freons 11 and 12 and as CO_2 propelled dusts on Hi-Sil® 233 and test them against as many pest species as is practical pursuing the following:

1. Encourages training of personnel for international vector control.
2. Stimulates research and development to improve techniques for international vector control and development of insecticide formulations for aircraft disinsection through WHO Collaborating Centres, consultations, and publications.
3. Advises member states on methods of assessment of vector infestation and of vector control in international vector control situations.
4. Encourages member states to fulfill their obligations under the IHR with regard to maintaining ports and airports free from mosquito vectors.
5. Advises the International Civil Aviation Organization (ICAO) and International Air Transport Association (IATA) of the continuing need for aircraft disinsection on vulnerable routes.

APPENDIX

A. *Some chronological records of mosquitoes detected in international ships and aircraft.*

1. In 1929 *Culex annulirostris* larvae were found in the hold of a ship arriving in Auckland, New Zealand, from Suva, Fiji. This species, which occurs in the Pacific islands and Australia, is absent from New Zealand (Graham 1939).
2. In 1931 28 *Culex quinquefasciatus** and one *Aedes aegypti* were collected from 102 aircraft landing at Miami, Florida, from the Antilles (Griffitts and Griffitts 1931).

---

*Throughout this book the name *Culex quinquefasciatus* Say is employed in accordance with recent taxonomic decisions, for the mosquito formerly widely referred to as *Culex pipiens fatigans* Wiedemann; without prejudice to the possibility that further revision may require further clarification of the taxon's status vis a vis other members of the *Culex pipiens* L. complex (see A. R. Barr 1981, 123-36 in *Cytogenetics and Genetics of Vectors*. Eds., R. Pal, J. B. Kitzmiller, and T. Kanda. Amsterdam: Elsevier and Tokyo: Kondansha)—Ed.

in our tractor trailers using d-phenothrin as a standard. We also include squares of wood and carpet for bioassay. We continue to encourage cooperation with APHIS, U.S. Department of Defense, our own research organization (ARS), and the Public Health Service; indeed, APHIS personnel cooperate actively in all phases of these tests. Data are collected in Miami in April; in Baltimore in late July we study primarily the Japanese beetle. The data are also stored into a computer using an optical reader; a program that allows for considerable flexibility is used in retrieving data (Schechter et al. 1977). Our tests today are conducted with insecticide applicators wearing protective clothing (see Figure 2-3).

In 1979-80, B. M. Cawley of LIL and J. Fons of APHIS (Fons et al. 1981) conducted studies on the efficacy of

Figure 2-3. USDA insecticide applicator wearing protective clothing.

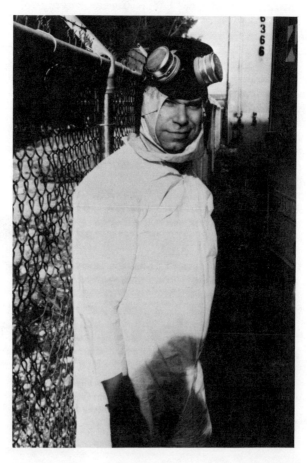

d-phenothrin in Hawaii on Mediterranean fruit fly, melon fly, and oriental fruit fly; their data indicated that we could use 2% d-phenothrin at 10 g/1000 cu ft against these pests.

At present we are investigating new propellent systems. All the water-based aerosols propelled with propane-isobutane that we have tested are flammable at some time during complete discharge of the contents of the can. Dimethyl ether and some other halogenated hydrogen are satisfactory propellents, but are also flammable.

A novel mechanism for dispersing an aerosol has recently been developed by the Envirospray firm, a subsidiary of Gro-group. This method is based upon slow release of carbon dioxide from citric acid and sodium bicarbonate contained within a plastic bag inside the aerosol can. The formulation to be propelled is in a separate compartment and must be prepared so that it does not attack the plastic bag. This eliminates a major problem in the use of CO_2 as a propellent, since if all the CO_2 were present initially as a gas, a container with heavier walls would be required. Also CO_2 propellent formulations usually produce particles that are larger than desired. Nevertheless, in our test this Envirospray formulation was comparable in efficacy to formulations using Propellents 11 and 12 (Fons et al. 1982). However, a more definitive assessment of this development cannot be made until data become available on formulation stability, resistance to heat and cold, and resistance of the containers to internal corrosion.

We plan to pursue the following avenues:

1. Search for new insecticides suitable for aircraft disinsection, and develop methods for formulation and delivery of these materials.
2. Conduct aircraft disinsection trials in Miami, Baltimore, and other suitable locations to evaluate newly developed aerosols and dusts against a wide spectrum of insects.
3. Work with industry to develop and evaluate suitable nonflurocarbon-propelled aerosol as satisfactory replacements for Freon.
4. Explore the possibility of residuals for long-term control in walkways and aircraft.
5. Study new methods for dispersing insecticides in enclosed spaces; these methods include ultralow volume (ULV) insecticides, commercial equipment, and new aerosol-can-dispersing systems.
6. Maintain and further develop present computer system

for information retrieval from the Miami and Baltimore trials.

Our cooperators have expressed a special interest in controlling Japanese beetles in the wheel wells and other external hiding spots on aircraft.

Because insects will get there any way they can, we need to work closely together with various countries. In spite of the prevailing winds, which have been invoked by some Pacific scientists as agents for insect dispersal (informal communication), there are still numerous (if often anecdotal) stories of introductions or possible introductions by means of aircraft.

We are attempting to participate in technological exchanges with other countries. Recently I traveled to Zimbabwe, one of the countries with which we interact with our agricultural technology exchange in the Office of International Cooperation and Development. Zimbabweans are interested in further exploring the concept of aircraft disinsection because they believe it can be beneficial to them as well as to us.

During the past 20 years two muscoid species of flies have been investigated by the laboratory. The face fly (*Musca autumnalis*), a cattle pest, was introduced to North America on aircraft in the early 1950s and is a major insect investigated by this group (Pickens and Miller 1980).

Recently the laboratory combined its aircraft disinsection activity and its other entomological capability. Two live specimens of *Musca vitripennis* were captured—in a warehouse and in an airplance—on McGuire AFB, NJ, last summer. This dipteran pest is common in Bulgaria and can be a vector of *Parafilaria bovicola,* a nematode that migrates through live animals and causes "green meat disease." The APHIS Veterinary Staff is interested in this problem. They led a trapping effort in which we participated. The team could not find the fly after extensive trapping, but we plan to study the biology and ecology of the fly further. If this insect were to become established, it might prove to be a problem for both animals and humans.

I have reviewed the history from our laboratory point of view of aircraft disinsection and have indicated that the research should continue in order to develop relevant procedures for disinsection in the 1980s. It seems to me that the symposium has provided much information supporting the need for such research.

REFERENCES

Cawley, B. M., H. J. Retzer, and R. E. Menzer. 1977. Performance of three insecticidal aerosols formulated with nonfluorocarbon propellants. *J. econ. Ent.* 70:675-77.

Cummings, H. S. 1938. Rapport sur les refuges pour moustiques dans les aeronefs. *Off. Internatl. d'Hyg. Publ.* 30:1997-2004.

Evens, M. E. 1955. The bomb that exploded into a $250 million business. *Dupont Mag.* 49:18-20.

Fales, J. H. 1973. A chronology of early aerosol development. *Proc. 60th Ann. Mtg. Chem. Specialties Mfctrs. Assoc.*

Fales, J. H., R. H. Nelson, R. A. Fulton, and O. F. Bodenstein. 1951. Tests with two insecticidal aerosols for use in aircraft. *J. econ. Ent.* 44:621-26.

Fons, J., B. M. Cawley, and D. K. Hayes. 1981. Evaluation of aerosols for quarantine control of three tephritid flies, 1979. *Insecticide and Acaricide Tests* 6:180.

Fons, J., S. Wood, B. M. Cawley, and N. O. Morgan. 1982. Candidate pesticide formulations for quarantine use, 1981. *Insecticide and Acaricide Tests* 7:230.

Fulton, R. A., O. C. McBride, and W. N. Sullivan. 1949. Toxicity of residues from carbon dioxide propelled insecticides. *J. econ. Ent.* 42:123-26.

Goodhue, L. D. 1942. Insecticidal aerosol production. Spraying solutions in liquified gases. *Industr. and Eng. Chem.* 34:1456-1460.

—————. 1965. How it all began. *Aerosol Age* 10:30.

Goodhue, L. D., and Sullivan, W. N. 1943a. Making and testing aerosols. In *Laboratory Procedures in Studies of the Chemical Control of Insects. AAAS Publs* 20:157-62.

—————. 1943b. Method of applying parasiticides. US Patent No. 2,321,023.

Griffitts, T. H. D., and J. J. Griffitts. 1931. Mosquitoes transported by airplanes. Staining methods used in determining their importation. USPHS *Publ. Hlth Reps* 46:2775-2782.

Hayes, D. K. 1976. Survival of the codling moth, the pink bollworm and the tobacco budworm after 90° phase-shifts at varied, regular intervals throughout the life span. *Shift Work and Health . . . A Symposium, July 12-13, 1975, Cincinnati, Ohio.* (P. G. Rentos and Sheppard, R. D., eds.).

Hayes, D. K., W. N. Sullivan, M. Z. Oliver, and M. S. Schechter. 1970. Photoperiod manipulation of diapause: a method of pest control. *Science* 169:382-83.

Hill, K. R., W. N. Sullivan, W. M. Jones, E. J. Miles,

G. G. Rohwer, and C. M. Amyx. 1970. Distribution and settling rate of CO_2-propelled micronized insecticidal dusts in Aircraft. *J. econ. Ent.* 63:1749-1752.

Iddings, C. 1973. Method of making liquid sprays. U.S. Patent No. 2,070,167.

Kisluik, M. 1929. Plant quarantine inspection of the dirigible *Graf Zeppelin. J. econ. Ent.* 22:594-95.

Knipling, E. B., and W. N. Sullivan. 1957. Insect mortality at low temperatures. *J. econ. Ent.* 50:368-69.

————. 1958. The thermal death point of several species of insects. *J. econ. Ent.* 51:344-46.

Leppla, N. C., T. E. Nelson, J. R. Peterson, and G. W. Adams. 1983. Insect flight and stress in continuous zero-gravity aboard the space shuttle. Submitted to *Bull. ent. Soc. Amer.*

McBride, O. C., W. N. Sullivan, and R. A. Fulton. 1950. Treatment of airplanes to prevent the transport of insects. *J. econ. Ent.* 43:66-70.

Morgan, N. O., and H. J. Retzer. 1981. Aerosol wind tunnel for vector insecticide evaluation. *J. econ. Ent.* 74:389-92.

Norris, K. H., F. Howell, D. K. Hayes, V. E. Adler, W. N. Sullivan, and M. S. Schechter. 1969. The action spectrum for breaking diapause in the codling moth, *Laspeyresia pomonella* (L.), and the oak silkworm, *Antheraea pernyi* Guer. *Proc. natl Acad. Sci.* 63:1120-1127.

Park Ross, G. A. 1938. La destruction automatique des moustiques dans les aeronefs et le vecteur de la fièvre jaune dans les tranversées aériennes en Afrique. *Off. Internatl d'Hyg. Publ.* 30:2002-2031.

Pickens, L. G., and R. W. Miller. 1980. Biology and control of the face fly, *Musca autumnalis* (Diptera: Muscidae). *J. med. Ent.* 17:195-210.

Porter, J. E., and J. H. Hughes. 1950. Insect eggs transported on the outer surface of airplanes. *J. econ. Ent.* 43:555-57.

Roheim, E. 1933. Method and apparatus for atomixing materials. U.S. Patent No. 1,892,750.

Sanders, P. A. 1970. Principles of aerosol technology. New York: Van Nostrand Reinhold Co.

Sasser, E. R. 1928. *Proc. 40th Ann. Mtg Amer. Assoc. econ. Entomol. J. econ. Ent.* 21:451-63.

Schechter, M. S., and W. N. Sullivan. 1972. 2. Test protocol. *J. econ. Ent.* 65:1444-1447.

Schechter, M. S., W. N. Sullivan, B. M. Cawley, D. K. Hayes, A. Baffoe, R. E. Menzer, and H. D. Burton. 1977. Computer storage and retrieval of insecticide test data. *J. econ. Ent.* 70:759–66.

Schechter, M. S., W. N. Sullivan, B. M. Cawley, N. O. Morgan, R. Waters, C. M. Amyx, and J. Kennedy. 1976. Gas-propelled aerosols and micronized dust for control of insects in aircraft and vans. *Israel J. Ent.* 6:133–45.

Schechter, M. S., W. N. Sullivan, J. F. Schoof, and D. R. Maddock. 1974. D-phenothrin, a promising new pyrethroid for disinsecting aircraft. *J. med. Ent.* 11:231–33.

Schechter, M. S., and D. Whittam. 1973. Double-nozzle dust gun. *J. econ. Ent.* 66:1335–1336.

Senior-White, R. A., and T. W. Kirkpatrick. 1949. Transport of insects on the exterior of aircraft. *Nature* 164:60–61.

Shepherd, R. H. 1961. *Aerosols: Science and Technology.* New York: Interscience Publishers.

Sullivan, W. N. 1971. The coupling of science and technology in the early development of the World War II aerosol bomb. *Military Med.* (Feb.):157–58.

————. 1976. Research to prevent the transport of insects on common carriers. Ph.D. Thesis, Tokyo University of Agriculture.

Sullivan, W. N., J. C. Azurin, J. W. Wright, and N. G. Gratz. 1964. Studies on aircraft disinsection at "blocks away" in tropical areas. *Bull. Wld Hlth Org.* 30:113–18.

Sullivan, W. N., F. R. DuChanois, and D. L. Hayden. 1958. Insect survival in jet aircraft. *J. econ. Ent.* 51:239–41.

Sullivan, W. N., L. D. Goodhue, and J. H. Fales. 1941. Insecticide dispersion. A new method of dispersing pyrethrum and rotenone in air. *Soap Sanit. Chem.* 17:98–100.

————. 1942. Toxicity to adult mosquitoes of aerosols produced by spraying solutions of insecticides in liquified gas. *J. econ. Ent.* 35:48–51.

Sullivan, W. N., D. K. Hayes, M. S. Schechter, and D. R. Morrison. 1977. Hatch of eggs and subsequent development of larvae of the gypsy moth, *Lymantria dispar,* during and after exposure to weightlessness in Skylab IV. *Proc. VII Int. Conf. Int. Soc. Chronobiol.* Washington, D. C.: The Publishing House I Ponte 643–46.

Sullivan, W. N., A. N. Hewing, M. S. Schechter, J. U. McGuire, R. M. Waters, and E. S. Fields. 1975. Further studies of aircraft disinsection and odor characteristics of aerosols containing resmethrin and D-*trans*resmethrin. *Botyu Kagaku* 40:5–13.

Sullivan, W. N., M. S. Schechter, C. M. Amyx, and E. E. Crooks. 1972. Gas-propelled aerosols and micronized dusts for control of insects in aircraft. 1. Test protocol. *J. econ. Ent.* 65:1442-1444.

Sullivan, W. N., and C. G. Thompson. 1959. Survival of insect eggs after stratospheric flights in jet aircraft. *J. econ. Ent.* 52:299-301.

Whittam, D., and M. S. Schechter. 1974. Double nozzle dust guns. *USDA, APHIS Publ.* 81-71.

WHO. 1961. Aircraft disinsection. *Wld Hlth Org Techn. Rep. Ser.* 206.

Chapter 3

Dispersal of Filth Flies through Natural and Human Agencies: Origin and Immigration of a Synanthropic Form of Chrysomya megacephala

H. Kurahashi

INTRODUCTION*

Chrysomya megacephala (Fabricius, 1784), the oriental latrine fly, has medical importance in transmitting various pathogens and eggs of intestinal parasites. It is commonly found in and around human dwellings in Southeast Asia and is widely distributed throughout the Australasian Region. In Australia this fly has not been recorded at any distance from the coast, where however it is prevalent in the larger towns down to Bateman's Bay. Zumpt (1965) considered that these pockets of infestation were evidence of recent introductions from elsewhere. Where did they originate?

*The study reported here was supported by a grant-in-aid to the Tokyo Medical and Dental University Overseas Scientific Research Project 1973, 1975, and 1977 from the Ministry of Education, Science and Culture, Japan. The author wishes to thank Professor Marshall Laird, Memorial University of Newfoundland, Canada, and Dr. Yoshito Wada, National Institute of Health, Japan, for their valuable guidance and critical review of the manuscript. He is also grateful to Prof. Dr. R. Kano, Dr. S. Shinonaga, and Dr. M. Iwasa, Tokyo Medical and Dental University, for their kind cooperation and valuable advice. Thanks are due to Dr. S. Asahina and Dr. T. Okada (Tokyo) for their encouragement given during biosystematic study.

Whence did this fly come? How did it achieve synanthropy? These questions stand in need of elucidation. Moreover, the species has recently become established in South and West Africa, also in Brazil and Peru in South America. Baez and I (1981) observed that *C. megacephala,* having been accidentally introduced by shipping, consequently became established in the Canary Islands. The synanthropic form of *C. megacephala* in new colonies is commonly found around garbage there. During an earlier survey (1982) I found feral forms in natural forests in New Guinea and other islands of the South Pacific. The phylogeny and geographical distribution of the oriental latrine fly suggest that its synanthropic form probably originated in New Guinea. It is accidentally transported from country to country through commercial activities, as well as being subject to natural dispersal.

IMMIGRATION: ACCIDENTAL
INTRODUCTION AND ESTABLISHMENT

Chrysomya megacephala (Fabricius) is a very common filth fly in Southeast Asia and is widely distributed over the Australasian Region including the Oceanian Subregion (Figure 3-1). Medical entomologists have generally assumed that the oriental latrine fly is found only in these areas. However, in 1977 and 1978, Kurahashi (1978) and Prins (1979) found it in South and West Africa. In 1978, too, Baez et al. (1981) reported an introduction of *C. megacephala* into the Canary Islands, and the first record to appear from the New World was that of Guimarães et al. (1978), following field work during 1977 to 1978 (Figure 3-1). More recently, Greenberg (1981) mentioned finding this Old World species in Peru. Discovery of this species in the New World and the Canary Islands was often accompanied by that of other Old World species such as *C. albiceps, C. putoria, C. chloropyga,* and *C. rufifacies.* Despite the numerous surveys that were made in the past to detect filth flies of medical importance, *C. megacephala* was not known from the Afrotropical and Neotropical Regions, nor from sections of the Palearctic Region (for example, Japan, Afghanistan) until so lately that recent invasion and colonization must be responsible for its presence there today. Tropical and subtropical climates most certainly favor such establishments following either accidental introductions through human agencies or involuntary dispersal by natural ones. In the Canary Islands (28°30'N, 15°10'W),

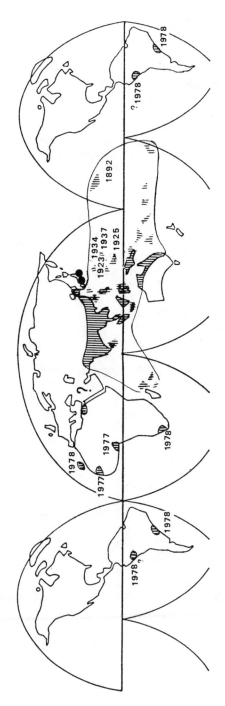

Figure 3-1. Geographical distribution of the oriental latrine fly, *Chrysomya megacephala* (Fabricius). Black spot: Occasional introduction into Honshu and Kyushu, not yet established.

megacephala

neither Baez and Santos-Pinto (1975) nor Hanski (1977)—who collected many flies during ecological studies of insect visitors to carrion—recorded *C. megacephala* before its discovery there in 1978, when, from the first moment of the relevant investigations by Baez et al. (1981), individuals of *C. megacephala* came to their trap situated in a garden of the capital, Santa Cruz. It is likely that the initial invasion of Santa Cruz by *C. megacephala,* and this fly's subsequent intra- and interinsular distribution, were effected via the maritime route. The insect's population has grown very considerably during its short period in the Canary Islands. Similar means of immigration and colonization are considered to have applied in the case of *C. chloropyga,* the Afrotropical filth fly (Hanski 1977; Baez et al. 1981), which was captured for the first time in the Canaries aboard a ship that had come from the island of Fernando Poo and moored in the harbor of Santa Cruz. Baez et al. (1981) now paid special attention to this Afrotropical species, and over the following months they duly found it at other sites on Tenerife, as well as on the islands of Fuerteventura and Lanzarote. The spread of foreign species through archipelagos as a consequence of increased commercial contacts with the major international port, must thus be expected once an introduction has been effected at the port. Some six decades ago Illingworth had suggested the possibility that *C. megacephala* (which he observed aboard a vessel bound for Hawaii from Shanghai) might extend its range through shipping. The fluctuation of the *C. megacephala* population in Santa Cruz during the following year is evident from Figure 3-2, which shows that the number of flies captured was greatest during the coldest and most humid months, and lowest in the dry season. This annual fluctuation is similar to that of other groups of Canarian flies previously known to have become established in the islands from elsewhere.

In the New World, the first published record of *Chrysomya* concerned *C. chloropyga,* which was caught in 1975 in Paraná, Brazil (Imbiriba et al. 1977). Following this, Guimarães et al. (1978) reported the discovery of *C. megacephala* and *C. albiceps* as well as *C. chloropyga* in São Paulo and Campinas in 1977-78. These species were found on meat and fish in markets and on garbage, carrion and faeces. The authors asserted that these exotic species were recently introduced because extensive collections in the same area in the early 1970s had netted only native species. All three species are not only now established but have also considerably extended their range in Brazil. Thus *C. megacephala* has been further reported from Rio de

Figure 3-2. Seasonal fluctuation of *C. megacephala* in Santa Cruz de Tenerife (Baez et al. 1981, modified).

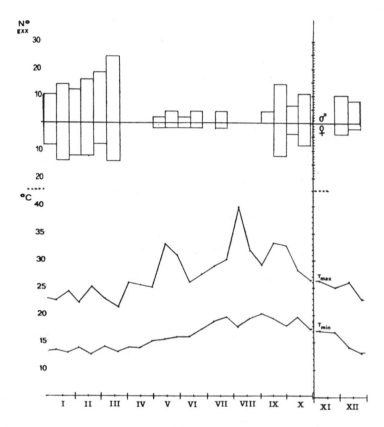

Canary Is.

Janeiro, *C. albiceps* is now known from Mato Grosso, and *C. chloropyga* has become widespread from northeastern to southern Brazil along the Atlantic Coast. Guimarães et al. (1979) have suggested the possibility that these flies were initially introduced into southern Brazil in 1975-76, during the great influx of Portuguese refugees from Angola.

Turning to Central America, Gagné (1981) examined a larva of *Chrysomya* sp., probably *C. albiceps,* which was collected in April 1974 from a wound on a goat in Puerto Rico. This specimen represents the earliest known record of a *Chrysomya* in Central America. Kurahashi (1980) reported *C. albiceps* (2 females) from Guatemala. Jirón (1979) recorded the Asian filth fly, *C. rufifacies,* from a human cadaver in Costa Rica in 1978. Gagné (1981) examined a long series of *C. rufifacies* caught in a liver-baited trap in Chiapas, Mexico, in January 1980. He believed that this Asian filth fly was established in Central America, too, and suggested the possibility that it had arrived there via one of the Pacific ports. The method of entry of *C. albiceps* into the American tropics is uncertain.

Commerce continues to increase by air, which may be the most effective route for *Chrysomya* introductions. In this connection, Laurence (1981) states that "Adult *Chrysomya* have been found in the luggage holds of aircraft and the sun-loving flies may well be attracted to the warm surface of aircraft standing on the airport apron." One, however, wonders why these flies did not reach Latin America sooner, and how is it that within only a few years they have dispersed so widely from several points of entry. Gagné (1981), however, reported two accidental importations of *Chrysomya sp.* (probably *C. chloropyga* from Nigeria) in dried shrimp and fish consignments intercepted by the Office of Plant Protection and Quarantine, APHIS, USDA, in Houston, Texas, in February 1980. Kusui (1980) noted two cases of the accidental introduction of *C. rufifacies* and one of *C. nigripes,* which were apprehended by quarantine inspectors, in aircraft arriving at Tokyo (at both the former international airport, Haneda, and its successor at Narita–New Tokyo International Airport) from Southeast Asia during 1975-79 (see pages 68, 69). He also reported seven cases of accidental importation of *C. rufifacies* and *Chrysomya* sp., probably *C. megacephala,* discovered aboard ships inspected at Shimotsu, Wakayama Prefecture, Honshu, during 1977-79. These ships arrived via the Southeast Asian maritime route. Synanthropic flies such as *Chrysomya* readily frequent ships, especially fishing boats, while they are tied up in harbor; and man may unintentionally transport them from country to country through commercial activities. Effective surveillance may intercept these filth flies at the airport or seaport of arrival, but should they escape detection there* little can be done to prevent their spread within a country.

In Japan three species of *Chrysomya* (*C. rufifacies, C. megacephala,* and *C. pinguis*) are commonly found in the Southwest Islands of Ryukyu. The last-mentioned species

---

*In this connection, it should be noted that some species of *Chrysomya* may be imported as larvae in ulcers of infected people, such as those on human toes (of a lady who had just flown from Sri Lanka to Malaysia) that harbored 30 maggots of *Chrysomya bezziana* (page 97).

is also found in mainland Japan and is considered to be indigenous. The former two have become established following arrival from abroad, and *C. megacephala* is also commonly found in the Bonin and Volcano Islands (Figure 3-3). While this species has become established from subtropical southern Japan to 30°N, it has not yet spread to the country's northern temperate region. The fly has, however, been recorded from Kagoshima, Nagasaki, Isahaya, Hyuga, Miyakonojo, Yamaguchi, Yonago, Kyoto, Yokohama, and Tokyo, as shown in Figure 3-3 (Kano 1958; Kato 1960; Fukuda 1960; Miyazaki 1960; Uemoto et al. 1962; Suenaga et al. 1964). Kano (1958) reported a third species, *C. rufifacies,* from Tokyo. These records of the filth flies include both occasional appearances caused by accidental introductions and natural invasions.

The latter have been frequently observed in Kyushu and Honshu, and even on these main islands *C. megacephala* has sometimes (indeed almost annually on occasion) appeared in the late summer and autumn (Figure 3-4). For instance, in 1982 large numbers of this fly were collected at this time of year in Southern Kyushu. Suenaga et al. (1964) concluded that *C. megacephala* became established in Nagasaki from 1953 to 1957, but was afterwards eradicated through improved sanitation, notably as regards sewage disposal. They concluded that the records from Kyoto and Tokyo are due to occasional incursions, not permanent establishments. I also investigated the occurrence of this fly in the late summer and autumn in Yumenoshima, a large man-made island deliberately constructed by an intensive garbage-dumping program in Tokyo Bay. A small number of adults having emerged from the garbage, at least one generation had bred there during the season. Nevertheless, I believe that this fly has so far failed to establish permanent populations in Honshu and Kyushu, where the climate is too severe in winter—this tropical species requires warmer conditions than 15°C mean temperature for normal larval development. It should be realized, too, that there is no record of *C. megacephala* from the Izushichito Islands, which lie between the Bonin Islands and Honshu.

To sum up, despite repeated arrivals in the main islands, the oriental latrine fly has so far proved unable to establish permanent colonies in Kyushu and Honshu. Its usual method of intermittent entry into Kyushu and Honshu is most probably via shipping, although natural agencies certainly contribute significantly. The maritime routes between Japan's main islands and the Southwest and Bonin Islands are rather busy ones. Various kinds of ships from the southern islands and Southeast Asia arrive in Tokyo

Figure 3-3. Known records of *Chrysomya megacephala* in Japan. Black: established. White: probably not established.

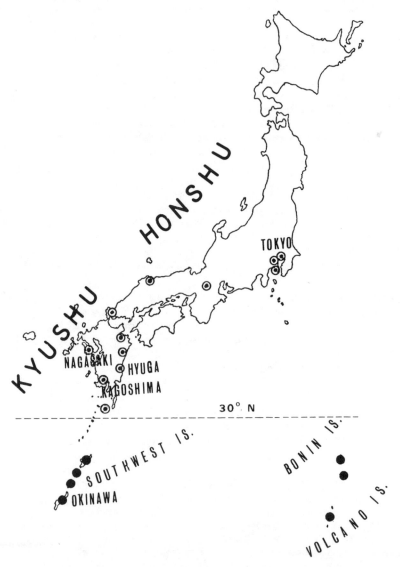

Bay throughout the year. Storms, particularly typhoons, are among the natural agencies displacing insects from the south to southern Japan. Many instances of the arrival of southern butterflies and dragonflies have been reported by local entomologists following typhoons. Surveys of naturally

Figure 3-4. Seasonal fluctuations of *C. megacephala* introduced into Kyushu and Honshu (Miyazaki 1960, modified).

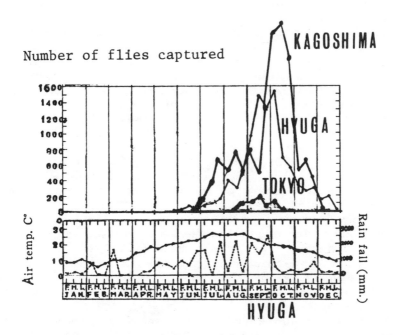

James (1962) suggested that the extension of this species' range to Micronesia took place by way of Japan—via the Bonin and Volcano Islands—prior to World War II. His records from Micronesia reached back to Hornbostel's collections on Guam in 1923 and on Rota in 1925. He also examined collections that were made by Okabe from Chichi Jima in 1934 and by Esaki from Saipan and Jaluit in 1937. *Chrysomya nigripes,* the only known representative of the subgenus *Microcalliphora,* is known only from Guam (Bohart and Gressitt 1951; James 1962). In Micronesia, *C. rufifacies* is apparently becoming widely established today, although its populations are much smaller than those of *C. megacephala.* James considered that the absence of

air-borne insects crossing the South China Sea have included several kinds of blowflies (Asahina 1970; Hayashi et al. 1979). However, the latter scientists failed to find *C. megacephala* among their collections. Kusui (1980) published an interesting report on insects found in aircraft entering Tokyo's international airports (both Haneda and Narita) from abroad, but the oriental latrine fly was not among his lists of species.

C. rufifacies from the Caroline Islands may simply reflect a lack of records, if not the fact that its introduction into those atolls has not yet taken place, or if it has, to the possible failure of the fly to establish itself—perhaps because of the difficulty of competing with the already-established *C. megacephala* under the restricted ecological conditions of the atolls.

Oceanic islands usually have a scanty endemic blowfly fauna. This undoubtedly reflects the scarcity of suitable breeding media in an area of small land masses separated by great distances and associated, until recent times, with a lack or scarcity of large animal carcasses. The arrival and establishment of ancestral stocks of blowflies and the subsequent evolution of forms that adapted to the native breeding media must have been hindered over the years by these factors. Obviously, most of the nonendemic fauna has resulted from the importation by man—at various times—of adaptable forms able to subsist on the atolls. In quite recent times, blowfly establishments must have been favored by profound changes in the economy and way of life, due to such happenings as introductions of larger mammals and development of garbage dumps. The transformed environment has permitted the development and survival of synanthropic forms that require large amounts of carrion and animal wastes for breeding purposes.

In 1982, I made a survey on Minami Iwo Jima, Volcano Islands, a small, isolated, virgin island of the Pacific (Kurahashi 1982). Four species of blowflies and one species of flesh fly were found breeding in bird carrion there: *Chrysomya megacephala, Lucilia snyderi, L. sericata, Stomorhina obsoleta,* and *Parasarcophaga misera.* It is believed that all of these could have reached the virgin island by natural agency. For example, *L. snyderi* is the single endemic blowfly known from the Bonin and Volcano Islands; breeding in the wounds of marine birds as well as avian carrion, it can probably be transported from island to island by migrating birds. However, this fly prefers a moist medium and is usually found at above 400 m in mountainous areas, characterized by fog and the development of moss forests. In the Bonin Islands, it is found only on the mountain of Chibusa (462 m) on Haha Jima. *L. graphita* is a native of the leeward Hawaiian Islands, Laysan, Ocean, and Midway, and has been intercepted from aircraft several times on Guam; however, there is no indication that it has as yet become established on any of the islands of Micronesia (James 1962). James also considered that aside from *L. snyderi,* the calliphorids of Micronesia fall into two groups, so far as geographical origin is concerned. First,

Hemipyrellia ligurriens, Stomorhina obsoleta, and *Lucilia sericata* invaded the area from the north, though apparently not very successfully. The first two are recorded only from the Bonin Islands, whereas the last-mentioned is known in this area from the Bonins, Volcano, Wake, and the Marshall Islands. The second group, which James considered as the true invaders, consists of seven species that have come from the south and west. These flies are tropical or subtropical elements and have been much more successful in having a wide distribution, with the exception of *C. nigripes.*

Among these invaders, *C. megacephala* has by far the most successful record, having become very abundant throughout the area. Hardy (1981) considered that this species probably reached Hawaii from the Orient during the early period of cattle, sheep, and goat introductions, although it is very common throughout the islands up to about 1500m above sea level. Grimshaw (1901) first reported this fly (under the name of *Calliphora azurea*) from material collected at Kona, Hawaii Island, in 1892. *C. rufifacies* was not recognized in Hawaii until 1918 (Illingworth 1918) and was also considered to be an early immigrant.

SPECULATION ON THE ORIGIN:
BIOSYSTEMATICS

Chrysomya megacephala gives its name to the *megacephala* group, which consists of seven species primarily from the Oriental and Australasian Regions. Some authors have chosen to relegate these flies to another genus (*Compsomyia,* Rondani 1875). *Chrysomya* is characterized by a fuscous mesothoracic spiracle, *Compsomyia* by a whitish one. The former genus is primarily indigenous in the Afrotropical Region, but *Chrysomya marginalis* enters the Oriental Region. *C. rufifacies* has been regarded by some as merely a subspecies of *C. albiceps*—an aberrant taxon found in the Oriental and Australasian Regions. In the *megacephala*-group, *C. bezziana* is known to be an obligatory producer of wound-myiasis in man and animals. It often causes major veterinary problems, whereas *C. megacephala* is a filth fly of medical importance. The latter normally breeds in faeces and carrion, and is characteristically found around garbage and lavatories, although its larvae are occasionally encountered as facultative parasites in traumatic myiasis. The other species seem to be primary scavengers and forest inhabitants.

The seven species of the *megacephala* group can be distinguished by the following key:

1. Base of upper squama whitish. 2
   Upper squama entirely fuscous; parafacialia and jowls fuscous 5
2. Upper and lower squamae largely fuscous to brown; parafacialia and jowls orange or reddish 3
   Upper and lower squamae largely whitish to pale gray; parafacialia and jowls fuscous to black or orange 4
3. Peristomal setulae yellow . . *C. saffranea* (Bigot)
   Peristomal setulae black, at least in part . . . .
   . . . . *C. megacephala* (Fabricius)
4. Parafacialia and jowls fuscous to black; setulae and hairs on parafacialia and facialia blackish; *ac* 0+2; venter of tergite 5 with black hairs only; male and female eyes dichoptic. . . . . .
   . . . . *C. phaonis* (Séguy)
   Parafacialia and jowls entirely orange; setulae and hairs on parafacialia and facialia yellowish; *ac* 0+1; venter of tergite 5 intermixed with yellow hairs; eyes in male holoptic, dichoptic in female. . . . . *C. bezziana* Villeneuve
5. Posthumeral bristle usually absent; body large, more than 12.0mm, purple in color. . . . . . .
   . . . *C. thanomthini* Kurahashi and Tumrasvin
   Posthumerals usually developed; body medium in size, bluish to greenish in color. 6
6. Body bluish; metacephala usually covered with yellowish hairs; length of jowls more than that of eye when viewed laterally; height of jowls about 3/10 in male, 4/10 in female of total head height; cerci elongate in male. . . . .
   . . . . *C. pinguis* (Wiedemann)
   Body greenish; metacephala usually covered with black and brown hairs; height of jowls as that of eye when viewed laterally; height of jowls about 2/10 of total head height in male, 3/10 in female; cerci stout, subequal to the length of surstyli. . . . . *C. defixa* (Walker)

POLYMORPHISM

Examination of the material obtained from New Guinea and South Pacific islands during my early survey in 1978

(Kurahashi 1982) has revealed the presence of two forms within the population of *C. megacephala*. These are differentiated by the size of the male eye facets (Figure 3-5). The typical form of *C. megacephala* has greatly enlarged upper facets; these are sharply demarcated from small ones on the lower third of the eye. This form is synanthropic and is commonly found around garbage in towns of various countries. The second form occurs in native forests of South Pacific islands from the Bismarck Archipelago to Samoa; its eyes exhibit almost uniform facets in both sexes. Feral examples of the typical form were also discovered by Dr. R. Kano (chief of the survey) and me in New Guinea. Such dimorphism has also been demonstrated in different populations of *C. pinguis, C. defixa,* and *C. saffranea.* The two forms are very similar to one another. However, the form of *C. megacephala* with normal eye facets can be distinguished from one having large demarcated facets by the following characteristics: body stout but not rounded, submetallic dark blue to green; squamae largely blackish; and vibrissaria, medianae, and facialia with black hairs. Male genitalia of the two forms are almost identical in the respective species. The condition of sharply demarcated large facets is considered to have arisen as a result of enlargement of the male eye associated with behavioral development. Imms (1957) stated in his textbook that the upper portion composed of large facets is adapted to give a superimposed image, the lower one of smaller facets giving an apposed image. The upper part probably perceives variations in the intensity of light from above produced by clouds, moving enemies, etc., without there being any necessity to perceive definite form. The lower part of the divided eye is clearly adapted for more acute vision and to receiving the more exact impressions produced by objects over which the insect may be flying or resting.

PHYLOGENY

To determine phylogenetic relationships, the seven species of the *megacephala* group, and their forms, have been submitted to taxonomic analysis on the basis of 16 characters, A-P. Each character is coded in 2 states—plesiomorphous (-) and apomorphous (+)—according to presumed deviation from generalized features of the genus *Chrysomya s. l.*

A: Jowls black (-) or orange (+)
B: Base of upper squama fuscous (-) or white (+)

Figure 3-5. Frontal view of male head. n.f.: feral normal form, from Solomon Islands. s.d.f.: synanthropic derived form, from Solomon Islands. f.d.f.: feral derived form, from New Guinea (*C. megacephala*).

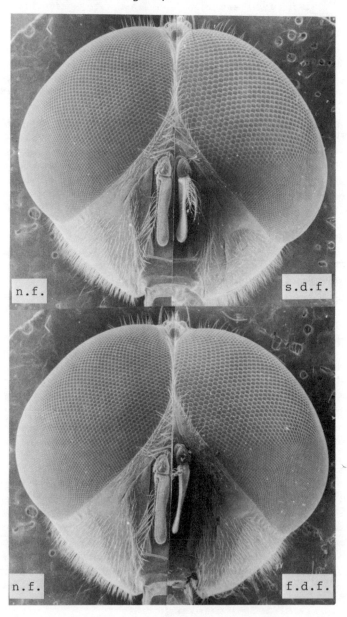

C: Base of upper squama with fuscous hairs (-) or with whitish hairs (+)
D: Peristomal setulae black (-) or yellow (+)
E: Vibrissaria and medianae with black hairs (-) or with yellow hairs (+)
F: Facialia with black hairs (-) or with yellow hairs (+)
G: Upper facets of male eyes normal (-) or large and distinctly demarcated from lower ones (+)
H: Antennae fuscous, entirely or dorsally (-) or entirely orange (+)
I: Tergite 5 with black hairs only (-) or intermixed with yellow hairs ventrally (+)
J: Cerci stout (-) or elongate (+)
K: Male eye dichoptic (-) or holoptic (+)
L: Upper most *ors* or prevertical bristle present (-) or absent (+) in male
M: Outer and inner vertical bristles present (-) or absent (+) in male
N: Spermatheca elongate oval (-) or globular (+)
O: Female tergite 6 of a single entire sclerite (-) or split into two lateral plates (+)
P: Types of male genitalia (a), (b), (c), (d), (e), (f), (g), (h)

The character P is used only for proximity analysis. The n × t matrix (Table 3-1) is prepared from the above list and is put in SCD (Sum of Character Difference) or SRR (Russell and Rao 1940) proximity analysis, and UPGA cluster analysis to obtain a dendrogram (Sneath and Sokal 1973). For each taxon (form), the percentage frequency of derived or apomorphous states (D%) is given in circles in the dendrogram. In calculating D%, intermediate entries (±) were counted twice, once as plesiomorphous, once as apomorphous (?); (NC) entries are disregarded.

$$D\% = \frac{\text{no. of } (+) + \text{no. of } (\pm)}{\text{no. of characters} + \text{no. of } (\pm) - \text{no. of } (?)} \times 100$$

A hypothetical ancestor whose characters all show plesiomorphous state was included for both phenetic and phyletic analysis. Figure 3-6 shows phenetic relationship of 12 taxa. Three subgroups can be easily distinguished in the dendrogram. *C. phaonis* is similar to the hypothetical ancestor. The group comprises three main branches: the first branch represents the ancestral stock; the second *defixa-thanomthini-pinguis;* the third *megacephala-bezziana-saffranea.* Figure 3-7 illustrates the numerical phyletics.

Table 3-1. The species and forms of _megacephala_ group: n (characters) × t (taxa) matrix.

t		A	B	C	D	E	F	G	H	I	J	K	L	M	N	O	P
1.	_Chrysomya_ saffranea, n.f.	+	+	+	+	+	+	-	+	+	-	+	+	+	+	-	a
2.	C. saffranea, d.f.	+	+	-	+	+	+	+	±	-	-	+	+	+	+	-	a
3.	C. megacephala, n.f.	+	+	+	-	±	-	-	-	-	-	+	+	+	+	-	b
4.	C. megacephala, d.f.	+	+	+	-	±	±	+	-	±	-	+	+	+	+	-	b
5.	C. defixa, n.f.	-	-	-	-	-	-	-	-	-	-	+	+	+	+	-	c
6.	C. defixa, d.f.	-	-	-	-	-	-	+	-	-	-	+	+	+	+	-	c
7.	C. pinguis, n.f.	-	-	-	-	-	-	-	-	-	+	+	+	+	+	-	d
8.	C. pinguis, d.f.	-	-	-	-	-	-	+	-	-	+	+	+	+	+	-	d
9.	C. thanomthini	-	-	-	-	-	-	+	-	-	-	+	+	+	+	-	e
10.	C. bezziana	+	+	+	±	+	+	-	-	-	-	+	+	+	+	-	f
11.	C. phaonis	-	+	±	-	-	-	-	-	-	±	-	-	-	-	+	g
12.	Ancestor	-	-	-	-	-	-	-	-	-	-	-	-	-	-	-	h

Figure 3-6. Phenetic dendrogram of the *megacephala* group.

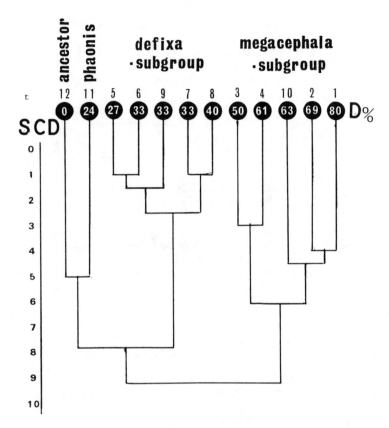

C. *phaonis* emerges as the most primitive (D% = 24), hence the most obvious choice as the closest taxon (from both phenetic and phyletic standpoints) to the hypothetical ancestor of this group. The normal form of C. *saffranea* (D% = 80) appears to be the most highly evolved taxon, hence the one differing most from the common ancestor. The dendrogram shows that a cluster "*defixa* and *megacephala* subgroup" has a sister-group relationship with an ancestral stock. The *megacephala* subgroup evolved from the *defixa* subgroup. The phylogenetic tree simplified after the Hennigian school is shown in Figure 3-8.

GEOGRAPHICAL DISTRIBUTION AND EVOLUTION

An ancestral stock, C. *phaonis,* is a rare species and seems to be relict in the West China Area as shown in Figure 3-9.

Figure 3-7.   Phyletic dendrogram of the *megacephala* group.

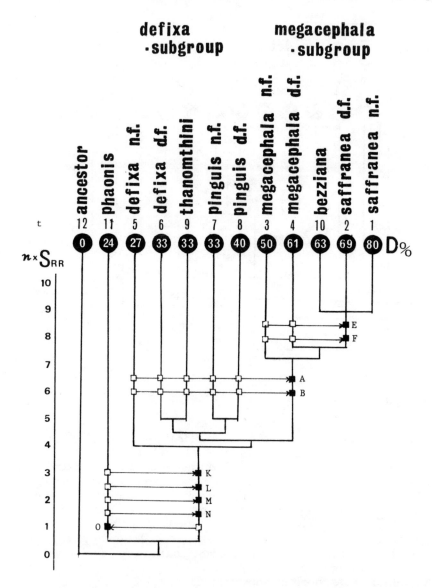

The *defixa* subgroup occurs mainly in the Oriental Region, and the derived forms of *C. defixa* and *C. pinguis* have more or less invaded Wallacea (Kurahashi 1982).   The d.f. of the latter species is also found in Palearctic China and Japan.   The n.f. of both species is restricted to the

Figure 3-8. Phylogeny of the *megacephala* group.

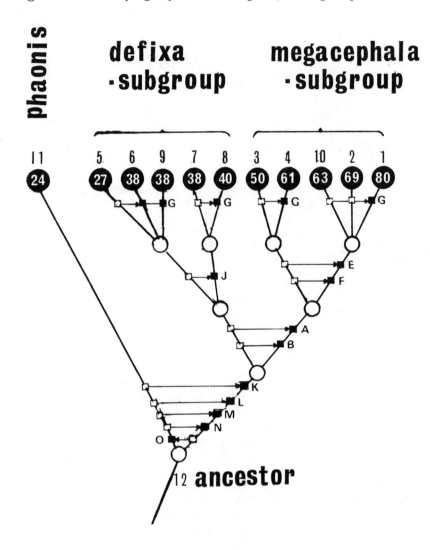

Malayan Subregion. *C. pinguis*, n.f. is also present in Palawan; but the fact that it does not predominate in that island's fauna suggests a relatively recent introduction. The *megacephala* subgroup is mainly in the Australasian area. The wide range of *C. megacephala* and *bezziana* may be due to recent introductions as mentioned above. The n.f. of *C. saffranea* occurs in southern parts of New Guinea and Queensland, and its derived form is found in

Figure 3-9. Geographical distribution of *Chrysomya phaonis* (Séguy).

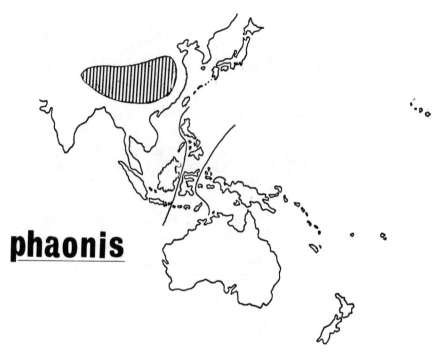

phaonis

New Caledonia. The normal form of *C. megacephala* is found from the Bismarck Archipelago to Samoa (Figure 3-10). Generally speaking, the derived form formerly occurred at the peripheries of the extent of its ancestral form n.f. This may suggests that even in the case of *C. megacephala,* the earlier isolation from the normal form probably occurred even along the margin of the distributional limit. It is likely that the d.f. of *C. megacephala* has evolved in New Guinea. The origin of *C. bezziana* remains obscure. If the close resemblance between *megacephala* and *bezziana* is not derived from a convergence, the same speculation may apply to the origin of this Old World screwworm. Evolution of the *C. megacephala*-group is schematized in Figure 3-11.

DEVELOPMENT OF SYNANTHROPY

Following the evolution of *C. megacephala* d.f., domestication of this form probably occurred also in New Guinea. Some relevant observations were made during my South

Figure 3-10. Geographical distributions of forms of *C. megacephala*. n.f.: normal form. d.f.: derived form. s.d.f.: synanthropic derived form.

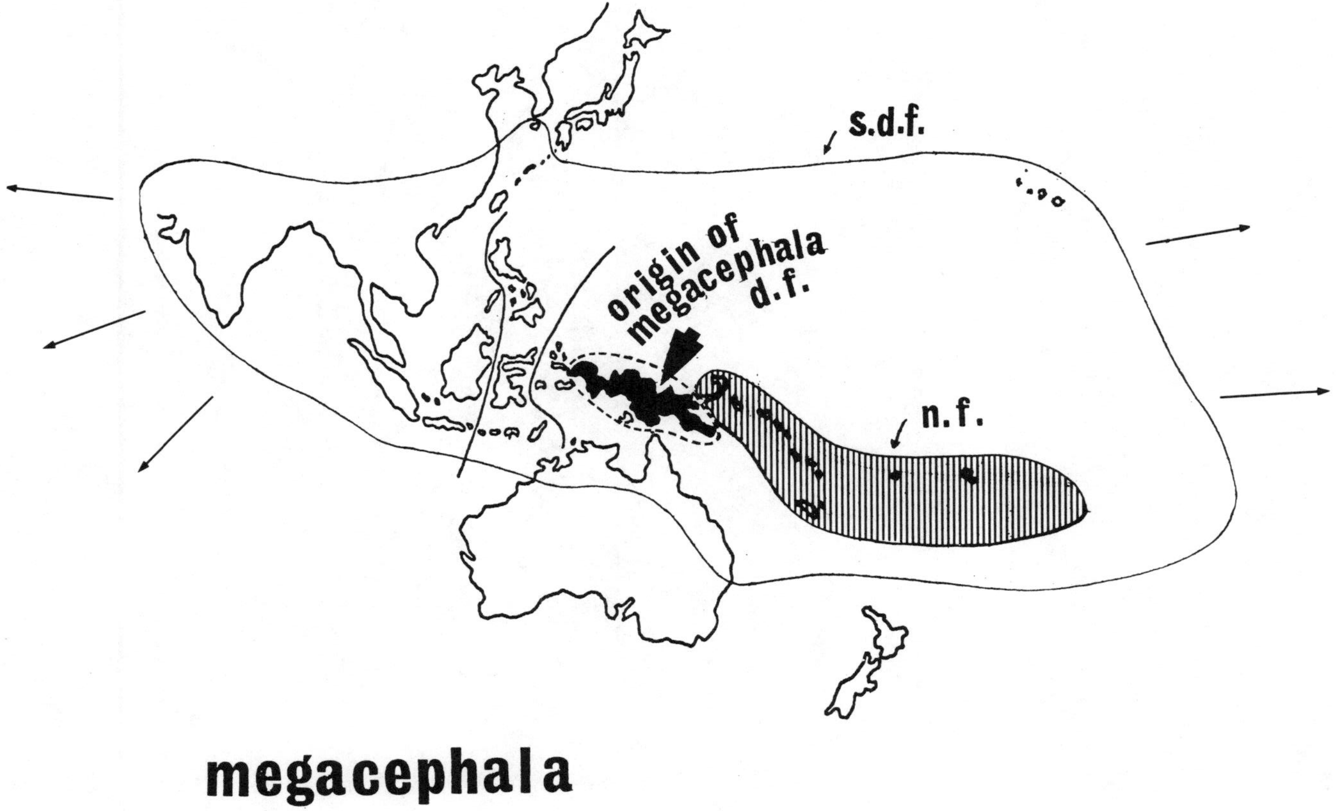

megacephala

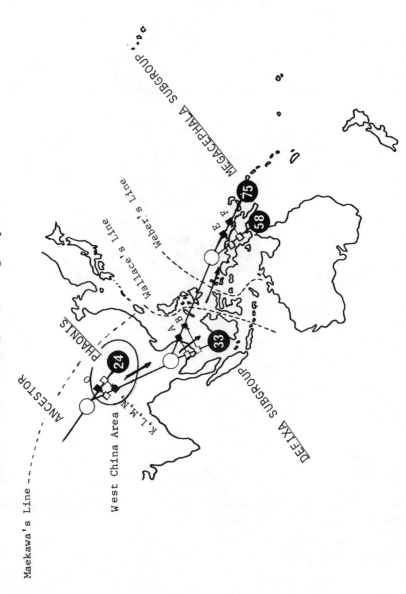

Figure 3-11. Evolution of the *megacephala* group.

Pacific surveys. Ecological information supports the theory that the d.f. originated in New Guinea, the synanthropic form having subsequently become widely distributed in the world. The primary habitat of the six related species is undoubtedly the native forest. In New Guinea, *C. megacephala* d.f. is feral and is commonly found in natural forests as well as secondary ones (Figure 3-12). However, the very similar synanthropic d.f. lives in villages and towns. The minor differences in the morphology of the male eyes of the two taxa consist in the frontal view of the eyes and the size of upper facets appearing intermediate between the n.f. of both forms and the synanthropic d.f. (Figure 3-5). While *C. megacephala* d.f. is feral, and found only in dense natural and seminatural forests, the synanthropic d.f. is observed around human dwellings and in secondary open forests from the Bismarck Archipelago to Samoa.

In the Oriental Region the synanthropic d.f. is usually domestic or peridomestic, although it is sometimes found in forests where it is not a dominant species in the forest fauna. It is likely that two feral forms have been established in the different types of environment characterizing New Guinea and other South Pacific islands. New Guinean d.f. is characteristic of relatively dry, sunny, clear, sparse, and rather hot forests. The natural forests of South Pacific islands where the n.f. occurs are characterized by dense, gloomy, highly humid conditions. Where secondarily modified environments occur, they contraindicate forest inhabitants. The new environment requires physiological and ecological changes for insects to establish themselves in it through microevolution. Such land modification as traditional slash-and-burn and shifting cultivation systems, are to be seen almost everywhere in New Guinea. People cut or burn away natural forests to produce sweet potatoes, yams, taro, maize, rice, etc. Shifting agriculture means that "bush fallow" plots of individuals or families are widely scattered, from near the village to a distance of several km. The New Guinean feral d.f. had to enter such secondary environments when man began to burn forests. It was likely that the New Guinean feral form had a potential adaptability to open land and survived even in grasslands that usually developed after shifting cultivation. The physiological and morphological differences became marked as a result of adaption to far-reaching land modification by man (Figure 3-13).

Once established (most probably) through agrobiocoenosis and finally in the anthropobiocoenosis, the synanthropic d.f.—being well adapted to severe environments in

Figure 3-12. Two forms found in different habitats in the South Pacific islands from Bougainville to Samoa.

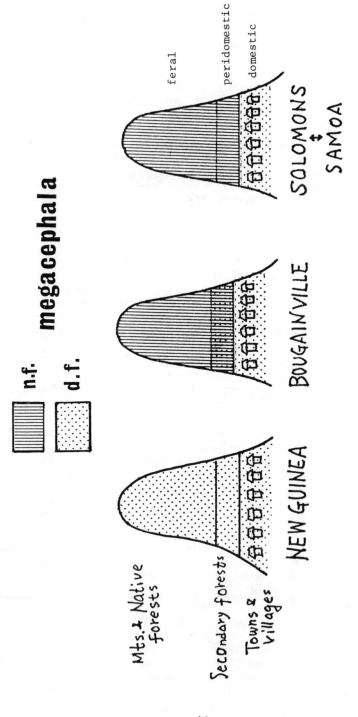

60

Figure 3-13. A scheme of the origin of synanthropic form of *C. megacephala* and its immigration.

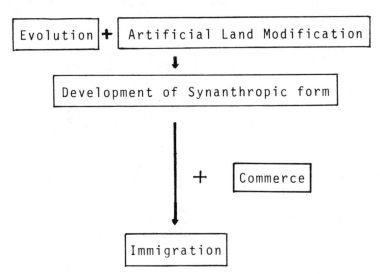

the anthropobiocoenosis—was in a position to accompany man to many other parts of the tropical and subtropical areas. The emigrant has thus become a dominant fly in urban and suburban areas of Southeast Asia, the South Pacific and Australia, and is currently succeeding in establishing colonies in Africa and South America. This emigrant form, however, finds cold winter conditions a severe barrier to its establishment in temperate countries.

REFERENCES

Asahina, S. 1970. Records of insects visiting a weather-ship located at the Ocean Weather Station "Tango" on the Pacific; V. Insects captured during 1968. *Kontyu* 38:318-30.

Baez, M., and E. Santos-Pinto. 1975. Dipteros de Canarias I: Calliphoridae. *Vieraea* 5:1-22.

Baez, M., G. Ortega, and H. Kurahashi. 1981. Immigration of the oriental latrine fly, *Chrysomya megacephala* (Fabricius) and the Afrotropical Filth Fly, *Ch. chloropyga* (Wiedemann), into the Canary Islands (Diptera, Calliphoridae). *Kontyu* 49:712-14.

Bohart, G. E., and J. L. Gressitt. 1951. Filth-inhabiting flies of Guam. *Bull. B. P. Bishop Mus.* 204:1-152.

Fukuda, M. 1960. On the effect of physical condition of

trap location upon the number of flies collected by fish-baited trap. *Endemic Dis. Bull. Nagasaki Univ.* 2:222-28 (in Japanese).

Gagné, R. J. 1981. *Chrysomya* spp., Old World blow flies (Diptera: Calliphoridae), recently established in the Americas. *Bull. ent. Soc. Amer.* 27:21-22.

Greenberg, B. 1980. Biology of Peruvian blow flies. Paper read at the XVI International Congress of Entomology, August 3-9, 1980, Kyoto, Japan.

Grimshaw, P. H. 1901. Part I. Diptera. In *Fauna Hawaiiensis* 3. Ed. D. Sharp, pp. 1-77. Cambridge: University Press.

Guimarães, J. H., A. P. do Prado, and A. X. Linhares. 1978. Three newly introduced blowfly species in southern Brazil (Diptera, Calliphoridae). *Rev. brasil. Ent.* 22:53-60.

Guimarães, J. H., A. P. do Prado, and G. M. Buralli. 1979. Dispersal and distribution of three newly introduced species of *Chrysomya* Robineau-Desvoidy in Brazil (Diptera, Calliphoridae). *Rev. brasil. Ent.* 23:245-55.

Hanski, I. 1977. Biogeography and ecology of carrion flies in the Canary Islands. *Ann. ent. fenn.* 43:101-7.

Hardy, D. E. 1981. Diptera: Cyclorrhapha IV. In *Insects of Hawaii,* 14. Honolulu: Univ. Hawaii Press.

Hayashi, K., H. Suzuki, Y. Makino, and S. Asahina. 1979. Notes on the transoceanic insects captured on East China Sea in 1976, 1977, and 1978. *Tropical Medicine* 21:1-10.

Illingworth, J. F. 1918. The Australian sheep fly in Hawaii. *Proc. Hawaii. Ent. Soc.* 13:429.

Imbiriba, A. S., D. T. Izutani, I. T. Milhoretto, and E. Luz. 1977. Introdução da *Chrysomya chloropyga* (Wiedemann, 1818) na região neotropical (Diptera, Calliphoridae). *Arch. biol. tecnol. Curitiba* 20:35-39.

Imms, A. D. 1957 (reprint of 1964). *A General Textbook of Entomology,* 9th ed. (rev. O. W. Richards and R. G. Davies), London: Methuen.

James, M. T. 1962. Diptera: Stratiomyidae and Calliphoridae. *Insects of Micronesia* 13:75-127.

Jirón, J. F. 1979. Sobre moscas califóridas de Costa Rica (Diptera, Cyclorrhapha). *Brenesia* 16:221-23.

Kano, R. 1958. Notes on flies of medical importance in Japan, Part XIV, Descriptions of five species belonging to Chrysomyinae (Calliphoridae) including one newly found species. *Bull. Tokyo med. dent. Univ.* 5:465-74.

Kato, Y. 1960. Flies in Nansatu District of Kagoshima Prefecture. *Igaku Kenkyu* 30:72-94 (in Japanese).

Kurahashi, H. 1982. Probable origin of a synanthropic fly *Chrysomya megacephala,* in New Guinea (Diptera: Calliphoridae). *Monogr. Biol.* 42:689-98.

——————. 1978. The oriental latrine fly: *Chrysomya megacephala* (Fabricius) newly recorded from Ghana and Senegal, West Africa. *Kontyu* 46:432.

——————. 1980. The Afrotropical filth fly, *Chrysomya albiceps* (Wiedemann) newly recorded from Guatemala, Central America. *Kontyu* 48:427.

——————. 1982. Calyptrate muscoid flies collected in Minami-Iwojima Island. In *Conservation Reports of the Minami-Iwojima Wilderness Area, Tokyo, Japan.* The Environment Agency, Japan: 349-51.

Kusui, Y. 1980. Study on the insect pests collected in aircraft and ships. *Ochanomizu Igaku Zasshi* 28:149-70 (in Japanese).

Laurence, B. R. 1981. Geographical expansion of the range of *Chrysomya* blowflies. *Trans. Roy. Soc. trop. Med. Hyg.* 75:130-31.

Miyazaki, T. 1960. On flies of medical importance in South Kyushu, I. Fly fauna in Hyuga City. *Kagoshima Daigaku Igaku Zasshi* 11:102-27.

Prins, A. J. 1979. Discovery of the oriental latrine fly *Chrysomya megacephala* (Fabricius) along the south-western coast of South Africa. *Ann. S. Afr. Mus.* 78:39-47.

Russell, P. F., and T. R. Rao. 1940. On habitat and association of species of anopheline larvae in South-eastern Madras. *J. Malar. Inst. India* 3:153-78.

Sneath, P. H. A., and R. R. Sokal. 1973. *Numerical Taxonomy: the principles and practise of numerical classification.* San Francisco: Freeman.

Suenaga, O., M. Shimogama, S. Kawai, M. Fukuda, and T. Tanikawa. 1964. Ecological studies of flies 9. Some notes on the flies trapped by fish baited traps in different places in middle and southwestern Japan. *Endemic Dis. Bull. Nagasaki Univ.* 6:39-47.

Uemoto, K., K. Matsuo, S. Kitamura, and K. Toita. 1962. Ecological studies on flies in Kyoto, I. Seasonal prevalences of adult flies. *Jap. J. Sanit. Zool.* 13:163 (in Japanese).

Zumpt, F. 1965. *Myiasis in Man and Animals in the Old World,* London: Butterworth.

Chapter 4

Survey on Accidental Introductions of Insects Entering Japan via Aircraft

S. Takahashi

INTRODUCTION

The number of international flights entering and leaving Japan has increased dramatically in recent years. For example, the number of aircraft on which a quarantine inspection was performed at Tokyo's former International Airport (Haneda) was only 3,711 in 1957; but by 1977, twenty years later, this number had grown sevenfold to 25,842. But the impact of the gradual replacement of older, smaller aircraft by new, larger planes has recently become apparent. In 1979, the year after the move to the New Tokyo International Airport (Narita), the number of landings was 27,136; but by 1981, it declined to 26,234 and a downward trend became apparent. The number of pas-

*I would like to express my deepest gratitude to Dr. Sakito Agata, Director of Narita Airport Quarantine Station, to Dr. Toshio Aida, former director of the station, for guidance and stimulation, and to Dr. Takeshi Kurihara, Professor, Department of Parasitology, Teikyo University School of Medicine, for his guidance in many ways in addition to mosquito identification. I would also like to thank my colleagues in the Health Bureau of the Quarantine Station for participating in this study. Finally, I would like to express my heartfelt thanks to Dr. Marshall Laird,

sengers carried, however, continues to increase yearly, and reached 4,772,916 quarantine examinees in 1981.*

It would seem inevitable from these figures that the number of opportunities for insect pests to be introduced via aircraft from overseas has also increased. As a result, the task of preventing the introduction of mosquitoes and other vectors of human disease has become more important for preventing epidemics internationally. WHO prescribes International Health Regulations (IHR) for enforcement in aircraft and airport areas and recommends the adoption of so-called "blocks-away" or in-flight vapor disinsecting systems to eliminate mosquito vectors of yellow fever, malaria, and other diseases of epidemiological significance in international traffic.

In order to clarify the circumstances surrounding the presence of insect pests within aircraft and, wherever necessary, to establish suitable countermeasures, inspections were conducted at Haneda Airport from May 1975 to May 1978 and at Narita Airport from June 1978 onwards. This chapter reports the results as of 1981 and describes the countermeasures now being implemented.

SUBJECTS AND METHODS

The insects of medical importance covered in this study included most importantly *Aedes aegypti* and *Xenopsylla cheopis,* vectors of yellow fever and plague, diseases subject to the regulations laid down in Japan's Quarantine Law and the IHR. The study also included species of mosquitoes that are epidemiologically important as international vectors of malaria, Japanese B encephalitis (JE), etc., as well as muscoid flies and cockroaches.

The aircraft searched for arthropods were primarily those on flights arriving at Haneda or Narita between 0900 and 1700. Particular attention was paid to flights originating from or with stopovers in tropical or subtropical

---

Director, Research Unit on Vector Pathology, and Research Professor (Parasitology), Memorial University of Newfoundland, for his concern and assistance in seeing this report published.

*This paper reports the results of a survey conducted into airport sanitary conditions by Dr. Sakito Agata, Director of Narita Airport Quarantine Station.

zones, but some flights originating elsewhere were included, too.

The study was conducted by quarantine officers who boarded the aircraft immediately after the passengers had left the cabin and baggage had been removed from the holds. Cabin and hold were examined with a flashlight in searching for live insects, which when found were secured by means of a collecting net and an aspirator. At the same time, flight attendants were questioned regarding the aircraft's point of origin and stopovers, including departure times, and performance of in-flight disinsecting between departure and arrival.

RESULTS AND OBSERVATIONS

A total of 928 aircraft were inspected between May 1975 and December 1981, live insects of medical importance being discovered on 400 (43.1%) of them. Totals of 840 mosquitoes were found on 168 aircraft, 955 flies on 295 aircraft, and 228 cockroaches on 54 aircraft; while one flea was found on a rat captured in the cargo hold of an aircraft. Species distribution is shown in Table 4-1.

Four genera and 13 species were represented in the mosquitoes captured. Those not present in Japan were:

> *Anopheles indefinitus*
> *Anopheles subpictus*
> *Anopheles vagus limosus*
> *Mansonia annulifera*
> *Aedes aegypti*
> *Aedes sollicitans*
> *Aedes v. vexans*
> *Culex gelidus*
> *Culex vishnui*

Furthermore, in most cases concerning the *C. pipiens* complex (which accounted for 96.7% of the total number of mosquitoes collected), specimens collected from planes coming from airports in tropical and subtropical zones were identified from abdominal markings and male genitalia as *C. quinquefasciatus* Say (= *C. pipiens fatigans* Wiedemann), a species the Japanese distribution of which is limited to Ogasawara, the Ryukyus, and the Amami Islands. Then, although found in some parts of Japan, *M. uniformis* (Table 4-1) is a species that is not present in the areas surrounding Haneda and Narita.

Table 4-1. List of collected insects of medical importance.

Mosquitoes

    Anopheles indefinitus (Ludlow)
    Anopheles sinensis Wiedemann
    Anopheles subpictus Grassi
    Anopheles vagus limosus King
    Aedes aegypti (L.)
    Aedes sollicitans (Walker)
    Aedes vexans vexans (Meigen)
    Culex pipiens L.
    Culex gelidus Theobald
    Culex tritaeniorhychus Giles
    Culex vishnui Theobald
    Mansonia annulifera (Theobald)
    Mansonia uniformis (Theobald)

Flies

    Musca domestica L.
    Chrysomya nigripes Aubertin
    Chrysomya rufifacies (Macquart)
    Lucilia cuprina (Wiedemann)
    Pollenia rudis (Fabricius)
    Aldrichina grapami (Aldrich)
    Boettcherisca sp.
    Sarcophaga peregrina Robineau-Desvoidy
    Fannia canicularis (L.)

Cockroaches

    Blattella germanica (L.)
    Supella longipalpa (Fabricius)
    Periplaneta americana (L.)
    Periplaneta australasiae (Fabricius)
    Periplaneta brunnea Burmeister
    Neostylopyga sp.
    Pycnoscelis surinamensis (L.)

Fleas

    Xenopsylla cheopis (Rothschild)

Four families, 8 genera, and 9 species of fly were identified. Since the most frequently captured muscoid fly, *M. domestica,* is distributed worldwide, it is difficult to determine where this species entered a particular aircraft. Nevertheless, by studying the frons/head width ratio and the width of color patterns on the abdomen of males using the method of my coworkers Kusui et al. (1980), and by performing the insecticide susceptibility test used by Ogata et al. (1974), it was possible to make an educated guess regarding each muscoid fly's place of introduction. It was determined as a result of the tests that almost all of the *M. domestica* captured aboard arriving aircraft were of foreign origin. The distribution area of *Chrysomya nigripes* and *Pollenia rudis* does not include Japan, and *Chrysomya rufifacies* is not found in Haneda Airport, Narita Airport, or their environs.

Three families, 5 genera, and 7 species of cockroaches were collected. Of these, the distribution of *Blattella germanica* is worldwide—and in many cases it appeared that these cockroaches inhabited the plane, so it was not possible to ascertain their point of introduction. Other species are normally rare or completely absent on Honshu.

Looking next at the combinations of insects recorded, we see from Table 4-2 that instances of muscoid flies alone being captured were the most frequent. One hundred ninety-six catches were made in 49% of the planes in which some insects of medical importance were found. Flies alone were followed in frequency of capture by the simultaneous capture of flies and mosquitoes with 76 cases (19%). Mosquitoes were captured in the absence of any other insects in 74 cases (18.5%) and cockroaches alone in 22 cases (5.5%). Flies and cockroaches were captured together in 14 cases (3.5%); and simultaneous captures of mosquitoes with cockroaches, and of mosquitoes with flies and cockroaches, were the least frequent, with 9 cases each (2.3%).

The breakdown by flight route is presented in Table 4-3. Of the total of 928 flights inspected, 654 flights from the south originated or had stopovers in tropical or subtropical zones (between 30°N and 30°S latitudes). Manila (MNL) flights were the most frequent with 229, followed by Taipei (TPE) with 171, Hong Kong (HKG) with 145, Honolulu (HNL) with 60, Bangkok (BKK) with 28, Guam (GUM) with 8, Saipan (SPN) with 8, Osaka (OSA) with 2, Singapore (SIN) with 2, and Noumea (NOU) with 1. A total of 274 flights originating from locations north of latitude 30°N were inspected. Moscow (MOW) flights were the most numerous with 69, followed by Los Angeles (LAX) with 51, Peking (now Beijing in Pinyin standard spelling; PEK) with

Table 4-2. Insects of medical importance captured on the arrival of international aircraft at Tokyo International Airport, Haneda (May, 1975-May, 1978) and New Tokyo International Airport, Narita (June, 1978-1981).

Year	No. of inspected aircraft	No. of aircraft in which live insect pests were captured							
		Total	(1) only	(2) only	(3) only	(1) & (2)	(1) & (3)	(2) & (3)	(1), (2) & (3)
1975	131	49	3	33	7	4	0	2	0
1976	104	38	11	13	2	6	2	2	2
1977	107	62	10	30	2	12	0	3	5
1978	89	50	7	20	3	17	1	2	0
1979	169	94	22	39	5	21	5	1	1
1980	144	58	12	27	3	11	0	4	1
1981	184	49	9	34	0	5	1	0	0
Total	928	400	74	196	22	76	9	14	9
	(100)%	(43.1)%							
		(100)%	(18.5)	(49)	(5.5)	(19)	(2.25)	(3.5)	(2.25)

(1) Mosquitoes; (2) Muscoid flies; (3) Cockroaches

41, Shanghai (SHA) with 35, Anchorage (ANC) with 28, Seoul (SEL) with 28, San Francisco (SFO)) with 7, Vancouver (YVR) with 5, Seattle (SEA) with 4, and Khabarovsk (KHV), New York City (NYC), Osaka (OSA), and Pusan (PUS) with one flight each.

Insects of medical importance were recorded for 162 flights from MNL (70.7%), 47 (27.5%) from TPE, 53 (36.6%) from HKG, 4 from HNL (6.7%), 21 from BKK (75%) and 1 from SIN. No insects were found in the flights from GUM, SPN, or NOU. On the northern flights, on the other hand, 26 flights (37.7%) from MOW contained insects, 8 from LAX (16.1%), 24 from PEK (58.5%), 23 from SHA (65.7%), 7 from ANC (25%), 16 from SEL (57.1%), 2 from YVR, and one flight from each of SFO, SEA, OSA, NYC, PUS AND KHV. The total then for southern flights is 288, for northern flights 112.

Insects were found on southern flights throughout the year, while with only two or three exceptions, discoveries of insects in northern flights were not made from mid-November through March.

Mosquitoes were found on 141 southern flights and 27 northern flights, flies on 202 southern and 93 northern flights, and cockroaches on 45 and 9 flights respectively.

Looking now at distribution by type of flight, we see that there were 909 passenger flights and 19 cargo flights, and captures were made in 391 (43.0%) and 7 (36.8%) cases respectively.

Then in Table 4-4, showing types of planes, we see that Boeing 707s were the most numerous with 233 planes, with insects collected from 146 planes (62.7%), followed by Boeing 747s with 55 cases out of 218 planes (25.2%), Douglas DC-8s with 110 out of 214 planes (51.4%), Douglas DC-10s with 39 out of 96 planes (40.6%), Lockheed L1011s with 9 out of 60 (15%), Airbus A300s with 19 out of 41 (46.3%), Ilyushin IL-62s with 15 out of 30 (50%), Vickers VC-10s with 4 out of 23 (17.3%), Boeing 727s with 1 out of 9 (11.1%), and the least frequent type, Tridents, with 2 out of 4 planes (50%).

The crews' answers to questions regarding the performance of in-flight disinsecting were positive in the case of 477 flights (51.4%) and negative in the case of 451 flights (48.6%). As insects were found in 194 (40.6%) of the planes in which disinsecting was said to have been performed and in 206 planes (45.7%) where it was not, hardly any difference is apparent.

As for the part of the plane where insects were discovered, by species discovered, a total of 568 females of C. pipiens s. l. (the most commonly found mosquito) were

Table 4-3. Number of aircraft investigated and insect pests captured by flight routings.

Flight routings	No. of aircraft investigated	No. of insect pests captured			
		Aircraft	(1)	(2)	(3)

Southern flights

Flight routings	No. of aircraft investigated	Aircraft	(1)	(2)	(3)
ATH-CAI-(AUH)-KHI-BKK	7	7	2	6	-
ATH-THR-KHI-BKK	7	3	-	1	2
BEY-BAH-DXB-KUL-TPE [C]	1	1	1	1	-
BEY-BOM-BKK-HKG-TPE [C]	1	-			
BEY-BOM-BKK-HKG-TPE-OSA [C]	1	-			
BEY-KUL-MNL-OSA [C]	1	-			
BGW-AUH-KHI-BOM-BKK	2	2	1	2	-
BGW-THR-KHI-BKK	2	-			
BGW-THR-KHI-BOM-BKK	10	9	5	7	-
BKK-HKG	2	-			
BKK-HKG-TPE	1	-			
BOM-CCU-BKK-HKG	28	22	15	15	5
BOM-DEL-BKK-HKG	5	4	3	3	-
BRU-ATH-DXB-BKK-MNL	1	1	-	1	-
CAI-BAH-BKK-MNL	23	20	11	17	1
CAI-BAH-BOM-BKK-MNL	22	19	17	18	3
CAI-BOM-BKK-MNL	6	3	3	3	-
CAI-SHJ-BOM-BKK-MNL	3	3	2	3	-
CMB-HKG	1	-			
FRA-ATH-KHI-BKK-HKG	4	2	1	1	-
GUM	8	-			
GUM-SPN	8	-			
GVA-ZRH-ATH-KHI-HKG	1	-			

Table 4-3. Continued

Flight routings	No. of aircraft investigated	No. of insect pests captured			
		Aircraft	(1)	(2)	(3)
HKG	51	14	3	12	1
HKG-TPE	75	12	7	4	-
HNL	58	4	1	3	-
JNS-SEZ-CMB-HKG	16	2	1	1	-
KHI-BKK-MNL	35	28	14	27	10
KUL-HKG-TPE	2	1	1	-	-
KUL-PEN-HKG-TPE	11	5	1	2	2
LAX-HNL	2	-			
LON-KRT-ADD-NBO-SEZ-CMB-HKG	10	3	1	1	1
LON-NBO-DAH-SEZ-CMB-HKG	1	-			
LON-DXB-HKG	2	-			
MNL	139	88	44	51	14
MNL-TPE	6	1	-	1	-
NOU	1	-			
NYC-LON-FRA-IST-BEY-THR-DEL-BKK-HKG	20	5	1	5	-
ROM-DEL-BKK-HKG	2	1	-	1	-
SIN	2	1	-	1	-
SIN-HKG-TPE	3	1	-	1	-
SIN-KUL-HKG-TPE	1	-			
TPE	70	26	6	15	7
ZRH-CVA-KHI-HKG	2	-			

Southern flights:

Total 44 routes	654	288	141	203	45

Table 4-3. Continued

		No. of insect pests captured			
Flight routings	No. of aircraft investigated	Aircraft	(1)	(2)	(3)

Northern flights

Flight routings		No. of aircraft investigated	Aircraft	(1)	(2)	(3)
AMS-ANC		3	-			
BRU-ANC		1	1	-	1	-
CPH-MOW		7	2	-	2	-
FRA-HAM-ANC		8	-			
FRA-MOW		2	1	-	1	-
KHI-RWP-PEK		11	10	5	9	4
KHI-RWP-PEK-SHA		6	4	2	3	1
LAX		1	-			
LAX	[C]	1	-			
LAX-SFO-ANC	[C]	1	-			
LON-ANC		2	1	-	1	-
LON-MOW		14	5	-	5	-
MEX-YVR		1	-			
NYC		3	1	-	1	-
NYC-ANC	[C]	3	1	1	-	-
NYC-CHI-SEA	[C]	1	-			
NYC-SEA		2	1	-	1	-
NYC-SFO		2	-			
PAR-ANC		2	-			
PAR-MOW		33	13	3	10	1
PEK		16	5	1	5	-
PEK-SHA		24	16	9	9	-
PEK-SHA-OSA		1	1	-	1	-

Table 4-3. Continued

Flight routings		No. of aircraft investigated	No. of insect pests captured			
			Aircraft	(1)	(2)	(3)
PUS		1	1	-	1	-
RIO-LIM-LAX-ANC	[C]	5	4	1	3	-
RIO-SAO-SJU-NYC-ANC		1	-			
ROM-FRA-MOW		1	-			
ROM-MOW		12	5	-	5	-
SAO-RIO-LIM-LAX		49	8	-	6	2
SEA	[C]	1	-			
SEL		26	15	3	12	1
SEL	[C]	2	1	1	-	-
SFO		5	1	-	1	-
SFO-ANC	[C]	1	-			
SHA		5	3	-	3	-
THR-PEK		14	9	1	9	-
WAW-MOW-KHV		1	1	-	1	-
YVR		4	2	-	2	-
ZRH-CPH-ANC		1	-			
Northern flights:						
Total	37 routes	274	112	27	92	9
All flights:						
Total	81 routes	928	400	168	295	54

[C] Cargo plane
(1) Mosquitoes; (2) Muscoid flies; (3) Cockroaches

75

captured, of which 102 were found in the cabin (18.0%) and 466 (82.0%) in the cargo space; and a tendency was observed for more to be found in holds carrying warm-blooded animals such as monkeys and birds. Common houseflies (*Musca domestica*) were the most frequently caught flies: 714 flies (85.1%) were found in passenger cabins and 125 (14.9%) in baggage-and-cargo compartments, showing a reverse tendency from that of mosquitoes, of which 5.7 times as many were found in passenger cabins as in holds. Two hundred three specimens of the most frequently found species of cockroach were found in passenger cabins (95.3%), while only 10 (4.7%) were found in holds.

Although this is not shown in the tables, one female rat (*Rattus rattus*) was found during mail-sorting at the airport post office. Having escaped from a package airmailed from Johannesburg, it was immediately sent to the Quarantine Station, where examination disclosed that it was carrying a female oriental rat flea, *Xenopsylla cheopis*.

Further examination of these results revealed first of all, in connection with the mosquitoes, that although specimens of *A. aegypti*–the yellow fever vector–had been captured in the past by Ogata et al. (1974), the origin of the flight in question (Manila) permitted the rejection of any association with yellow fever. Prudence is necessary, however, with respect to other vector-borne diseases carried by *A. aegypti,* such as dengue haemorrhagic fever (DHF), which is known to be prevalent in the Philippines. Furthermore, with respect to *Anopheles subpictus,* one cannot preclude the possibility pointed out by Ogata et al. (1974) that malaria may enter Japan via malaria-carrying mosquitoes carried aboard aircraft. Consideration must also be given to the association between *Culex gelidus* and *C. tritaeniorhynchus* and JE.

There has been a tendency for the number of insect captures per aircraft searched to decline in recent years. This phenomenon is especially noticeable for mosquitoes and cockroaches. A possible explanation could be the increased use of jumbo jets and the rapid increase in the number of relatively new planes. Incidentally, this is confirmed by Table 4-4, where we see that the incidences of insect capture are 62.7% for the B-707 and 51.0% for the DC-8 but less for the newer models: 40.6% for the DC-10, 25.2% for the B-747, and 15% for the L1011.

With regard to the utility of in-flight disinsecting in the passengers' section, our study revealed that insects were found on 96 out of 345 southern flights that had been disinsected (27.8%) and in 87 out of 304 that had not (28.6%). The same figures for the northern flights were 31

Table 4-4. Insect pests by type of aircraft.

Aircraft	1975	1976	1977	1978	1979	1980	1981	Total	(%)
B-707	17/35	14/33	25/36	22/31	36/45	18/30	14/23	146/233	(62.7/100)
B-727	-	1/1	-	-	-	0/2	0/6	1/9	(11.1/100)
B-747	15/47	2/22	5/16	3/12	5/20	12/33	13/68	55/218	(25.2/100)
DC-8	9/26	9/24	20/35	18/24	36/65	17/32	1/8	110/214	(51.4/100)
DC-10	4/9	5/8	5/7	5/9	10/17	5/17	5/29	39/96	(40.6/100)
L-1011	0/4	3/7	3/6	1/5	1/6	0/14	1/18	9/60	(15/100)
IL-62	4/5	4/6	2/4	1/5	0/3	1/2	3/5	15/30	(50/100)
VC-10	0/5	0/2	0/1	0/3	4/11	0/1	-	4/23	(17.3/100)
A-300	-	0/1	1/1	-	1/1	5/12	12/26	19/41	(46.3/100
TRD	-	-	1/1	-	1/1	0/1	0/1	2/4	(50/100)
Total	49/131	38/104	62/107	50/89	94/169	58/144	49/184	400/928	(43.1/100)

77

out of 132 (23.5%) and 49 out of 147 (33.3%) respectively. Judging only from these results, it would be difficult to say that in-flight disinsecting is effective. Whether the cause lies in the ineffectiveness of the insecticide used or in the inappropriateness of the method of disinsectization is unclear, however.

As for measures taken to remedy this situation, we have decided to notify the crew and/or airline employees each time insects of medical importance are discovered on board, alerting them to the significance of the presence of insects on board during flight and instructing them to perform disinsecting appropriately before arrival at the airport whenever insects are found. We also inform the airlines and related enterprises at Narita Airport of the results of our regular inspection into sanitary conditions on aircraft and point out measures that need to be taken, stressing the particular importance of eliminating insects of medical importance when discovered in planes.

In addition to checks of incoming planes, the Narita Airport Quarantine Station is carrying out a survey in accordance with IHR into the presence of medically important insects in the airport perimeter and protective area to find out the situation in the airport's immediate vicinity; where needed we take such necessary measures as spraying and recommending structural improvements to eliminate the breeding of insect pests and vertebrates harboring insect ectoparasites.

As a result, there are as yet no cases of mosquito species known to have been introduced from overseas establishing themselves in Japan. However, from the similarities between *Culex pipiens pallens,* a species known to inhabit the airport area, and *C. quinquefasciatus,* the mosquito most frequently captured in aircraft, it can be inferred that transformations may occur in the future by hybridization with species introduced from other countries (the presumed explanation for the Japanese variant, *C. pipiens pallens*). We thus think it necessary to continue morphological observations of vector species on a long-term basis to elucidate this point.

REFERENCES

Bailey, J. 1977. Guide to hygiene and sanitation in aviation. Geneva: WHO.
Kusui, Y., S. Shinonaga, R. Kano, M. Kato, Y. Hayashi, Y. Arisaowa, and T. Suzuki. 1980. Note on houseflies entering Japan on international aircraft. *Jap. J. Publ.*

Hlth 27-10:604 (in Japanese).

Ogata, K., I. Tanaka, Y. Ito, and S. Morii. 1974. Survey of the medically important insects carried by the international aircraft of Tokyo International Airport. *Jap. J. sanit. Zool.* 25:177-84.

Rajapaksa, N. 1980. The global spread of insect disease vectors by aircraft. Communicable Diseases Intelligence, Commonwealth Dept. Hlth, Australia.

WHO. 1974. International Health Regulations (1969), Second annotated edition. WHO, Geneva.

Chapter 5

Recent Introductions of Some Medically Important Diptera in the Northwest, Central, and South Pacific (including New Zealand)

J. S. Pillai and S. Ramalingan

The main patterns of distribution of mosquitoes in the South Pacific were determined by the early migrations of the Pacific peoples in pre-European times and by the Europeans and other immigrants in the more recent past. The salt-tolerant *Aedes polynesiensis,* which is the main vector of subperiodic filariasis over a wide region of the South Pacific, probably owes its present distribution to man's early migrations by sailing craft across the oceanic barriers. By the end of the seventeenth century, distribution patterns were already well established. In the 1800s, the increase in shipping activity associated with European colonization brought the introduction of such cosmopolitan species as *Aedes aegypti*. Once introduced, this vector quickly became widespread within the region. Further to the west *A. albopictus* and other species of mosquitoes have now become established in areas where they were not previously known to be present. Nor are sea- and aircraft the only means of dispersal of undesirable species: human travelers also can be directly involved in the transportation of insects through personal infection. The most striking example is of movement of people with myiasis due to sarcophagid Diptera. Two such cases were lately detected at the University Hospital, Kuala Lumpur, in recent arrivals in Malaysia. Clearly, all kinds of insect introductions due in one way or another to transportation are a continuing

81

process. This chapter examines some of the more recent introductions, and speculates on their possible origins.*

THE DISCOVERY OF *AEDES AEGYPTI* IN TOKELAU

According to Christophers (1960), *Aedes aegypti* is almost the only mosquito that has spread around the world through human agency. Its natural distribution is strictly limited by latitude; it rarely occurs north of 45°N or south of 35°S. It is a domestic species that, after its introduction to the South Pacific, has not spread inland and remains mainly in and around the larger seaports associated with commercial activity. Despite its early and widespread dispersal in the region, some of the remoter and less frequented islands were known to have escaped invasion by *A. aegypti*. The Tokelau Islands are one such group, where the occurrence of this mosquito was only recently reported.

The Tokelaus comprise a group of three atolls situated between latitudes 8-10°S and longitudes 179-173°W, approximately 625 km north of Western Samoa. Each atoll consists of a ring of surf-beaten coral reef encircling a largish lagoon 6-15 km across. The atolls are infrequently visited by outsiders, though they have been the subject of recent entomological investigations, which enables one to speculate on a possible timeframe for the introduction to have occurred.

In the 1920s O'Connor (1923) and Buxton and Hopkins (1927) carried out studies of the mosquito fauna of Tokelau. They reported the presence of only one species, *Aedes variegatus* var. *pseudoscutellaris,* as *Aedes polynesiensis* was known at the time. About 30 years later, Dr. Marshall Laird undertook a detailed study of mosquito ecology of the three atolls, visiting them three times from 1954 to 1960. In 1958, he and Dr. Donald H. Colless found an additional species, *Aedes vexans nocturnus,* on Fakaofo (Laird and Colless 1962). Hinckley (1969), who carried out an entomological survey in Tokelau in 1966, also reported the occurrence of only *Aedes polynesiensis* and *Aedes vexans nocturnus.*

---

*We are grateful to Dr. E. J. Reye of the University of Queensland for his permission to quote from his extensive investigations on *Culicoides belkini* in the South Pacific. Our studies were supported by funds from the New Zealand Medical Research Council, UNDP/World Bank/WHO Special Program for Research and Training in Tropical Diseases, and the WHO Western Pacific Regional Office.

Aedes aegypti was first discovered on Fakaofo Atoll breeding in artificial containers in May 1978. Two months later when the remaining two atolls (Nukunono and Atafu) were visited, large numbers of *A. aegypti* larvae proved to have become established there, too, in artificial containers on the village islets. Another well-known cosmopolitan species, *Culex quinquefasciatus* was also found for the first time in a domestic effluent ditch on Fakaofo (Urdang and Pillai 1978; Pillai and Urdang 1979).

It seems very unlikely that the earlier investigators from O'Connor to Hinckley would have overlooked the presence of the distinctive *Aedes aegypti*. It is thus highly probable that the species reached the Tokelaus and became established between the late 1960s and mid-1970s. The most likely vehicle of entry seems to be through shipping, as until very recently there were no air services to Tokelau; although from World War II until the aftermath of the 1966 hurricane, Royal New Zealand Air Force flying boats visited all three atolls intermittently. As the administering authority, the New Zealand government provides a charter shipping service four to six times a year. Starting from Apia in Western Samoa, a round trip takes usually about 10 days during which all three atolls are visited, unloading and loading supplies and passengers. As there are no berthing facilities, the vessel heaves to outside the reef, while its boats and shore-based outboards run a shuttle service to the village islet. Larvae of *Aedes aegypti* could thus have been carried to the three atolls by such contacts. Uncovered lifeboats or barrels of water on board the ship during the Pacific voyage to the Tokelaus may have provided a suitable environment for *Aedes aegypti* breeding in the accumulations of rain water, especially if the drain plugs were left in place. Under these conditions it is not unlikely that an adequate population of the mosquito can be supported for prolonged periods during the voyage, with the crew providing the blood meal for adults. Once the colony is established, it becomes a relatively easy matter for the species to reach ashore and become established (Figure 5-1). Rainwater collected from corrugated iron roofs and stored in a variety of storage tanks constitutes an ideal breeding habitat for *Aedes aegypti* and other domestic species.

The Recovery of *Culex quinquefasciatus* on Fakaofo Atoll

Culex quinquefasciatus is also presumed to have achieved its circumtropical distribution largely through human intervention. Although it was discovered on Fakaofo about the

Figure 5-1. Introduction of *Aedes aegypti* and *Culex quinquefasciatus* into Tokelau.

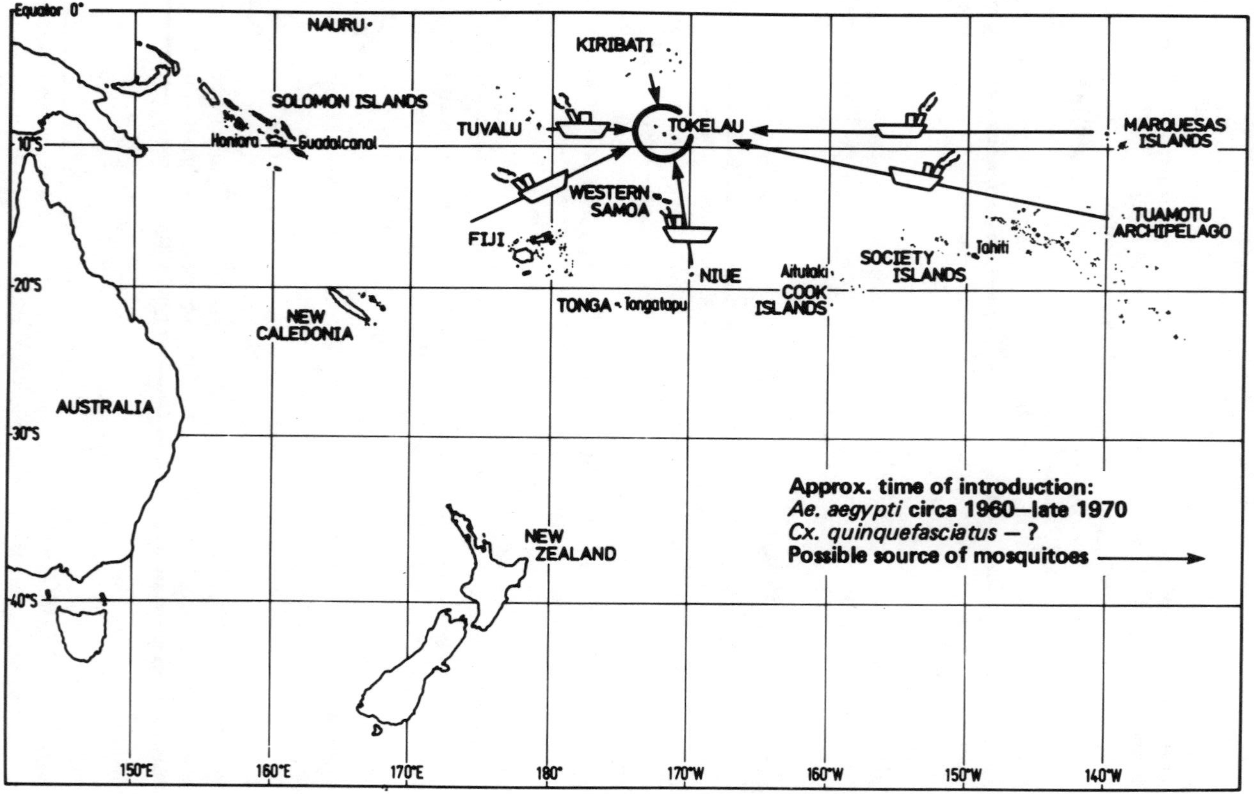

84

same time as *Aedes aegypti* (Pillai and Urdang 1979; Urdang and Pillai 1978), it is possible that it may have been present for a longer period; but because of its limited occurrence, it had escaped detection by earlier investigators. Ground pools are rarely formed on coral atolls, and opportunities for the establishment of the species is rather limited. It is interesting to note that it was found breeding in one of the few domestic wastewater drainage channels on the village islet of Fakaofo. Again it is highly likely that the species gained entry aboard visiting ships (Figure 5-1).

INTRODUCTION OF *AEDEOMYIA CATASTICTA* AND *AEDES VIGILAX* INTO FIJI

Aedeomyia catasticta was until quite recent years believed to be confined to Australia; while *Aedes vigilax* was thought to be restricted to coastal regions of Australia, New Guinea, the Solomons, and New Caledonia. Both species are now established in Fiji.

Laird (1956) suggested that *A. catasticta* may have entered Fiji via the international airport at Nadi, situated on the western side of the main island of Viti Levu. During the war years, the airport also catered for a substantial volume of military aircraft movement linking Fiji, Australia, the Solomons, and New Caledonia, which also may have provided an opportunity for the introduction of the mosquito species.

Burnett (1960) disagreed with Laird's suggestion, expressing the view that it reached Fiji from the northwest by island hopping. This also implies that shipping may have been involved and the likely source appears to be the Solomons, whose *A. catasticta* population is indistinguishable from Fijian examples of the mosquito according to Belkin (1962).

There is also a considerable amount of conjecture regarding the introduction of *Aedes vigilax* into Fiji. Lever (in Paine 1943) claimed that adults were captured in buildings on the southeast coast of Viti Levu in 1940, these specimens being afterwards identified as *A. vigilax* by the late F. W. Edwards of the British Museum.

Paine undertook extensive mosquito collections from 1927–1935 that formed the basis of his bulletin "An introduction to the mosquitoes of Fiji," first published in 1935. Despite his painstaking surveys, *Aedes vigilax* was not recorded; it was thus generally assumed that the mosquito was introduced after 1935, but before 1940. However, this view has been disputed by Symes (undated), who undertook investigations of the natural history of human filariasis in Fiji from 1954-1956; he suggested that the earlier citation was based on a misidentification by Edwards, but did not elaborate further on the correct identity of the species. Burnett (1960) suggested that the species had entered Fiji "probably sometime before November 1957" by air through Nadi International Airport (Figure 5-2).

DISPERSAL OF *CULICOIDES BELKINI* IN THE SOUTH PACIFIC

Culicoides belkini is a biting midge that appears to have reached pest status in several islands of the south Pacific in recent years. Although the species was first described from Tahiti's Faáa Airport with a doubtful record from Tutuila Naval Station, American Samoa (Wirth and Arnaud 1969), the midge is thought to be endemic to Fiji (E. J. Reye pers. comm. 1982). The upsurge in activity is linked to large scale disruptions to the coastal ecosystems, undertaken to provide facilities for an expanding tourist industry. The species is considered to be indigenous to Fiji, and the rapid spread to other areas of the South Pacific appears to have been aided by aircraft movements. Following the construction of an airport on Bora Bora in eastern Polynesia, its presence there was first reported in 1959. With the expansion of air links in French Polynesia, the midge began to disperse in a southeasterly direction, eventually reaching Tahiti in 1961. From Tahiti it spread to the Tuamotus, the eastern extremity of French Polynesia, through air contact points on Rangiroa and Hao; by 1973 it was present throughout the whole group. Later (1968) it reached the Cooks and was found six years later on Guadalcanal not far from Honiara, which is a regular stopover point for Air Pacific, Fiji's international airline* (Figure 5-3).

MOSQUITO INTRODUCTIONS INTO NEW ZEALAND

The mosquito fauna of New Zealand comprises some 16 species, most of which are representatives of an ancient

---

*According to Dr. Reye, Brisbane in Queensland is threatened with invasion by this insect, as Brisbane is the terminating point for the Air Pacific flight.

Figure 5-2. Introduction of *Aedeomyia catasticta* and *Aedes vigilax* into Fiji.

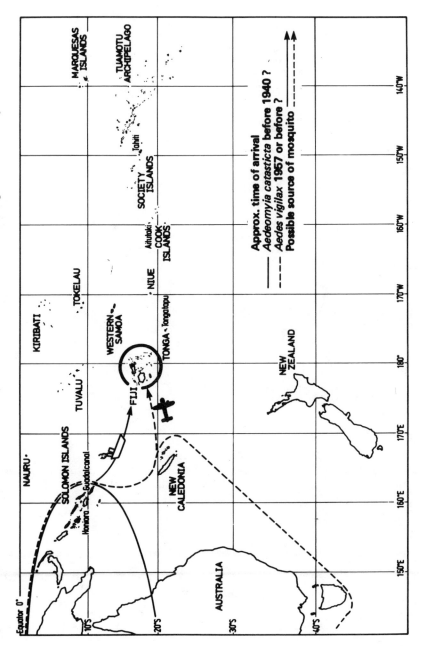

87

Figure 5-3. Dispersal pattern of *Culicoides belkini* in the South Pacific.

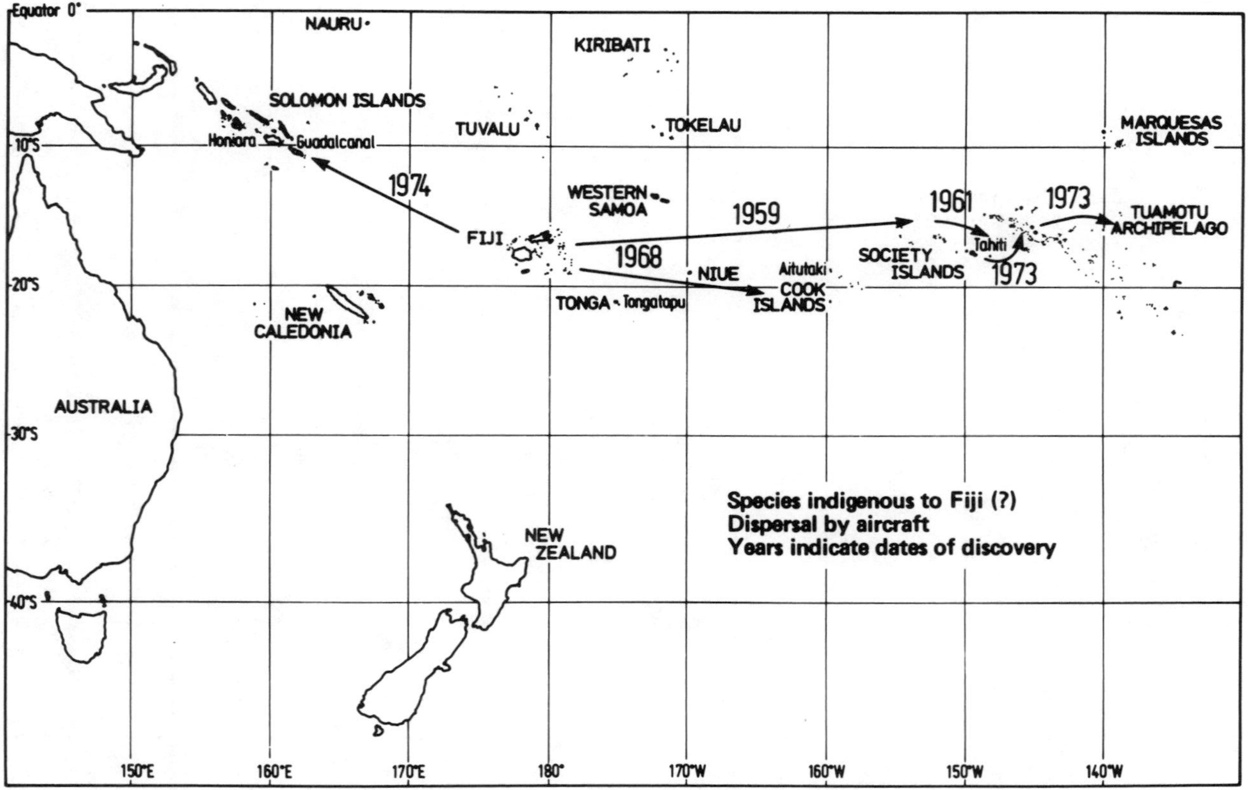

continental fauna with close affinities to SE Tasmania and mainland Australia. Belkin (1968) refers to three waves of dispersal as having led to the present composition of the New Zealand culicid fauna, the earliest (comprising the *Nothodixa-Neodixa* line) having occurred at the time of the classical southern hemispheric dispersal of plants. This was later followed by a wave of Australian culicid faunal elements, and recently by a second such wave. The last category includes at least three species that appear to have been introduced through human agency.

The Introduction of *Aedes australis*

Aedes australis is a brackish-water breeder, its aquatic stages utilizing supralittoral pools. It is endemic to the southern and eastern coasts of mainland Australia, Tasmania, and Lord Howe and Bass Strait Islands. The presence of the mosquito in New Zealand was first detected in 1961, when larvae were collected in a derelict boathull on Stewart Island, situated a little south of the South Island (Nye 1962). Its distribution was subsequently investigated, and it was found that the species also occurred along the southeastern coast of the South Island (Pillai 1971). This distribution pattern still appears to be holding (Pillai, unpublished data). Belkin (1968) suggested that the presence in New Zealand of *A. australis* represents a natural eastward extension of the migration of an Australian species. However, this theory remains unconvincing in view of the mosquito's absence from the west coast of both main islands of New Zealand, where suitable conditions exist for colonization by *Aedes australis*. If it were a case of natural dispersion, it is highly probable that the species would have been able to reach and indeed become established on the west coast. Its presence on the east coast only suggests that its arrival here was influenced by other events. The most likely explanation is that trans-Tasman shipping might have been involved. This speculation is supported by the facts that *A. australis* is well established around Bluff, Dunedin, Oamaru, and Timaru—ports that are regularly visited by vessels from Australia (Figure 5-4).

Introduction of *Culex quinquefasciatus* into New Zealand

The presence of *Culex quinquefasciatus* in New Zealand was first reported by Belkin (1968). It occurs in relatively low numbers in isolated pockets around Auckland and Whangarei

Figure 5-4. Introduction of *Aedes australis* into New Zealand.

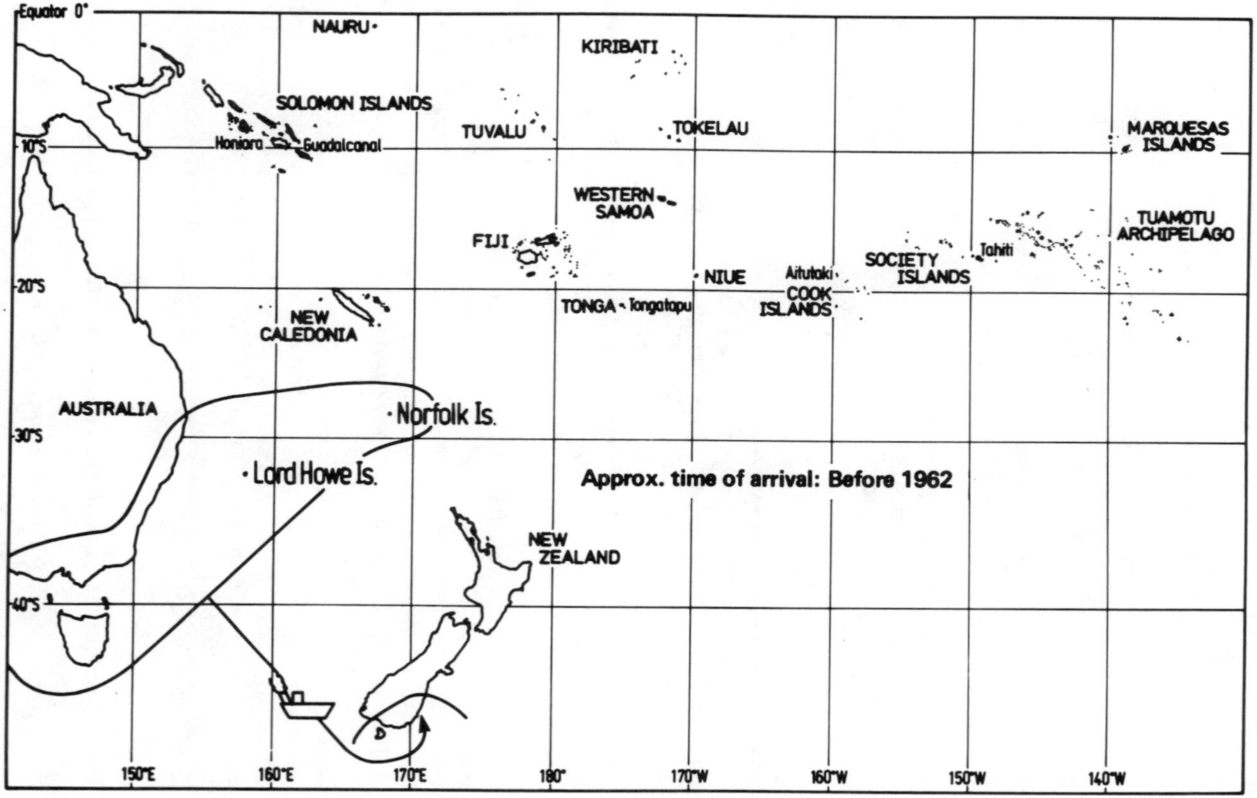

(Pillai 1978). According to Belkin, the species was "un-doubtedly introduced by ships." However, aircraft dispersal should not be discounted. Interceptions by the Plant Health Diseases Division of the Ministry of Agriculture show that in the period 1970-74, a large number of live specimens among the four species of mosquitoes identified were *Culex quinquefasciatus* from Hawaii (Table 5-1). The species could have reached New Zealand from any number of sources sometime before 1968. Having arrived there, it is now confined to isolated pockets in the north of the North Island (Figure 5-5).

Table 5-1. Mosquitoes intercepted on aircraft 1970-74 (Plant Health Diseases Division, Levin).

Species	No. times intercepted	No. intercepted (adults)	Country of Origin
Culicidae			
Aedes vexans nocturnus	1	1	Fiji
Culex bitaeniorhynchus	4	3	Fiji/Hong Kong
Culex quinquefasciatus	1	many	Hawaii/USA
Culex sp.	1		Hong Kong

Introduction of *Aedes notoscriptus* into New Zealand

Aedes notoscriptus is widely distributed in Australia, New Caledonia, the Loyalty Islands, New Britain, New Ireland, New Guinea, and the Moluccas. Adults of the New Zealand populations show some variations from other populations, due possibly to a colder environment (Belkin 1968). The introduction of this species into New Zealand through shipping appears plausible, though natural dispersal via the prevailing wind current from Australia cannot be ruled out. Graham (1939) reported having taken it more than once on vessels arriving at Auckland from Sydney; it is therefore not surprising that the species occurs mainly around the seaports of Auckland, Whangarei, and Nelson (Figure 5-5).

Figure 5-5. Introduction of *Aedes notoscriptus* and *Culex quinquefasciatus* into New Zealand.

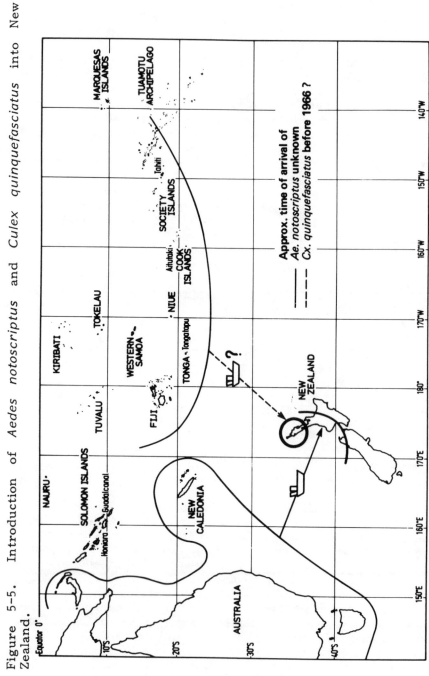

INTRODUCTION OF *AEDES ALBOPICTUS*
AND *CULEX ANNULIROSTRIS* INTO THE
CAROLINE AND MARSHALL ISLANDS,
MICRONESIA

Aedes albopictus has a widespread distribution in the Oriental Region, where it is one of the most abundant day-biting species. It is an established vector of dengue virus and has been incriminated during outbreaks of dengue haemorrhagic fever (DHF) in both Thailand (Gould et al. 1968) and Singapore (Rudnick and Chan 1965). Within the Oriental Region, it extends from Pakistan on its western limits, through the Indian subcontinent, and throughout Southeast Asia to Japan in the northeast and to Papua New Guinea (PNG) in the southeast. In the Indian Ocean, *A. albopictus* occurs in Madagascar, Mauritius, and the Seychelles; and it is known to have been introduced through human agency to the Hawaiian, Bonin, and Mariana Islands in the North Pacific.

Aedes albopictus was unknown in the South Pacific east of PNG until Elliott (1980) reported it as occurring on Guadalcanal in the Solomons and on Ndendi Island in the Santa Cruz group. In 1982, eight mosquito specimens from Honiara, Guadalcanal, was sent to one of the authors (SR) for identification. Six of these specimens were identified as *A. albopictus,* thus confirming its presence on Guadalcanal. Elliott speculated that this mosquito had entered the Solomons from the west, probably from PNG, by shipping.

During March–May 1981, several islands in the South and Central Pacific were visited by one of us (S.R.) on behalf of WHO. In surveys carried out on these islands, *Aedes albopictus* was collected on Ponape in the Carolines and on Majuro in the Marshalls. On the latter atoll, a collection of the immature stages of *A. albopictus* was made from a coconut and these were reared to adults. In Ponape, a single adult female was collected while attempting to feed. In his publication on the mosquitoes of Micronesia, Bohart (1957) reported *A. albopictus* as being abundant in Guam and Saipan and stated that this species was not known from the Carolines. These records of the species from Ponape and Majuro are therefore new, and extend its known range into the Central Pacific. This dispersal was probably brought about through the agency of interisland shipping. It is also possible that adult *A. albopictus* may have been transported by aircraft. Continental Air Micronesia, for example, island hops from Saipan to Guam/Truck/Ponape/Kwajalein/Majuro/Johnston/Honolulu. It is possible that *A.*

albopictus entering the aircraft at either Saipan or Guam may have been carried to Ponape and Majuro.*

Culex annulirostris, a vector of Ross River virus (RRV) was collected during the survey in March–May 1981 from Majuro. This is also a new record from the island and entry could have been by shipping or aircraft.

THE INTRODUCTION OF *AEDES AEGYPTI* AND *ANOPHELES LITORALIS* INTO SABAH, MALAYSIA

For nearly five decades it was believed that *Aedes aegypti* was absent from Sabah, despite an earlier report of its presence there (Stanton 1920). In 1965 Chow reported that *A. aegypti* had not been encountered during the previous seven years in Sabah; and again in 1970 that it had not been found in Sabah. In 1970 Ramalingam reported the occurrence of this species in the port of Semporna on the east coast of Sabah. Five breeding collections were obtained from drums and from wooden boats that were still under construction. In a following survey that same year, Macdonald (1970) reported *A. aegypti* from Tawau, Sandakan, and Kudat on the east coast and from Labuan Island off the west coast of Sabah. As there is regular sea traffic between the Philippines and several ports on the east coast of Sabah, it is likely that this species was introduced thereby. This is supported by the collection of a late-instar larvae of *A. aegypti* in a boat, which had arrived from the Balbac Islands (Philippines) just six days earlier (Macdonald 1970).

Anopheles litoralis also appears to have been introduced into Sabah from the Philippines through shipping. This species, which breeds in brackish waters along the coast, was not definitely known to occur in Sabah until reported by Ramalingam (1974). It is a common coastal species in the Philippines.

---

*As Air Nauru now operates flights between Majuro and Tarowa (Kiribati), from where there are services westward to Nauru and southward to Funafuti (Tuvalu) and Fiji (see Figure 8-1), this poses further aviation-borne dispersal hazards into island groups already suffering from dengue and DHF problems—Ed.

THE PRESENCE OF *AEDES TOGOI* IN PENINSULAR MALAYSIA

Aedes (Finlaya) togoi was regarded as being essentially a temperate species, occurring in Japan, Korea, Siberia/USSR, China, and Taiwan, and extending to about the Tropic of Cancer at its southern limit. However, in 1966 it was collected from Cam Ranh Bay and Con Son Island on the east coast of Vietnam. It was also identified from four localities on the east coast of Thailand (Figure 5-6) between the years 1965–68 (Gould et al. 1968). In 1968 it was collected from four localities over a stretch of 175 km between Juantan and Kuala Trengganu on the east coast of peninsular Malaysia (Ramalingam 1969).

Following its description in 1907, *Aedes togoi* was not collected outside the temperate region for some 60 years. It is of medical importance, being a vector of *Brugia malayi* in Japan, and it is an excellent experimental vector of several species and subspecies of filarial parasites. It is also a vector of Japanese B encephalitis (JE). As *A. togoi* readily attacks man, it is unlikely that it was present all along in Southeast Asia without being noticed. In Malaysia especially, many collections had been made in the past from rock pools along the east coast, without its being reported. It is more likely that this species was introduced into Southeast Asia by ships from Japan. During the 1950s, Japanese ships frequently visited the east coast of Malaysia in connection with trade in iron ore and timber. In fact an adult female, *Aedes togoi* was actually collected on board a ship between Iwo and Agrihan islands in the Central Pacific (Bohart 1956).

TRANSPORT OF DIPTERA WITHIN A HUMAN HOST

A novel method of introduction of an arthropod of medical importance into a country is when man himself acts as a host and transports the arthropod within his tissues. Arthropods that are internal parasites such as *Sarcoptes scabiei, Demodex folliculorum, Tunga penetrans,* and the larvae of myiasis-causing flies may be transported in this manner.

There are two well documented cases (Ramalingam, unpublished data) of the larvae of myiasis-causing flies being introduced into peninsular Malaysia within the flesh of patients. In the first of these, a 40-year-old Chinese male was referred to the University Hospital in Kuala Lumpur from the Queen Elizabeth Hospital, Sabah, Borneo, for

Figure 5-6. New Records of Aedes (F.) togoi from Southeast Asia.

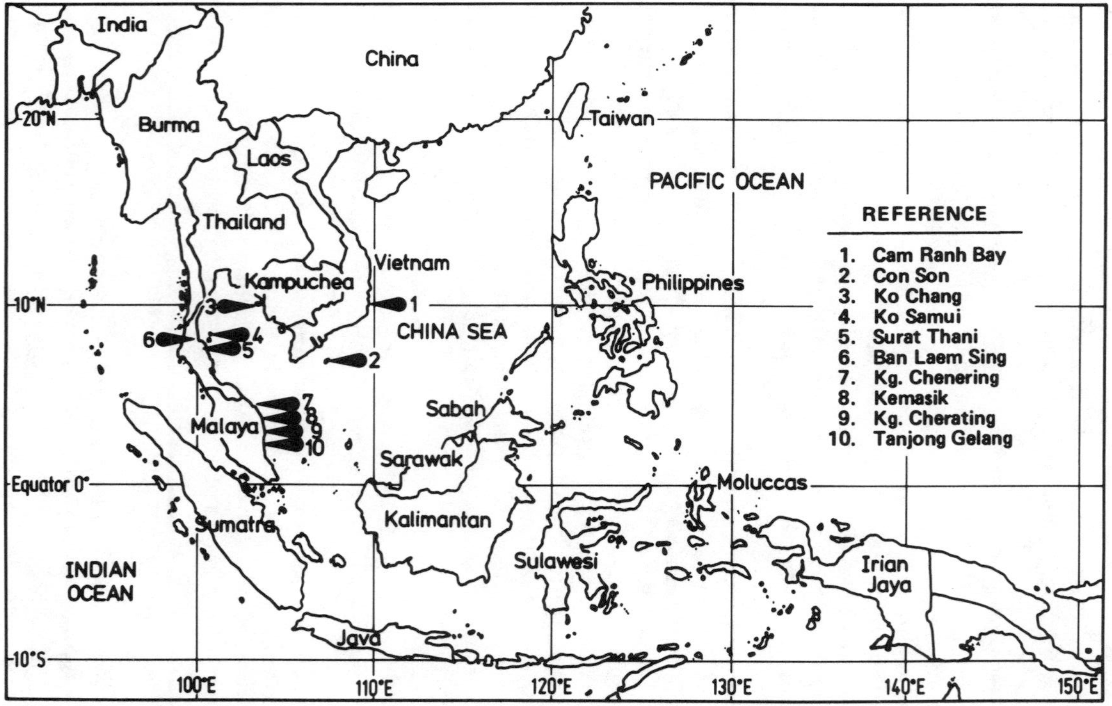

REFERENCE

1. Cam Ranh Bay
2. Con Son
3. Ko Chang
4. Ko Samui
5. Surat Thani
6. Ban Laem Sing
7. Kg. Chenering
8. Kemasik
9. Kg. Cherating
10. Tanjong Gelang

96

hypertension and nonspecific arteritis. On admission, he was seen to have a wet gangrene of the fourth left toe, with blackened skin. During the next two days, 16 mature maggots of *Lucilia sericata* were recovered from the wound. The second case involved a 69-year-old Indian female who returned to Kuala Lumpur after a year's stay in Sri Lanka. Two days after returning she was admitted to the University Hospital, Kuala Lumpur, with ulcers on the outer aspect of the third toe and on the median aspect of the fourth toe. Thirty large maggots of *Chrysomya bezziana* at least 5-6 days old, were recovered from these ulcers.

In both cases, there appears to be no doubt that the fly larvae were introduced into peninsular Malaysia within the wounds of patients. Both of them arrived at Kuala Lumpur on commercial flights and neither were aware that they were harboring maggots. Fortunately, in both cases, the fly species was still within its known range of distribution. However, with the present-day mode of fast, mass transportation, it is entirely possible that a myiasis-causing fly might use this method to extend its range into a country where it did not previously occur.

DISCUSSION

It seems probable that the species discussed in this chapter owe their present distribution to human intervention in one form or another. There is certainly a considerable amount of circumstantial evidence to support this view, though the precise time of dispersal of the species is a matter for speculation.

An argument against this is the possibility of wind currents transporting mosquitoes over long distances during atmospheric disturbances during the West-East flow of the prevailing wind. This is particularly so in the migrating patterns of some Australian insects to New Zealand across the Tasman Sea. Fox (1978), who studied the migratory behavior of lepidopterous insects from 1968-76, recorded the movement of 36 Australian species to New Zealand. His analysis showed that the insects concerned were on a migratory flight within Australia, before somehow being blown off course, and that they may thus "get caught up by various meteorological conditions and thereafter get transported to New Zealand." He went on to state that while the journey across the Tasman might therefore be purely passive, the flight within Australia is not.

There is no evidence to suggest that any of the mosquito species referred to in this chapter are capable of forming migratory swarms—or that they multiply in large numbers—for mass migrations across an ocean barrier of some 2000 km and thus become established in New Zealand. Human intervention seems more likely than this.

The prevailing winds in the Tokelau Islands, Fiji, and French Polynesia are the North East and South East Trades. The two species of mosquitoes referred to in Fiji were presumably derived from a westerly source opposite to the prevailing wind direction. The eastward dispersal of *Culicoides belkini* has also been against the prevailing wind currents. Of course, one cannot rule out altogether the possible role of cyclonic depressions, which do not necessarily follow the established wind patterns and which could serve to bring about the long-distance displacement of insects, including mosquitoes. However, the dispersal of *C. belkini* in eastern Polynesia and western Melanesia and of *Aedes aegypti* and *Culex quinquefasciatus* to the Tokelau Islands does not demand such an exceptional explanation. Thus, closely associated airport construction and tourism were contemporary with the spread of *C. belkini* throughout the Pacific. Turning to *Aedes aegypti* and *Culex quinquefasciatus,* these mosquitoes owe their global distribution mainly to human intervention, and there is no reason to suppose that their introduction to the Tokelau Islands has been through any other means.

Aedes aegypti, the main vector of dengue and DHF, has now been dispersed widely in the South Pacific, where dengue has become virtually endemic. Despite its wide distribution, though, *A. aegypti* has not so far penetrated several isolated islands (Rotuma, Northern Cooks, Marquesas [Belkin 1962]), and New Zealand. Even though New Zealand is situated in a temperate climatic zone, the possibility of this mosquito's introduction and establishment cannot be disregarded. According to Christophers (1960), the world distribution pattern of the species is determined by the 10° winter isotherm line. This line runs just south of Auckland city and includes most of the Auckland peninsula. A field survey carried out in this region during 1977-79 showed that the species was not present (Pillai 1978). However, the threat of introduction from sources in Australia or from the Pacific Islands in the north is very real and requires the utmost vigilance. Quarantine services must always remain alert to the possibility and meet the challenge of diversification and increase in the various communication links.

Another important consideration, is the absence of anopheline vectors of malaria in parts of Melanesia and the whole of Polynesia, except for a few western outliers in

Melanesia such as Rennell and Ontong Java. At present the disease occurs west of Buxton's Line, which separates the malarious Vanuatu from the nonmalarious New Caledonia. There is always a danger that Vanuatu's only malaria vector, *Anopheles farauti,* may one day cross this barrier, possibly through human intervention, and become established in New Caledonia, Fiji,* Samoa, or even New Zealand. Ideal habitats for the species are known to exist on New Caledonia, Fiji, and possibly Tonga. With further reference to Buxton's Line, Laird (1956) commented: "This line should not be regarded as indicative of a barrier beyond which anophelines are destined never to advance, but rather as an ever present reminder of the proximity of a dangerous species of *Anopheles* to a zone in which it would flourish; for following its introduction into such groups, as Fiji, Samoa and the Cook Islands *An. farauti* would not be subject to the attacks of any parasites to which it is not already exposed in its present area of distribution and would furthermore be favored by a generally lower degree of competition and a higher degree of freedom from predators consequent upon the decreasing utilization of larval habitats by aquatic animals."

Although spread of anophelines probably constitutes the most serious threat to the region, the possibility of the introduction of other Diptera should not be overlooked. There is now an urgent need to upgrade quarantine services throughout the region, so that these and other undesirable introductions are prevented. This also implies a stringent check on man himself, who may unwittingly transport unwanted species through personal infection, for example, in the form of myiasis.

REFERENCES

Belkin, J. N. 1962. *Mosquitoes of the South Pacific.* Berkeley and Los Angeles: University of California Press, 2 vols.
————. 1968. Mosquito studies (Diptera: Culicidae) VII. The Culicidae of New Zealand. *Contr. Am. Ent. Inst.* 3, 1.
Bohart, R. M. 1956. Diptera, Culicidae. *Insects of Micronesia* 12:1-85.

---

*A danger nowadays increased by direct aviation links between Port Vila, Vanuatu, and Nadi, Fiji—Ed.

Burnett, G. F. 1960. *Filariasis Research in Fiji 1957-1959.* A report to the Secretary of State to the Colonies.

Buxton, P. A., and G. H. E. Hopkins. 1927. *Researches in Polynesia and Melanesia* pts I-IV. *No. 1 Mem. Ser. Lond. Schl. Hyg. Trop. Med.*

Chow, C. Y. 1965. *Aedes aegypti* in the Western Pacific Region. Wld Hlth Org. Seminar on *Aedes aegypti.* Geneva: WHO.

————. 1970. Report on a field visit to Sabah, East Malaysia. WHO/WPR/MAL/18.3. Mimeographed.

Christophers, S. R. 1960. *Aedes aegypti* (L.). *The Yellow Fever Mosquito: Its Life History, Bionomics, and Structure.* Cambridge: University Press. 739 pp.

Elliott, S. A. 1980. *Aedes albopictus* in the Solomon and Santa Cruz Islands, South Pacific. *Trans Roy. Soc. Trop. Med. Hyg.* 74:747-48.

Fox, K. J. 1978. Transoceanic migration of Lepidoptera to New Zealand: A history and a hypothesis on colonization. *N.Z. Ent.* 6:368-79.

Gould, D. J., T. M. Yuill, M. A. Moussa, P. Simasathian, and L. C. Rutledge. 1968. An insular outbreak of dengue haemorrhagic fever: 111. Identification of vectors and observation on vector ecology. *Amer. J. Trop. Med. Hyg.* 17:609-18.

Graham, D. H. 1939. Mosquito life in the Auckland District. *Transactions Roy Soc in N.Z.* 69:210-24.

Hinckley, A. D. 1969. Ecology of terresterial arthropods on the Tokelau atolls. *Atoll Res. Bull.* 124.

Laird, M. 1956. Studies of mosquitoes and freshwater ecology in the South Pacific. *Roy. Soc. N.Z. Bull.* 6.

————. 1967. A coral island experiment. *WHO Chronicle* 21:18-26.

Laird, M., and D. H. Colless. 1962. A field experiment with a fungal pathogen of mosquitoes, in the Tokelau Islands. *Proc XI. Intl Congr Entomol* (Vienna 1960) 2:867-68.

Macdonald, W. W. 1970. A survey of the distribution and relative prevalence of *Aedes aegypti* in Sabah, Brunei and Sarawak. WHO/VBC/70.233. Mimeographed.

Paine, R. W. 1943. An introduction to the mosquitoes of Fiji. 2nd Ed., revised by R. J. W. W. Lever. *Dept. Agric., Fiji. Bull.* 22.

Nye, E. R. 1962. *Aedes* (*Pseudoskusea*) *australis* Erichson (Diptera, Culicidae) in New Zealand. *Trans. Roy. Soc. N.Z.* 3:33-34.

O'Connor, F. W. 1923. Researches in the Western Pacific. *Res. Mem. Lond. Schl. Trop. Med.* IV.

Pillai, J. S. 1971. *Coelomomyces opifexi* (Pillai and

Smith). *Coelomomycetaceae: Blastocladiales* 1. Its distribution and ecology of infection pools in New Zealand. *Hydrobiologia* 38:425-36.

——————. 1978. A report to the N.Z. Health Dept. on a mosquito survey of the northern half of North Island. Unpublished document.

Pillai, J. S., and J. Urdang. 1979. The discovery of the mosquito *Aedes aegypti* in Tokelau. *N.Z. Med. J.* 87:212-13.

Ramalingam, S. 1969. New record of *Aedes (Finlaya) togoi* (Theobald) in West Malaysia. *Med. J. Malaya,* 23:288-92.

——————. 1970. The occurrence of *Aedes (Stegomyia) aegypti* in Sabah. *Med. J. Malaya* 25:73-74.

——————. 1974. Some new records of *Anopheles* from Sabah, Malaysia. *S.E. Asian J. Trop. Med. Pub. Hlth.* 5:147-48.

Rudnick, A., and Y. C. Chan. 1965. Dengue Type 2 virus in naturally infected *Aedes albopictus* mosquitoes in Singapore. *Science,* 149:638-39.

Stanton, A. T. 1920. The mosquitoes of Far Eastern parts, with special reference to the prevalence of *Stegomyia fasciata. Bull. Ent. Res.* 10:3.

Symes, C. B. (undated). Observations on the natural history of human filariasis in Fiji. A report to the Secretary of State to the Colonies on investigations conducted over the period 1954-56.

Urdang, J., and J. S. Pillai. 1978. Recovery of *Aedes aegypti* from Tokelau. *South Pacific Commn., Dengue News,* 6:9.

Wirth, W. W., and P. H. Arnaud, Jr. 1969. Polynesian biting midges of the genus *Culicoides* (Diptera: Ceratopogonidae). *Pacific Insects* 11:507-20.

Chapter **6**

An Introduction of Aedes aegypti into California and Its Apparent Failure to Become Established

D. Jewell and G. Grodhaus

In May 1979, an unfamiliar fourth-instar larva of the genus *Aedes** was collected from a site adjacent to the San Francisco International Airport, San Mateo County, California. Identification of the specimen could not be made using the keys to California mosquitoes. The specimen was submitted to the California Department of Health Services, Vector Biology and Control Branch, where it was tentatively identified as *Aedes aegypti*. Since this species is not known to occur in California, and because of its vector potential, confirmation of the identification was sought and received from the United States National Museum, Medical Entomology Project.

The location of the *A. aegypti* find was at the freeway interchange at the passenger terminal entrance to the San Francisco International Airport. This location is approximately 1,500 m from the nearest docking facility for international air carriers. The specimen was taken during a routine inspection of the interchange area by a staff technician of the San Mateo County Mosquito Abatement District.

---

*The larva was initially determined to be *Aedes aegypti* by Lucia T. Hui, Vector Biology and Control Branch, California State Department Health Services. Her identification was confirmed by E. L. Peyton and Yiau-Min Huang.

103

The preferred habitats of this species are artificial water holding containers. This specimen, however, was taken by dipping from a rainpool on the ground. Larvae in the sample had been combined from several separate rainpools, so it is impossible to identify the exact site of the find. The rainpools of this region are associated with winter and spring precipitation, have the same general characteristics and tend to be short-lived. The occurrence of *A. aegypti* in California, and especially its development in a rainwater pool, is a most unusual occurrence. It is likely that an egg or eggs had been deposited in an artificial container and that the contents of the container were subsequently washed into the rainpool. A large amount of debris, suitable as habitat, existed in the area. These items included cups, cans, tires, bottles, and pails. The containers were subject to periodic filling and drying as a result of precipitation.

Table 6-1 shows the species of mosquito larvae collected from the pools in the interchange area during the 1978-79 rainfall season (July 1 to June 30). Other than *A. aegypti,* the mosquitoes collected were all cool weather species and expected to occur in this location at this time of year.

Table 6-1. Mosquito species collected at terminal entrance, San Francisco International Airport, January-June 1979.

	January	February	March	April	May	June
Aedes bicristatus Thurman and Winkler	X					
Aedes increpitus Dyar	X	X				
Aedes aegypti (L.)					X	
Culiseta inornata (Williston)		X	X	X		
Culiseta incidens (Thomson)		X				
Culex tarsalis Coquillett			X	X	X	

Table 6-2 shows temperature and rainfall during the early months of 1979.

Table 6-2. Weather data, San Francisco International Airport, January-June 1979.

Month	Temperature		
	10 year average	Mean daily average 1979	Deviation from average
	C°	C°	C°
January	8.9	8.5	- 0.4
February	10.8	10.1	- 0.7
March	11.6	12.4	+ 0.8
April	12.2	13.5	+ 1.3
May	14.4	16.2	+ 1.8
June	14.4	16.0	+ 1.6
	Precipitation		
	cm	cm	cm
January	10.9	16.8	+ 5.9
February	20.3	14.9	- 5.4
March	7.1	7.0	- 0.2
April	3.1	1.8	- 1.4
May	0.2	0.3	+ 0.1
June	0.2	0	- 0.2

At the beginning of the 1979-80 rainfall season, all artificial containers in the interchange area were inspected. Each container was transferred to the State Vector Control Laboratory, flushed with water and the contents were examined under the microscope. The results are shown in Table 6-3. Only Culex and Culiseta eggs, larvae, and exuviae were found.

Table 6-3. Water-holding containers examined for evidence of Aedes aegypti and other invertebrates, terminal entrance, San Francisco International Airport, 1979.

Category of container	Number examined	Results (Negative unless otherwise noted)
Plastic cups and cartons (incl. plastic-lined paper)	19	1 cup with ostracods and Psychoda exuviae
Plastic trays	4	1 48-oz. bottle with amphipods, copepods, and Cladocera
Plastic bottles	2	
Plastic pails	1	1 50-gal. pail with Culex and Culiseta exuviae, Psychoda larvae
Miscel. plastic containers	2	1 ice chest with aquatic Oligochaeta
Metal cans	7	
Metal pails	2	1 5-gal. tar bucket with ostrocods and Cladocera; 1 5-gal. paint bucket with culicid (probably Culiseta) egg shells
Misc. metal containers	3	1 auto air filter with Cladocera
Glass bottles	4	1 4/5-gal. bottle with Cladocera
Glass jars	1	1 gal. jar with Cladocera
Rubber tires	3	1 auto tire with culicid (probably Culiseta) egg shells; 1 motorcycle tire with Psychoda and Eristalis larvae

Thirty-six black-jar "ovitraps" (Fay and Eliason 1966) were distributed at random throughout the interchange area. Each jar was inspected weekly for presence of eggs or larvae. No mosquito activity was observed in any of the jars throughout the sampling period.

Three thousand meters north of the airport, an aircraft tire firm maintained an outdoor stockpile of new and used aircraft tires, some of which had been imported from countries with endemic *A. aegypti* populations. Repeated inspection of the tires at this site were negative for mosquitoes. Two tree holes in the interchange area were monitored, but failed to yield *A. aegypti*. In the spring of 1982, after the *A. aegypti* surveillance program was terminated, one of the tree holes that was being monitored for *A. aegypti* began producing another aedine mosquito, *Aedes sierrensis* (Ludlow).

Removal and sampling of water-holding containers in the interchange area was carried out throughout the study, a practice that depleted the potential habitat for *A. aegypti*. The rainpools were drained by the California Department of Transportation (Cal-Trans), which further reduced habitats of the other *Aedes* species.

Three years have elapsed without additional collections of *A. aegypti*. The black jars that remain in the area are occasionally sampled during routine surveillance, as are other artificial water holding containers. We suspect that this singular occurrence of *A. aegypti* was a result of a gravid female that escaped from an aircraft and deposited an egg or eggs before its own demise. Based upon climatic conditions of the known habitats of *A. aegypti,* the authors feel that the survival and reproduction of this species in San Mateo County, California, would be remote.

REFERENCES

Fay, R. W., and D. A. Eliason. 1966. A preferred oviposition site as a surveillance method for *Aedes aegypti*. *Mosquito News* 26:531-35.

Chapter 7

Mosquito and Other Insect Introductions to Australia Aboard International Aircraft, and the Monitoring of Disinsection Procedures

R. C. Russell, N. Rajapaksa,
P. I. Whelan, and W. A. Langsford

INTRODUCTION

The idea of protecting a community from the introduction of disease—the concept of quarantine—dates from the Middle Ages with the efforts aimed at preventing outbreaks of plague in Europe. Australia, from its establishment in 1788, quickly became quarantine-conscious, for smallpox was soon recorded, and imported cases of plague, cholera, dysentery, typhoid fever, and venereal disease threatened the early colony. (Anonymous 1978; Chapter 10).

Today, however, the solutions to these problems are rarely so simple as those formerly employed, such as having ships stand off for a specified period to allow diseases to become apparent for recognition or to allow infective periods to pass. The problems have indeed become more complex; the rapid development of air transport in the past few decades has made the use of incubation periods for infectious diseases (a main criterion for quarantine) virtually obsolete. Moreover, the spread of tourism has created new travel links between different parts of the world far removed from the former traditional exchange routes and opened the way for new imported diseases. Likewise, the difficulties in administering any international regulations in this matter have also multiplied with the increasing number of independent countries (Bruce-Chwatt 1980).

These changing patterns of disease and travel have demanded changes in quarantine strategies. Australia* is seen to be very much at risk. The natural quarantine protection that our geographic location, and relatively recent development, may have afforded us in the past is being continually eroded, and our concern with quarantine in human health, together with relevant animal and plant interests is well founded.

Australia was the first country in the world to apply the quarantine code to aircraft, when in 1920 it extended the definition of a "vessel" subject to quarantine procedures to include aircraft (Anonymous 1933). Since that time each arrival by air has been subjected to the usual quarantine examination and surveillance.

In animal and plant quarantine fields, we depend critically on our comparative freedom from serious pests and disease for inter- and intra-national trade. As regards human disease, developments in public health, advances in technology, and more enlightened and better informed bureaucracies—all balanced against an increasing emphasis on individual freedoms in modern society—have led to recent changes in the philosophies and strategies of human quarantine in Australia.

Quarantine in Australia is the responsibility of the Commonwealth Department of Health that, in conjunction with officers of the Department of Agriculture in each state, endeavors to maintain the effective quarantine by which Australia remains free of the devastating human, animal, and plant diseases that afflict many other countries of the world. The situation as detailed a generation ago

---

*Quarantine officers at all Australian airports mentioned contributed to the study and their assistance was greatly appreciated. Staff members of Qantas facilitated the investigations also and their contribution is gratefully acknowledged. Entomology technical staff of the N. T. Department of Health, particularly Mr. K. Hodder and Ms. P. Roberts; and Messrs. L. Smee, A. Catley, R. Paton and B. Read of Plant Quarantine Branch were involved in some aspects reported here. Technical assistance was provided by staff of the Commonwealth Institute of Health and is also gratefully acknowledged. Dr. Chan Kai Lok, Director of the Vector Control Division, Ministry of the Environment, Singapore, was of great assistance in the trial from that country, as were officers of the New Zealand Health, Agriculture, and Customs Departments.

(Lee 1951) has not changed substantially in this regard.

However, with quarantine it is not only disease that has become important. As has been pointed out, the risk of aircraft introductions of insects leading to the establishment of new foci of potential vectors of disease organisms is greater than that of the introduction of insects actually infected with such organisms (Magath 1945; Soper and Wilson 1943).

The spectacular epidemic of malaria in Brazil in the 1930s following the introduction of *Anopheles gambiae* is well known (Soper and Wilson 1943), as are also the outbreaks of malaria caused by the same species in Egypt in the 1940s within a few years of its being recorded there for the first time (Chapter 1).

Potentially dangerous quarantine situations in medical entomology for the Pacific region have been discussed in the literature, and the spread of malaria and/or its vectors (especially the *Anopheles punctulatus* group of mosquitoes); yellow fever and dengue viruses or their vectors, including *Aedes aegypti;* or other arboviruses or their vectors such as Murray Valley encephalitis, Japanese B encephalitis (JE), and Ross River virus (RRV) with *Aedes* and *Culex* species around the Pacific has either been shown to occur, or is of great concern. As well, there is the possibility of introducing infected vectors into a country where a disease eradication campaign has been successful, or importing insecticide resistant strains (Basio 1973; Bruce-Chwatt 1973; Eads 1972; Laird 1956b, 1961; Nowell 1977).

To protect a country or community from the introduction of undesirable insects, quarantine measures should take two principal forms: airport sanitation and surveillance, and aircraft disinsection (Bruce-Chwatt 1973). The first line of defense should be airport sanitation—effective insect control at and around the airport, prevention of conditions suitable for insect establishment, and an insect surveillance program to detect insect introductions; the second option—the disinsection of incoming aircraft—being used to prevent insects that may be aboard from entering the protected area.

The procedures for vector control in international health have been developed by the World Health Organization (WHO) and have been in operation since the 1950s (Chapters 1, 10, and 15). However, the increasing complexity of the situation calls for continuing upgrading of procedures and the coordination of these with the aircraft industry, the International Civil Aviation Organization (ICAO), and the International Air Transport Association (IATA) (Bruce-Chwatt 1973).

IMPORTATION OF INSECTS ABOARD AIRCRAFT

The first recorded interception of insects in aircraft occurred in 1928 when a quarantine officer boarded the dirigible *Graf Zeppelin* after a trans-Atlantic flight to the United States (Chapter 2; Laird 1961). Since that time an extensive literature has been generated about the transport of insects in aircraft.

Various reviews and synopses of interest have appeared (Basio 1973; Denning et al. 1947; Carnahan 1938; Hughes 1949; Laird 1951a, 1956a, 1956b; Whitfield 1939; WHO 1961; Welch 1939), as well as reports less general in coverage and pertaining to collections from more specific regions (Aziz 1948; Basio et al. 1970; Basio and Reisen 1971; Dethier 1945; Highton and van Someren 1970; Laird 1951b; Mendonça and Cerqueira 1947; Pemberton 1944; Porter 1958). One report (Hughes 1949) gave in considerable detail the entomological findings (106,106 specimens) from a large number of aircraft (80,716) entering various airports in the United States from other countries for the period 1937-47. Other reports include one from Hawaii (Pemberton 1944) of 11,448 specimens collected, one from Africa (Dethier 1945) with more than 2,000 specimens, one from Brazil (Mendonça and Cerqueira 1947) with 40,168, and another from New Zealand (Laird 1951b) with 548 insects.

Apart from simply collecting insects from arriving aircraft, several studies were made on the ability of certain species to survive air travel. Early observations (Griffitts and Griffitts 1931) showed that some insects could not only survive an air journey, but also that they would not necessarily leave the aircraft at intermediate stops. Further reports indicated that other than in really extreme conditions of heat or cold, free-flying insects could easily withstand the aircraft environment (Griffitts 1933; Hicks and Chand 1936; Knipling and Sullivan 1958; Laird 1948; McMullen 1933; Sullivan et al. 1958). If able to survive in the more "primitive" conditions of the unpressurized aircraft of some of the above tests, how much more acceptable would be the "comfortable" environment of today's modern international aircraft!

In accord with the concern of many other countries, Australia had become interested in the transport of insects by aircraft in the 1930s, and in 1937, the Director General of Health instructed that every airplane arriving in Darwin, NT, from overseas be inspected and that any insects found be collected for identification. The inspections involved aircraft arriving at either the Darwin airport or the flying-boat base.

For the period July 1937 to November 1938 the records are incomplete; few searches seem to have been recorded and most identifications were done in Darwin. Cockroaches predominate in the existing records, although it is interesting to note that the very first insect captured was a male *Anopheles* mosquito.

Between December 1938 and August 1939, collections were more assiduous. All specimens were sent to Sydney to the School of Public Health and Tropical Medicine (now the Commonwealth Institute of Health) for identification, and our records show 177 aircraft inspected with more than 480 insects recovered. It is not recorded whether the insects were dead or alive when captured; but from September 1939, careful records were kept in this regard. From this date to October 1941, inspections totaled 337 aircraft with more than 290 insects recovered and identified. A summary of these collections is presented in Table 7-1, and the medically important taxa are listed in Table 7-2.

After October 1941 the collection program at Darwin ceased and only ad hoc submissions of insects for identification came from Darwin and Cairns until 1974. Our records for this intervening period show the identification of mosquito specimens to be predominantly *Culex quinquefasciatus,* or *Aedes vigilax* in some instances. Few insects other than mosquitoes were submitted to this Institute during those years.

Table 7-1. A summary of insect collections from overseas aircraft arriving in Darwin, NT, between December 1938 and October 1941.

Dates	Aircraft inspected	Insects recovered	Avg. No. insects per aircraft
12/38 - 8/39	177 (average 20 aircraft per month, with range of 12-25)	481 ++	2.7
9/39 - 10/41	337 (average 13 aircraft per month, with range of 6-16)	291 ++ (205 alive, 86 ++ dead)	0.9 (0.6 alive)

Table 7-2. Insects of public health interest recovered from overseas aircraft arriving in Darwin, NT, between December 1938 and October 1941.

Members of the following families were recorded:

Culicidae (mosquitoes): various species including:

Aedes	aegypti
Aedes	vigilax
Anopheles	? barbirostris
Anopheles	maculatus
Anopheles	sundaicus
Anopheles	vagus
Culex	quinquefasciatus
Culex	sitiens
Mansonia	? sp.

Ceratopogonidae (biting midges): Culicoides sp.

Phlebotomidae (sandflies): ? Phlebotomus sp.

Tabanidae (horse flies)

Muscidae: Musca domestica (housefly)
      : Stomoxys calcitrans (stable-fly)
      : Haematobia exigua (buffalo-fly)

Calliphoridae (blowflies)

Tachinidae

Phoridae

Chloropidae (eye-flies)

Hippoboscidae (louse-flies)

Siphonaptera (fleas): Ctenocephalides canis

Blattidae (cockroaches): including Blattella germanica

With the introduction of Indonesian Airlines flights into Darwin in 1973 (from Surabaya, Denpasar, and Koepang) and the finding of a number of malaria cases among passengers on these flights, the Commonwealth Department of Health decided to institute an insect recovery program once more. Searches of these aircraft were made on a regular basis for insects, especially those of medical importance. The aims were to determine the numbers and types of insects arriving on the aircraft and to monitor the effectiveness of disinsection procedures.

The program received early impetus when *Anopheles* mosquitoes were detected regularly, with some specimens being freshly blood-fed, and it was decided to extend the activity to other international airports in Australia.

Collection techniques were standardized as far as practicable. Only aircraft cabins and cockpits (not cargo holds) were searched, with two collectors entering the aircraft after the "knockdown" insecticide spray and after the passengers had left the aircraft. Every part of the cabin and cockpit was searched, within the time limitations, with special attention being paid to lighting panels/conduits, luggage racks, and other undisturbed areas. Search time was limited in all instances, but averaged about 15-20 minutes per plane. Collections were by entomologists of the Health Department or by quarantine officers under entomological direction. Collection sheets gave details of aircraft registration, flight route, date, collection time, and number of specimens recovered.

The insect recovery program began in Darwin in February 1974 and continued until March 1979. During this period systematic collections were also carried out at Brisbane, Sydney, and Perth; Tables 7-3 and 7-4 summarize the results.

Overall, 307 aircraft were inspected, with 5,517 specimens (including 686 mosquitoes) collected, an average of 18 insects per aircraft (Table 7-3). An obvious criticism of this type of study is that it is difficult, if not impossible, to know accurately where and when the insects entered the plane. They could have been on the aircraft for some time, possibly months, particularly in the case of large airliners of foreign companies that may visit Australia only infrequently (also in the case of those specimens taken from lighting panels or bays that were obviously very inadequately or infrequently cleaned). In some instances, it was clearly evident that the above was in fact the case, and dust-covered specimens bore this out.

We were able to investigate this facet with the program in Darwin and aircraft on the Indonesian route. Here B707, BAC111, VC9, and Hawker-Sidley aircraft were limited to the route, and individual aircraft could be followed through the program and regularly checked. Thus

Table 7-3. Summary of Insect Recovery Program*.

Airport/Date	No. of aircraft inspected	No. of insects collected	Avg. No. of insects per aircraft	No. of insect orders represented
Darwin				
21.2.74 - 11.11.74	59	557	9.4	9
8.6.75 - 31.7.75	5	196	39.2	7
5.1.76 - 13.9.76	18	234	13	9
29.11.76 - 3.10.77	19	245	12.9	9
10.10.77 - 24.7.78	17	161	9.5	6
14.8.78 - 13.3.79	12	87	7.3	8
Sydney				
31.7.74 - 9.8.74	49	810	16.5	10
7.11.74 - 11.11.74	32	1005	31.4	11
14.3.75 - 16.3.75	34	892	26.2	10
28.10.75 - 1.11.75	28	399	14.3	9
Brisbane				
3.9.75 - 8.9.75	25	733	29.3	9
Perth				
18.4.75 - 20.4.75	9	198	22.0	6
Totals	307	5517	18.0	14

*The numbers of insects collected will in many cases represent an accumulation of dead insects over a period of time prior to aircraft searching, as well as some instances where regular aircraft searches allowed an appreciation of weekly or even daily flight insect numbers.

the presence of insects, particularly mosquitoes, could be reliably associated with site and date of origin in some cases. For instance, consecutive searches of the one BAC111 aircraft, using the same search sites, resulted in continuous recoveries of mosquitoes, some freshly knocked down and not dead.

Table 7-4. Order of insects* collected from aircraft.

Order	No. of specimens	Percent of identified total
Diptera	3563	64.6
(Family Culicidae)	(686)	(12.4)
Hemiptera	781	14.2
Hymenoptera	381	6.9
Lepidoptera	288	5.2
Coleoptera	285	5.2
Blattoidea	98	1.8
Ephemeroptera	48	0.9
Neuroptera	27	0.5
Orthoptera	24	0.4
Odonata	9	0.2
Psocoptera	6	0.1
Thysanoptera	4	0.08
Dermaptera	2	0.04
Phthiriaptera	1	0.02
Total	5517	

*A small number of spiders were collected and are not included in the results.

To attempt to gain an idea of the actual numbers of insects being introduced with individual flights, the information presented in Table 7-5 has been derived from Darwin searches. These results show remarkable similarity between the different planes followed over the period, when the numbers of insects collected were reduced to an average number per day.

Table 7-5. Insects recovered from individual aircraft consecutively searched when entering Darwin from Indonesian route.

B707 (Registration No. N107BN): 15 fortnightly searches over 34 weeks

Total insects	Average/Darwin flight	Average/day
137	9.1	0.6

BAC111 (Registration No. PK-PJC): 21 fortnightly searches over 52 weeks

Total insects	Average/Darwin flight	Average/day
136	6.5	0.4

VC9 (Registration No. PK-MVE): 14 searches over 54 weeks

Total insects	Average/Darwin flight	Average/day
210	15	0.6

If we return to the overall collection figures and compare the Darwin 1974-79 collections to the 1938-41 collections (Table 7-5a), we see the apparently large increase.

Table 7-5a. Comparison of 1974-79 to 1938-41 collection figures.

	Aircraft inspected	No. insects	Average/aircraft
1938-41	514	772 ++	1.50 +
1974-79	130	1480	11.38

However, if we could separate current flight insects from the accumulated test individuals, we might see less of a difference; for example, the "daily" values for Darwin 1976-79 from B707, BAC111, VC9 on the Indonesian routes were 0.4-0.6 insects/flight. What may actually be represented is an increase in the accumulated numbers of insects in modern planes, for several reasons, including that modern aircraft have more sites likely to accumulate insects.

It is tempting to compare these figures with those quoted for earlier studies. The 1937-47 report from the United States (Hughes 1949) showed a total of 80,716 aircraft inspected; 28,752 (35.6%) harbored arthropods, and 3,873 (4.8%) harbored mosquitoes. The total number of arthropods collected was 106,106, including 16,846 that were alive; this total included 12,825 mosquitoes representing 10 genera and 73 species, 25 of which were considered truly exotic. These records would indicate a rate of 1.3 insects per flight (0.2 live insects per flight), and the Australian studies reported from 1938-41 (Table 7-1) show an average of 1.5 insects per aircraft with 0.6 live insects per aircraft for the period September 1939 to October 1941.

Few such investigations have been recorded in the literature in more recent years but WHO (1971) reported spot checks between 1964 and 1968 on aircraft arriving in Hawaii wherein 373 insects (including 65 mosquitoes) were collected (from an unknown number of aircraft). During the same period Philippine collections (Basio et al. 1970) resulted in 14,246 aircraft being searched to provide 708 insects (534 mosquitoes), which is an average of 0.05 insects per aircraft, while American collections (Evans et al. 1963) recorded averages from 0.81 to 19.2 insects per aircraft.

Whether all or even any of these insect recovery figures can be compared is arguable, but if the Australian figures are indeed high in comparison to other studies, the reasons may be very complex and not beg explanation.

However, the majority of aircraft arriving in this country refuel or stop at night at foreign airports before flying the final sector of their route to Australia. The aircraft thus, particularly if "standing off" on the tarmac for loading, can act as giant light traps to attract local insect populations. This might be even more so in the case of the larger aircraft with their wide doorways and brighter lighting.

Most of the specimens were collected in or near the interior lighting panels. They are undisturbed areas and are reasonably accessible, and for this reason they are also more liable to be productive, as are luggage rack areas.

Because of the different interior conformations and designs of the various aircraft, collection experience revealed "profitable" sites according to aircraft type:

B707: most insects were located behind the removable lighting panels.

B747: the front and rear aisle lighting bays and the flight deck gave the best results.

DC8: the uncovered lighting panels proved productive.

DC10: the lighting conduits around the front of the aircraft provided most specimens.

It is also difficult to draw conclusions from some of the collections because of the varying collection times. It was not practicable to conform to a particular collection time per aircraft, let alone type of aircraft based on size; but the study does not appear to have suffered because of this for within the data sheets, there is not an overall obvious relationship between number of insects and amount of time spent collecting. More important was the search pattern in the aircraft, with the various types of aircraft affording optimal collection sites as mentioned above. Even here however, this was soon obvious to the collectors and incorporated into standard collection technique. With the Darwin collections in particular, the places searched and time spent became routine procedure.

Of the insects collected, we were most interested in those of medical importance, particularly the mosquitoes. A report from the United States (Evans et al. 1963) listing mosquitoes recovered from aircraft arriving at Miami, New Orleans, and Honolulu airports showed a diverse collection of species, as did reports from the Philippines (Basio 1973; Basio et al 1970). Our collection program also produced an interesting assortment of species (Table 7-6) with a number of vectors included (Table 7-7).

The collection of the malaria vectors *Anopheles subpictus, A. sundaicus, A. barbirostris,* and *A. vagus* on flights from Southeast Asia in general—and the Indonesian area specifically—indicate a potential for reintroduction of malaria, since there were instances where clinical cases of malaria have arrived on the same aircraft as the exotic vectors. The presence of male anophelines on some flights and the finding of 32 and 26 *Culex quinquefasciatus* on two BAC111 aircraft arriving in Darwin from Denpasar in 1977 indicates that the breeding sites are not too far removed from the aircraft loading zone, a situation that should not be tolerated on an international airfield.

The northern part of Australia is of particular concern in this regard. Even though WHO has recognized that Australia has eradicated malaria with the last indigenous transmission on the mainland being in 1962, the presence of vectors arriving on aircraft along with passengers who could be suffering from parasitaemia (or viraemia in the

Table 7-6. Species of mosquitoes (Family: Culicidae) collected during
program.

Species	Ports collected
Aedes albopictus	Darwin, Perth
Aedes vigilax	Darwin, Brisbane, Sydney
Aedes ? campestris/dorsalis	Sydney
Aedes ? spp.	Darwin, Sydney
Anopheles barbirostris	Darwin
Anopheles subpictus	Darwin
Anopheles sundaicus	Darwin
Anopheles vagus	Darwin
Culex annulirostris	Perth, Darwin, Brisbane, Sydney
Culex ? barraudi/edwardsi	Sydney
Culex bitaeniorhynchus	Darwin
Culex quinquefasciatus	Brisbane, Perth, Darwin, Sydney, Melbourne*
Culex gelidus	Darwin, Sydney
Culex perplexus	Sydney
Culex pipiens gp.	Sydney
Culex sitiens	Darwin, Melbourne*
Culex sitiens gp.	Darwin, Sydney, Melbourne*
Culex tritaeniorhynchus	Darwin, Sydney
Culex ? spp.	Darwin, Sydney
Culiseta ? sp.	Sydney
Mansonia uniformis	Perth, Darwin, Sydney, Brisbane

*Some ad hoc collections made at Melbourne are not included in the
overall results (Tables 7-4 and 7-5), but mosquito species identified are
listed here.

case of a virus disease such as dengue) is worthy of
serious concern.

There are disturbing recent records of malaria and other
disease vectors being transported by aircraft in the Pacific
(Eads 1972; Nowell 1977; Chapters 1, 4, 5, 6, 9, 10, 13,
and 15), and we would be most concerned to exclude those
anopheline species recovered during this program as well as
others not taken, but posing a similar risk and hazard,

Table 7-7. Some insect vectors of human diseases collected from aircraft in Australia.*

Species	Airport	Vector status
Aedes albopictus	Darwin, Perth	Dengue fever, DHF, Chikungunya virus
Aedes vigilax	Darwin, Brisbane, Sydney	RRV, Edge Hill virus, Sindbis virus
Culex quinquefasciatus	Darwin, Perth, Brisbane, Sydney	Bancroftian filariasis, Arboviruses
Culex tritaeniorhynchus	Darwin, Sydney	JE, Chikungunya virus, Sindbis virus, Getah virus, Tembusu virus
Culex gelidus	Darwin, Sydney	JE, Getah virus, Chikungunya virus, Sindbis, Tembusu virus
Culex annulirostris	Darwin, Brisbane, Sydney, Perth	RRV, Kunjin, Australian encephalitis, Sindbis viruses
Mansonia uniformis	Darwin, Brisbane, Sydney, Perth	Malayan filariasis, Bancroftian filariasis, Chikungunya virus
Anopheles subpictus	Darwin	Malaria
Anopheles sundaicus	Darwin	Malaria

*Of these, Aedes vigilax, Culex quinquefasciatus, C. annulirostris and Mansonia uniformis are known to be present in Australia.

such as Anopheles punctulatus from New Guinea. Moreover, although Aedes aegypti was not found on aircraft (somewhat surprisingly) during this survey, Aedes albopictus was, and both species being vectors of dengue fever, are distinctly unwelcome. A. albopictus does not exist in Australia (although it is close by in Southeast Asia, New Guinea, and the Pacific) and A. aegypti appears to be now confined to Queensland and its reestablishment in areas from which it has disappeared is not desirable.

Despite the facts that vector insects can be imported by aircraft, there is no clear evidence concerning the magnitude of the epidemiological risk (WHO 1971). However, even without the establishment of breeding populations of potential vectors there may be need for concern here because of recent reports of people who had never been to a malaria endemic area, but lived or worked in the vicinity of European airports handling aircraft coming from Africa, and who contracted malaria (Anonymous 1979; Chapter 1), presumably from imported infective vectors.

The total insect collection has also been tabulated against type of aircraft (Table 7-8) although it should be appreciated that within this grouping some aircraft represent limited and specialized air routes (for instance, B727 only flew Port Moresby to Brisbane, and the Hawker Sidley aircraft only flew the Indonesian route to Darwin).

If we consider the types of aircraft associated with the insect recoveries made during 1974-79 (Table 7-8), the smaller B727/VC10 ranked well with the larger B747/DC10, although the two former samples are very small and probably not comparable. The B727s also came from the one route, New Guinea. The Darwin series collections on B707/BAC111/VC9 showed similar collection figures on same route and aircraft type displayed only minor variation. For the larger aircraft, DC10/B747 yielded more insects/search because the undisturbed area was greater and led to easy collection of larger numbers of insects in one place/unit time.

It would appear that the route may be the more important (Table 7-9), but again it is extremely difficult to interpret the figures for comparison.

Although the Indonesian route provided anopheline vectors, it was not the source of most insects on an average number per aircraft basis. That dubious distinction lay with New Guinea, although involving a small sample only, followed by the United States/Pacific or New Zealand routes (Table 7-9).

Ovitrap Surveillance

As a further means of monitoring mosquito importations, particularly that of *Aedes aegypti* (now only known to be present in one Australian state, Queensland), ovitraps were set up at Darwin, Sydney, and Brisbane airports. The traps consisted of a black jar, half-filled with water, with a wooden paddle placed inside. The ovitraps were serviced

Table 7-8. Insect recoveries from aircraft by type of aircraft.*

Type of aircraft	No. of aircraft inspected	Total No. of insects recovered	Avg. No. insects/ aircraft
Beechcraft 18	1	0	0
Cessna 402	1	9	9.0
Heron	1	5	5.0
Mooney Ranger	1	0	0
DC3	1	2	2.0
Hawker Sidley	38	368	9.7
F28/Fokker Friendship	8	67	8.4
VC9	23	329	14.3
VC10	4	108	27.0
BAC111	22	146	6.6
B707	91	1004	11.0
B707 (wide-look)	12	129	10.8
B727	7	495	70.7**
B747	47	1308	27.8
DC8	28	510	18.2
DC10	20	1037	51.9
Total	307	5517	18.0

*This table takes no account of accumulation of dead insects on individual aircraft over time before or between searches.

**The 7 flights involved here for B727 were all from one route--Port Moresby to Brisbane--and 2 aircraft contributed 309 of the 495 insect total.

Table 7-9. Insect recoveries from aircraft by route into Australia.*

Route	No. of aircraft	No. of insects	Average/ aircraft
1 Southeast Asian (Bombay, Kuala Lumpur, Singapore, Djakarta, Surabaya, Denpasar, Koepang, Bacau, Tamika)	178	2745	15.4
2 Asian (Tokyo, Hong Kong, Manila)	35	554	15.8
3 USA/Pacific (USA, Honolulu, Nadi, Papeete, Noumea, Norfolk Island)	31	722	23.3
4 PNG (Port Moresby)	8	507	63.4**
5 New Zealand (Auckland, Wellington, Christchurch)	37	867	23.4
6 South Africa (Johannesburg, Mauritius)	7	113	16.1

   *This table takes no account of accumulation of dead insects before or between searches. Because of this unknown accumulation factor, as well as the various airlines involved, no hard conclusions can be drawn from these results; yet apart from the New Guinea route, the other routes returned reasonably comparable figures.
   **Two of the 8 flights contributed 309 of the 507 insects collected.

regularly and, although maintained for only relatively short periods in Sydney and Brisbane, they have been used continuously in Darwin since 1974.

   In Sydney the ovitrap program was conducted for 8 months from July 1974, but at no time did any of the traps exhibit mosquito eggs or larvae. The Sydney international terminal docking area is, however, not conducive to mosquito survival and the lack of positive results was not surprising.

The Darwin program, in contrast, for the 3 month period from June 1974, yielded 1771 larvae of various local mosquito species, although no exotic species. No *Aedes aegypti* have been detected from 1974 to the present. Similarly, no *A. aegypti* were found at Brisbane airport during the program.

AIRCRAFT DISINSECTION

Initial provisions for the disinsection of aircraft appeared in the International Sanitary Convention for Aerial Navigation of 1933 (Laird 1961), and in that same year the Director-General of Health in Australia stated that it was considered advisable that from the commencement of regular air traffic to Australia the practice of disinsection immediately before departure, to free each aircraft from mosquitoes, should be instituted (Cumpston 1933).

Inflight spraying of aircraft bound for U.S. ports was in practice by 1937 using pyrethrum; and DDT with pyrethrins was introduced in 1944 (Laird 1952), although it was not until 1951 that International Sanitary Regulations (ISR) were adopted covering international transport by air as well as land and sea. Among other obvious quarantine concerns, ISR incorporated special provisions for disinsection of aircraft (WHO 1957).

WHO (1951) recommended that disinsection on departure should be undertaken prior to take-off, before passengers boarded but after baggage and freight had been loaded. Spraying during the flight was disapproved, and this procedure was later endorsed (WHO 1957).

The techniques for aircraft disinsection have been changed and amended over the years since an early report (Williams and Dreessen 1935) recommended the use of pyrethrum and prescribed dosage requirements for complete disinsection, leading to a number of papers on the subject prior to the 1951 Regulations (David and Tew 1949; Duguet 1949; Dunnahoo 1942, 1943; Garnham 1946; Mackie and Crabtree 1938; Sullivan et al. 1942; Whittingham and Galley 1949).

WHO (1961) reemphasized that insect quarantine should take two main forms, namely airport sanitation (noting that too many international airports fell far short of the ideal) and aircraft disinsection (seen to be only a compromise involving the relative risks of disease introduction, entomological efficiency, passenger comfort, aviation facilitation, and aircraft safety), and made recommendations on protection of airports from vectors and on aircraft disinsection with aerosols. Quoting reports that many mosquitoes were surviving "in-the-air" aerosol treatments, WHO now recommended disinsection following passenger embarkation and before take-off ("blocks-away" disinsection) to overcome these inadequacies. The opportunities for vectors to reinfest aircraft after a predeparture treatment, and the disadvantages associated with postarrival treatments, were considered in the recommendations, as was the need to cause the least possible interference to air traffic.

A standard reference aerosol of DDT (3.0%) and pyrethrum extract (1.6%) as active ingredients with xylene, petroleum distillates, and Freon 11 and 12 as propellents was proposed. However, because of the numerous problems associated with aerosol disinsection, including concerns about effectiveness, passenger acceptance, security of compliance, and air-traffic delays, WHO (1961) recommended a move to a vapor treatment using DDVP (Dichlorvos) via an automatic dispensing system that was under study in the United States at that time. A WHO resolution subsequently recommended that from 1971 either aerosol disinsecting before take-off, in-flight vapor disinsection, or aerosol disinsection on the ground on arrival be used in pressurized international aircraft. The vapor (DDVP) disinsection system underwent much investigation (Jensen et al. 1965; Jensen et al. 1961; Pearce et al. 1961; Schoof et al. 1961), but because of detrimental reactions on aircraft components the system had to be abandoned.

Further studies in the 1960s had supported the concept of "blocks-away" disinsection (Sullivan et al. 1964; Sullivan et al. 1962) using the DDT/pyrethrins standard reference aerosol. With DDT becoming less acceptable worldwide, and concern over DDT resistance, the search for alternative aerosols (Schechter and Sullivan 1972; Sullivan et al. 1972) resulted in the approval of synthetic pyrethroids resmethrin and bioresmethrin (as 2.0% solutions in Freon 11 and 12) by WHO in 1972 (WHO 1974).

Australia, which to this time had used a DDT (2.0%)/ Pyrethrins (1.2%) formulation, now adopted the use of 2.0% bioresmethrin "on arrival," but this preparation was soon to be discontinued—and replaced by a pyrethrins (1.2%) preparation—due to unfavorable reaction from passengers. Such a situation had been indicated by earlier studies; and with long-term use, photodecomposition of insecticide residue created an unacceptable odor problem, widely recognized but also disputed (Sullivan et al. 1975).

A further series of studies investigated the use of other compounds, particularly d-phenothrin (Cawley et al. 1974;

Liljedahl et al. 1976; Schechter et al. 1974)—which had no discernible odor and did not require solvents other than the propellent materials—and 2.0% d-phenothrin was duly approved by WHO (1977).

The next step in the continuing investigations came about because of the prohibition in the United States of the halogenated chlorofluoroalkanes (Freon 11 and 12) as propellents in aerosols in order to reduce the risk of ozone depletion, and water-based preparations of d-phenothrin were compared with the normal Freon-based aerosols (Sullivan et al. 1978, 1979). The results indicated that, although the water-based aerosols were as effective as the Freon-based counterparts, the propellents used (propane, iso-butane) posed a possible fire risk. This risk was seen as being reducible by refinements in aerosol construction and care in handling, but the formulations required further assessment before they could be recommended for aircraft.

In 1974 the Commonwealth Department of Health in Australia convened meetings to discuss the problems posed by modern international aircraft, particularly the wide-bodied aircraft such as the B747 and the DC10. The restrictions on landing times at Sydney Airport, which see most of the aircraft arriving from the areas to the north of Australia being loaded at night with the added risk of insects being attracted to the aircraft lights, was the main cause for concern. The insect recovery program then instituted soon showed the concern to be well founded, particularly for those aircraft entering Darwin from the Indonesian routes.

Prior to 1974, the cabins of all arriving aircraft in Australia were sprayed with the pyrethrins (1.2%)/DDT (2%) formulation at the rate of 10 grams per 1000 cubic feet of space and the doors opened after two minutes; when the passengers and crew had disembarked, the cabins were resprayed with 30 grams per 1000 cubic feet and the doors kept closed for five minutes.

By 1974, the aerosol formulation had changed to bio-resmethrin (2.0%), but the procedure for disinsection involving the double treatment was maintained. Later that year the bioresmethrin spray was replaced by a pyrethrins (1.2%) formulation because of the former's odor problem. However, passenger complaints of eye and nasopharynx irritation led to a reduced-concentration formulation (0.4% pyrethrins/1.6% piperonyl butoxide) being introduced in 1975.

The double-spraying procedure was still being maintained when d-phenothrin (2.0%) was introduced as the insecticide. However, in 1978 a problem was raised when electronic equipment components on Qantas B747 aircraft were found to be affected by a residue build-up attributable to the insecticide. A trial was conducted to assess the efficacy of a single spray of 10 grams per 1000 cubic feet; this proved acceptable and the second cabin spray was dropped from the normal disinsection procedure.

AIRCRAFT DISINSECTION TRIALS

The insect recovery surveys had highlighted the importance of disinsection of cabins of overseas aircraft but the system of "on-ground" spraying—with the double-spray technique—was delaying aircraft movements. To facilitate the disembarkation of passengers and expedite the quarantine and customs procedures, Qantas requested the Department to assess and carry out trials on in-flight disinsection on the two different types of aircraft that the airline operated at that time, namely Boeing 707s and 747s.

On a trial conducted in November 1975, on a B707 aircraft on the Auckland/Sydney route, live mosquitoes were used as test insects for an in-flight disinsection (0.4% pyrethrins, 1.6% pip. butoxide). The results showed a 100% knockdown and 100% mortality at 24 hours of all mosquitoes. However, two trials aboard B747 aircraft (November 1975 Auckland/Sydney and March 1976 Melbourne/-Sydney) failed to produce 100% knockdown of test mosquitoes (*Culex quinquefasciatus*) at all test stations within the aircraft passenger cabin and flight deck.

Examination of the results of these in-fight tests revealed areas, such as the forward end of the first class cabin, which the insecticide apparently did not reach either because of inadequate spraying technique or through the venting of the cabin atmosphere.

In consultation with Qantas, a precision format was devised to overcome the above problems. The exact position and movements of crew members while disinsecting, the timing, the zones that each member should handle, the control of air movements by the flight deck, and control of the operation by the flight service director were all put together as part of a Qantas operational procedure.

It was decided to test this procedure on a B747 on the Singapore/Sydney route on 9-11 May 1976, and the results have been reported in detail elsewhere (Langsford et al. 1976). In summary, 33 test cages (cylindrical cardboard cups, approximately 170 cc, with cloth netting tops and bottoms), each containing ten mosquitoes (*Culex quinquefasciatus*), were allocated among seven test stations on the aircraft. The cups were placed in groups of five for six of the seven positions and in a group of three for the seventh (the lower lobe galley in the cargo hold area), which would be subjected only to the initial spray. For each group one cup was sealed inside a plastic bag at the time of positioning within the aircraft to act as a control.

The spray trial was carried out during taxiing after touchdown at Sydney airport, and immediately prior to landing all cups were examined and all test insects were alive.

After spraying, all test stations were examined for knockdown, and half of each group were sealed in plastic bags before the second spray.

After the second spray, the remaining cups were sealed, all cups were removed to a laboratory where they were maintained under favorable conditions and observed for possible recovery at two hours, 12 hours, and 24 hours post-spray.

All cups subjected to the "in-flight" spray showed 100% knockdown with no recovery after 24 hours. All controls were satisfactory and the amount of insecticide actually dispensed was determined from weighing the cans after the trial and found to be 2.6% less than the prescribed dosage of 10 grams per 1000 cubic feet.

The in-flight procedure had proven successful in test kill, efficiency of operation, and cabin environment control, but for other reasons it was not introduced and the two-spray "on-arrival" procedure continued at Australian international airports.

Not long after this, the new formulation aerosol containing d-phenothrin (2.0%) was introduced; but Quarantine Assistants at the various airports expressed concern regarding its effectiveness as a knockdown agent. A disadvantage of d-phenothrin, albeit a minor one, is that it has relatively slow knockdown properties and although it gives excellent kill, knockdown could be enhanced by the addition of a compound with faster knockdown properties, such as bioresmethrin (Sullivan et al. 1978), if this feature gave cause for concern.

As a result, a trial was carried out using a Merpati BAC111 in Darwin on November 14, 1977. Test mosquitoes (*Culex quinquefasciatus*) were used at 9 test stations throughout the aircraft. Zero knockdown was observed at all stations immediately after spraying; but within a 30 minute holding period, 100% knockdown occurred with all insects, and there was no recovery after 24 hours.

In November 1978, Qantas advised that they were experiencing problems with the electronic equipment on B747 aircraft, which appeared to be attributable to the d-phenothrin formulation currently used for cabin disinsection.

It was considered that because of the improved efficiency of the modern synthetic pyrethroids, the practice of using a second disinsection spray might be foregone, thus reducing the amount of spray used in the aircraft, and therefore the amount of residue deposited.

Accordingly, a series of trials was set up to investigate this proposal. Because of the particular requirements for aircraft operation, the only insecticides considered were among those recommended by WHO. These included pyrethrum, resmethrin, bioresmethrin, and d-phenothrin. Resmethrin and bioresmethrin were excluded because of known side effects, namely production of offensive odors.

The insecticide formulations used in these trials were:

1. 2% d-phenothrin at 10 grams per 1000 cubic feet.
2. 0.4% pyrethrins/1.6% piperonyl butoxide at 10 grams per 1000 cubic feet.
3. 2% d-phenothrin at 5 grams per 1000 cubic feet.
4. 0.4% pyrethrins/1.6% piperonyl butoxide/0.4% d-phenothrin at 10 grams per 1000 cubic feet.

The test insects again were *Culex quinquefasciatus* and the cages and techniques used were similar to those of the Singapore trial (Langsford et al. 1976). The aircraft used were parked at hangars and had arrived in Sydney up to a day previously; controls showed no effect from residual insecticide.

In all cases following the spraying, the test mosquitoes were immobilized by the time they were transferred to clean cups. With one exception, 100% mortality was observed after 18 hours. All treatments thus gave virtually 100% mosquito mortality. However, the two pyrethrin-based sprays had a highly irritant respiratory effect on personnel, and the d-phenothrin at 5 grams per 1000 cubic feet did not produce satisfactory mortality with fruit flies (*Dacus tryoni*), also run as test insects.

It was recommended therefore that the disinsection procedures as used in Australia be amended to use a single spray of 2% d-phenothrin at the rate of 10 grams per 1000 cubic feet, in line with WHO recommendations. Such became the practice and has been maintained until the present time.

In 1980, Qantas again requested the Department to consider the blocks-away procedure, this time suggesting an assessment of a single treatment with 2% d-phenothrin to be established as standard disinsection procedure on the trans-Tasman route between New Zealand and Australia, the former being considered a low risk country.

Three trials were subsequently undertaken on the Auckland/Sydney route in May-July 1980 on B747-standard and B747-"Combi" aircraft.

The protocol for the trial was essentially the same as that established for the earlier trials (Langsford et al. 1976), but in these 1980 trials three categories of test cup were used:

1. Controls: Four control trials were designated:
   a) Insectary Controls: cups were left under favorable conditions in the CIH insectary at Sydney.
   b) Travel Controls: cups travelled in sealed, insulated containers for the whole exercise.
   c) Aircraft Atmosphere Controls: cups were distributed throughout the aircraft and left for 15 minutes prior to placement of test cups, then sealed in plastic bags, and kept to monitor effects of residual insecticides.
   d) Fixed Station Controls: cups, sealed in plastic bags, placed at each of the standard fixed test stations aboard the aircraft.

2. Fixed Station Trials: Four cups placed at each of the seven standard fixed stations and exposed to the insecticide spray for the duration of the flight (approximately 4 hours).

3. Wild Cup Trials: Eleven single cups placed "randomly" throughout the cabin to monitor less accessible situations and various "nooks and crannies."

After the passengers had boarded at Auckland, the disinsection spray took place. After arrival in Sydney, all cups were sealed, removed to an insectary, trial mosquitoes were transferred to uncontaminated holding cups, and all specimens were held under favorable conditions with sugar solution for up to 48 hours for observation.

The knockdown qualities of the spray were recorded by observing the reactions of test specimens at a number of the Wild Stations and an example of results (Table 7-10) reflects the delayed knockdown for the d-phenothrin, 100% mortality eventuated.

The results for the overall trial (Table 7-11) confirmed that d-phenothrin is indeed efficient. The controls showed no significant mortality, and virtually 100% mortality at all

Table 7-10. B747 Auckland/Sydney Trial: Knockdown monitoring of Wild Station cages after "blocks-away" spray.

Time	Wild Station 1: knockdown percent
Spray	--
Spray + 5 minutes	50
Spray + 10 minutes	90
Spray + 15 minutes	90
Spray + 20 minutes	100
Spray + 25 minutes	100
Spray + 30 minutes	100
Spray + 35 minutes	100
Spray + 65 minutes	100

test stations was achieved (of the 1500 specimens used, only 3 individuals survived).

One comment on the methods used in all the trials is that in setting up the test mosquitoes in cylindrical-type cages with only top and bottom mesh openings the individual insect is somewhat more protected than a "free-flying" individual in an aircraft (although possibly less so than one secreted in clothing or carry-on baggage). Previous studies (Tew et al. 1951), however, indicated that a 50% mortality for caged mosquitoes in the presence of aerosols may be equivalent to a kill approaching 90-100% for free-flying insects. Neither are such caged specimens subject to "flushing out" by the insecticide from areas of possibly sublethal concentration to areas of higher concentration (McGovern and Fales 1946); and thus our levels of mortality in these trials indicate excellent control.

This final series of trials indicated that a blocks-away spray of d-phenothrin (2.0%) at 10 grams per 1000 cubic feet should be sufficient to conform to quarantine require-

Table 7-11.   B747 Auckland/Sydney Trial: Effects of "blocks-away" disinsection procedure on Culex quinquefasciatus.

Mortality (% Effect-Knockdown/Mortality)

Fixed Station	5 hrs.					24 hrs.				
	Control	(i)	(ii)	(iii)	(iv)	Control	(i)	(ii)	(iii)	(iv)
TRIAL 1--B747 Standard Aircraft										
FS 1	10	100	100	100	100	10	100	100	100	100
2	0	100	100	60	80	0	100	100	100	100
3	0	100	100	100	100	0	100	100	100	100
4	0	100	100	100	100	0	100	100	100	100
5	10	100	100	100	90	10	100	100	100	90
6	0	100	100	100	100	0	100	100	100	100
7	0	100	100	100	100	0	100	100	100	100
TRIAL 2--B747 "Combi" Aircraft										
FS 1	0	100	100	100	100	0	100	100	100	100
2	0	100	100	100	100	0	100	100	100	100
3	0	100	100	100	100	0	100	100	100	100
4	0	100	100	100	100	0	100	100	100	100
5	0	100	100	100	100	0	100	100	100	100
6	0	100	100	100	100	0	100	100	100	100
7	0	100	100	100	100	0	100	100	100	100
8	10	100	100	100	100	30	100	100	100	100
TRIAL 3--B747 "Combi" Aircraft										
FS 1	0	100	100	100	100	10	100	100	100	100
2	0	100	100	100	100	0	100	100	100	100
3	0	100	100	100	100	0	100	100	100	100
4	0	100	100	100	100	0	100	100	100	100
5	0	100	100	100	100	0	100	100	100	100
6	0	100	100	100	100	0	100	100	100	100
7	0	100	100	100	100	0	100	100	100	100
8	0	100	100	100	100	20	100	100	100	100

ments, particularly with regard to the trans-Tasman route to Australia. However, the blocks-away technique has not as yet been introduced as standard procedure for the trans-Tasman, or any other international flight route into Australia, due to other considerations.

These studies have not included the cargo holds of the aircraft, either for insect recovery or for disinsection trials. Quarantine officers normally undertake disinsection of holds under a standard procedure whereby the insecticide (2% d-phenothrin) is sprayed through the "portholes" in the hold doors for 90 seconds; then two containers are removed, and the officers enter this space and spray for 2 minutes in all directions. The hold is then shut for 10 minutes before the rest of the cargo containers are removed. As each container is subsequently opened, it is sprayed for 10 seconds before unpacking.

However, Qantas has developed an automatic device that has been fitted to all B747 aircraft in its fleet. The device is attached to the inside surface of the cargo doors, and aerosol cans of insecticide are fitted into brackets at the last airport before take-off for Australia. The instrument is activated automatically by the pilot during take-off; quarantine officers at the Australian port of arrival can verify from the ground that the cans have discharged by observing indicators through the pressure relief hatches. The insecticide used is a formulation of pyrethrins (2.5%), d-phenothrin (2.0%), and piperonyl butoxide (1.25%).

CONCLUSIONS

The distribution of many insect species is changing and developing throughout the world, and the role played by aircraft in disseminating species cannot be denied or lightly dismissed.

In the Pacific we need to look no further than Guam to see evidence of the effects of breakdown of quarantine against insects of public health concern (Basio and Reisen 1971; Nowell 1977, 1980; Chapter 8). While only seven mosquito species are indigenous to Guam, this total had doubled by 1969 and quintupled by 1972, according to Nowell. However, the latter's dramatic figures (including 34 rather recent introductions) are challenged by Ward (Chapter 8), who recognizes an introduced mosquito fauna of only half that size, namely 17 species. Nevertheless, the recent introduction rate is clearly alarming, especially as no less than five species of *Anopheles* are involved, and there is at least one known instance of local malaria infection due to *Plasmodium falciparum,* which could have been due to the bite of a locally bred anopheline that had previously fed from a hospitalized patient with malaria, or of an already-infected vector that had arrived in an aircraft, while JE and dengue fever have occurred also, apparently associated with introductions of either infected vectors or human carriers (Nowell 1977).

Whether this situation threatens many other Pacific countries is, of course, arguable, but the risk certainly exists for some. Australia would appear to be at risk of the introduction of vector mosquitoes, particularly the brackish-water-breeding anophelines *Anopheles subpictus* and *A. sundaicus* from Indonesia; for the Darwin Airport surrounds may well be receptive to these and other species too.

Airport sanitation, both at foreign and Australian airports, should still be a high priority consideration in attempts to prevent introduction of these insects, while continuing aircraft disinsection would appear to be justified in the current circumstances.

The current WHO/IHR (1974) recommend the maintenance of a 400 m mosquito-free zone for international airports. This, however, is based on the flight range of *Aedes aegypti* and is aimed at quarantine against that species. Other vector species have greater flight ranges, and 400 m should be regarded as inadequate to prevent the entry of such vectors into the transit area. A more practical recommendation designed to take into account the anopheline and culicine vectors other than *A. aegypti,* such as those listed in this paper as having been taken from aircraft arriving in Australia, could be a mosquito-free zone of at least one kilometer around an international transit area where mosquito control measures would be pursued.

REFERENCES

Anonymous. 1933. Disease risks from oversea air traffic. *Health* (Feb. 1933):12-16.
————. 1978. Director-General of Health, Commonwealth of Australia. *Ann. Rep.,* 1977-78.
————. 1979. Malaria—the phoenix with drug resistance. *Lancet* (1):1328-1329.
Aziz, M., Jr. 1948. *Anopheles* eradication in Cyprus. *J. R. Sanit. Inst.* 67:498-513.
Basio, R. G. 1973. The mosquito control program at the Manila international airport and vicinity (Philippines) with comments on problems encountered on the aerial transportation of mosquitoes. In *Vector Control in Southeast Asia,* Proc. First SEAMEO workshop, eds. Y. C. Chan, K. L. Chan, and B. C. Ho, pp. 78-84.
Basio, R. G., M. J. Prudencio, and I. E. Chanco. 1970. Notes on the aerial transportation of mosquitoes and

other insects at the Manila international airport. *Philipp. Ent.* 1:407-8.

Basio, R. G., and W. K. Reisen. 1971. On some mosquitoes of Guam, Mariana Islands (Diptera: Culicidae). *Philipp. Ent.* 2:57-61.

Bruce-Chwatt, L. J. 1973. Global problems of imported disease. In *Advances in Parasitology* Vol. 11, ed. B. Dawes, pp. 75-114. London: Academic Press.

—————. 1980. Jet-borne pestilences: Today and tomorrow. In *Environmental Medicine,* eds. G. M. Howe, and J. A. Loraine, pp. 339-56. London: Heinemann.

Carnahan, C. T. 1938. Activities of the U.S. Public Health Service in mosquito control for airplanes. *Fla. Anti-Mosq. Assn. Rep.* 12:1-7.

Cawley, B. M., W. N. Sullivan, M. S. Schechter, and J. U. McGuire. 1974. Desirability of three synthetic pyrethroid aerosols for aircraft disinsection. *Bull. Wld Hlth Org.* 51:537-40.

Cumpston, J. H. L. 1933. Aeroplane traffic and the protection of Australia from disease. *Med. J. Aust.* (2):326-32.

David, W. A. L., and R. P. Tew. 1949. Disinsectisation of aircraft. *Month. Bull. Min. Hlth. Pub. Hlth Lab. Ser.* 8:166-72.

Denning, D. G., J. J. Pratt, Jr., A. E. Staebler, and W. W. Wirth. 1947. A tabulation of insects recovered from aircraft entering the United States at Miami, Florida, during the period July 1943 through December 1944. *U.S. Dept. Agric., Foreign Plant Quarantine Memorandum* No. 474.

Dethier, V. G. 1945. The transport of insects in aircraft. *J. econ. Ent.* 38:528-31.

Duguet, J. 1949. Disinsectisation of aircraft. Study made in connexion with the revision of international conventions. *Bull. Wld Hlth Org.* 2:155-91.

Dunnahoo, G. L. 1942. The control of insects transported by aircraft. *Fla. Anti-mosq. Assn. Rep.* 16:10-13.

—————. 1943. Insect control of aircraft. *Soap and Sanit. Chem.* 19:111-13.

Eads, R. B. 1972. Recovery of *Aedes albopictus* from used tires shipped to United States ports. *Mosq. News* 32:113-14.

Evans, B. R., C. R. Joyce, and J. E. Porter. 1963. Mosquitoes and other arthropods found in baggage compartments of international aircraft. *Mosq. News.* 23:9-12.

Garnham, P. C. C. 1946. The efficacy of insecticidal sprays in aircraft. *East Afr. med. J.* 23:272-77.

Griffitts, T. D. H. 1933. Air travel in relation to public health. *Amer. J. Trop. Med.* 13:283-90.

Griffitts, T. D. H., and J. J. Griffitts. 1931. Mosquitoes transported by airplanes. Staining methods used in determining their importation. *U.S. Publ. Hlth. Reps.* 46, 47:2775-2782.

Hicks, E. P., and D. Chand. 1936. Transport and control of *Aedes aegypti* in aeroplanes. *Rec. Malar. Serv. India* 6:73-90.

Highton, R. B., and E. C. C. Van Someren. 1970. The transportation of mosquitoes between international airports. *Bull. Wld Hlth Org.* 42:334-35.

Hughes, J. H. 1949. Aircraft and Public Health Service foreign quarantine entomology. *U.S. Publ. Hlth. Repts.* Suppl. 210.

Jensen, J. A., V. P. Flury, and H. F. Schoof. 1965. Dichlorvos vapour disinsection of aircraft. *Bull. Wld Hlth Org.* 32:175-79.

Jensen, J. A., G. W. Pearce, and K. D. Quarterman. 1961. A mechanical system for dispensing known amounts of insecticidal vapours. *Bull. Wld Hlth Org.* 24:617-22.

Knipling, E. B., and W. N. Sullivan. 1958. The thermal death points of several species of insects. *J. econ. Ent.* 51:344-46.

Laird, M. 1948. Reactions of mosquitoes to the aircraft environment. *Trans. roy. Soc. N.Z.* 77:93-114.

————. 1951a. The accidental carriage of insects on board aircraft. *J. roy. aeronaut. Soc.* 55:735-43.

————. 1951b. Insects collected from aircraft arriving in New Zealand from abroad. Wellington: *Zool. Publs Victoria Univ. Coll.* No. 11.

————. 1952. Insects collected from aircraft arriving in New Zealand during 1951. *J. Aviat. Med.* 23:280-85.

————. 1956a. Wartime collections of insects from aircraft at Whenuapai. *New Zealand J. Sci. Tech.* (B) 38:76-84.

————. 1956b. Studies of mosquitoes and freshwater ecology in the South Pacific. *Roy. Soc. N.Z. Bull.* 6.

————. 1961. Quarantines and zoologists. *Med. Serv. J.* (Canada) 17:563-70.

Langsford, W. A., N. Rajapaksa, and R. C. Russell. 1976. A trial to assess the efficacy of inflight disinsection of a Boeing-747 aircraft on the Singapore/Sydney sector. *Pyrethrum Post* 13:137-42. (also WHO/VBC/76.636)

Lee, D. J. 1951. The problems of insect quarantine. *Proc. Linn. Soc. N.S.W.* 76:v-xix.

Liljedahl, L. A., H. J. Retzer, W. N. Sullivan, M. S. Schechter, B. M. Cawley, N. O. Morgan, C. M. Amyx, B. A. Schiefer, E. J. Gergerg, and R. Pal. 1976. Aircraft disinsection: the physical and insecticidal characteristics of (+) - phenothrin applied by aerosol at "blocks away." *Bull. Wld Hlth Org.* 54:391-96.

McGovern, E. R., and J. H. Fales. 1946. *Soap and Sanitary Chemicals* 22:127-29.

McMullen, J. 1933. Observations et experiences nouvelles sur le transport des moustiques par les aeroplanes. *Bull. Off. Int. Hyg. Publ.* 25(6):1024-1027.

Mackie, F. P., and H. S. Crabtree. 1938. The destruction of mosquitoes in aircraft. *Lancet* 235:447-50.

Magath, T. B. 1945. Quarantine procedures with special reference to air travel. *J. Aviation Med.* 16:165-74.

Mendonca, F. C. de, and N. Cerqueira. 1947. Insects and other arthropods captured by the Brazilian Sanitary Service on landplanes or seaplanes arriving in Brazil between January 1942 and December 1945. *Bol. Ofic. Sanit. Panamer.* 26:22-30.

Nowell, W. R. 1977. International quarantine for control of mosquito-borne diseases on Guam. *Aviation, Space, and environ. Med.* 48:53-60.

—————. 1980. Comparative mosquito collection data from the southern Mariana Islands (Diptera: Culicidae). *Proc pprs ann conf Calif Mosq Vector Contr Assn* 48:112-16.

Pearce, G. W., H. F. Schoof, and K. D. Quarterman. 1961. Insecticidal vapours for aircraft disinsection. *Bull. Wld Hlth Org.* 24:611-16.

Pemberton, C. E. 1944. Insects carried in transpacific airplanes. *Hawaii. Plant. Rec.* 48:183-86.

Porter, J. E. 1958. Further notes on Public Health Service quarantine entomology. *Florida Ent.* 41:41-44.

Schechter, M. S., and W. N. Sullivan. 1972. Gas propelled aerosols and micronized dusts for control of insects in aircraft. 2. Pesticide formulations. *J. econ. Ent.* 65:1444-1447.

Schechter, M. S., W. N. Sullivan, H. F. Schoof, D. R. Maddock, C. M. Amyx, and J. E. Porter. 1974. d-Phenothrin, a promising new pyrethroid for disinsecting aircraft. *J. med. Ent.* 11:231-33.

Schoof, H. F., J. A. Jensen, J. E. Porter, and D. R. Maddock. 1961. Disinsection of aircraft with a mechanical dispenser of DDVP vapour. *Bull. Wld Hlth Org.* 24:623-28.

Soper, F. L., and D. B. Wilson. 1943. *Anopheles gambiae* in Brazil 1930-1940. New York: *Rockefeller Foundation*.

Sullivan, W. N., L. D. Goodhue, and J. H. Fales. 1942.

Toxicity to adult mosquitoes of aerosols produced by spraying solutions of insecticides in liquefied gas. *J. econ. Ent.* 35:48–51.

Sullivan, W. N., F. R. DuChanois, and D. L. Hayden. 1958. Insect survival in jet aircraft. *J. econ. Ent.* 51:239–41.

Sullivan, W. N., J. Keiding, and J. W. Wright. 1962. Studies on aircraft disinsection at "blocks away." *Bull. Wld Hlth Org.* 27:263–73.

Sullivan, W. N., J. C. Azurin, J. W. Wright, and N. G. Gratz. 1964. Studies on aircraft disinsection at "blocks away" in tropical areas. *Bull. Wld Hlth Org.* 30:113–118.

Sullivan, W. N., R. Pal, J. W. Wright, J. C. Azurin, R. Okamoto, J. U. McGuire, and R. M. Waters. 1972. Worldwide studies on aircraft disinsection at "blocks away." *Bull. Wld Hlth Org.* 46:485–91.

Sullivan, W. N., A. N. Hewing, M. S. Schechter, J. U. McGuire, R. M. Waters, and E. S. Fields. 1975. Further studies of aircraft disinsection and odor characteristics of aerosols containing resmethrin and d-transresmethrin. *Botyu-Kaguku* 40(1):5–13.

Sullivan, W. N., B. M. Cawley, M. S. Schechter, D. K. Hayes, K. Staker, and R. Pal. 1978. A comparison of freon- and water-based insecticidal aerosols for aircraft disinsection. *Bull. W.H.O.* 56(1):129–32.

Sullivan, W. N., B. M. Cawley, M. S. Schechter, N. O. Morgan, and R. Pal. 1979. Aircraft disinsecting: the effectiveness of freon-based and water-based phenothrin and permethrin aerosols. *Bull. W.H.O.* 57(4):619–23.

Tew, R. P., W. A. L. David, and J. R. Busvine. 1951. *Monthly Bull. Min. Hlth. Lab. Serv.* 10:30.

Welch, E. V. 1939. Insects found in aircraft at Miami, Florida, in 1938. *Publ. Hlth. Rep.* (US) 54:561–66.

Whitfield, F. G. S. 1939. Air transport, insects and disease. *Bull. ent. Res.* 30:365–442.

Whittingham, H., and R. A. E. Galley. 1949. The disinsectisation of aircraft: recent progress of work in the United Kingdom and colonies. *Month. Bull. Min. Hlth. Pub. Hlth. Lab. Ser.* (UK) 8:186–87.

WHO. 1951. WHO Expert Committee on Insecticides. *WHO Tech. Rep. Ser.* 34.

————. 1957a. International Sanitary Regulations. Geneva: WHO.

————. 1957b. WHO Expert Committee on Insecticides. *WHO Tech. Rep. Ser.* 125.

————. 1961. Aircraft disinsection. *WHO Tech. Rep. Ser.* 206.

————. 1971. Vector quarantine in air transport. *WHO Chronicle* 25:236-39.

————. 1974. International Health Regulations (1969). Second Annotated Ed. Geneva: WHO.

————. 1977. Official Records No. 240. Geneva.

Williams, C. L., and W. C. Dreessen. 1935. The destruction of mosquitoes in airplanes. *Publ. Hlth Rep.* (US) 50:663-71.

Chapter 8

Mosquito Fauna of Guam:
Case History of an Introduced Fauna

R. A. Ward

INTRODUCTION

Guam is the largest and southernmost of the Mariana Islands located in the Pacific Ocean, 5,000 km west of Hawaii. The climate is tropical and annual rainfall is about 1,780 mm. The island is a territory of the United States and the populace is largely dependent upon federal sources for revenue, although a growing tourist trade is developing with Oriental nations.

An analysis of the mosquito fauna of Guam serves to document a dramatic change in a faunal component of an isolated island during a time span of less than 40 years. Although as many as 41 species and subspecies of mosquitoes have been reported from Guam, only 24 have been verified on the basis of museum specimens or larval rearings. Of the 24 species, seven are restricted to the Mariana Islands. The remaining species have largely been introduced since the end of World War II in 1945. Certain of the introductions have been a normal consequence of commerce, while others were associated with military activities.

For this review,* the mosquito fauna of Guam is restricted to the established species. These in turn have been

*Wesley R. Nowell has been most supportive of my interest in the Guam mosquito fauna and has provided many

separated into two components: the endemic group of seven species and an introduced fauna comprising 17 species. This is essentially a conservative approach as Nowell (1980) has listed 41 species with recorded collection dates on Guam. The reasons for the deletion of 17 reported species will be discussed later.

MOSQUITOES ENDEMIC TO GUAM

The seven endemic species,* comprising 29% of the 24 species on Guam, are not yet recorded from locales outside the Mariana archipelago.** Each of them, however, occurs on other islands in the Marianas in addition to Guam. This is not surprising due to the relative proximity of the islands and now-constant flow of air traffic among Guam, Rota, and Saipan (Nowell and Sutton 1977).

Discussions of the relationships of these seven species are primarily based upon comparative studies of the external anatomy of the adult and larval stages and zoogeographical analysis of distribution patterns. This type of analysis should also involve genetic studies and examination

---

useful suggestions towards preparation of this paper. Unpublished collection records from the USAF School of Aerospace Medicine have been provided by Dennis D. Pinkovsky and Jerry T. Lang. Similar records from the Bernice P. Bishop Museum were furnished by Wallace A. Steffan. Adela C. Ramos and Robert J. McKenna offered constructive advice on the status of many of the early species records. Marshall Laird provided the needed stimulus for the completion of this study. Appreciation is expressed to the *South Pacific Bulletin* for its standing permission to republish such material as reproduced herein in Figure 8-1.

Aedes (Stegomyia) guamensis Farner and Bohart; *Aedes (Stegomyia) pandani* Stone; *Aedes (Stegomyia) rotanus* Bohart and Ingram; *Aedes (Stegomyia) saipanensis* Stone; *Aedes (Aedimorphus) oakleyi* Stone; *Culex (Culex) annulirostris marianae* Bohart and Ingram; *Culex (Culex) litoralis* Bohart.

**The alleged introduction of *Culex litoralis* to Singapore Harbor (Colless 1957) was based upon a misidentification of *C. alis* Theobald (Sirivanakarn 1976).

of other life history stages. However, this type of material is not available for all species.

The single endemic species of the subgenus *Aedimorphus, Aedes oakleyi,* is a member of group C (Alboscutellatus Group of Knight and Hurlbut [1949]). Group C contains 10 or 11 species that are restricted to the Australian, Papuan, Oriental, Indomalayan, South Pacific, and Western Pacific areas.

Aedes oakleyi, which occurs on Anatahan Island in the northern Marianas and Saipan and Guam in the southern Marianas, is most closely allied to *A. senyavinensis* Knight and Hurlbut (1949)—known only from Ponape Island in the Carolines. Group C may contain a third Micronesian species, *A. trukensis* Bohart (1957), described from Truk in the eastern Carolines. Since only the female of this species is known, confirmation of its placement requires collection of male individuals for study of the palpi and male genitalia. However, the general appearance of female *A. trukensis* is very similar to the two other Micronesian species of the group.

Three of the four endemic species of the subgenus *Stegomyia* on Guam (*Aedes pandani, A. rotanus* and *A. saipanensis*) are members of the Pandani Group of species. The Pandani Group (Group F of Bohart [1957]) contains only the above three species plus *A. agrihanensis* Bohart and *A. neopandani* Bohart. This group is restricted to Micronesia and is apparently without close relatives. The medial golden yellow scale pattern on the adult scutum and stellate setae on the abdomen of the larva are very characteristic of this group. Bohart (1957) indicates that the Pandani Group may be distantly related to the Scutellaris Group. The latter, containing about 40 species, is extremely widespread throughout the Pacific region, Asia, and the Indonesian islands.

The immature stages of the Pandani Group primarily develop in the leaf axils of various *Pandanus* species, though they are also encountered in taro axils, tree holes, and occasionally coconut shells. Stellate setae have evolved independently in several groups of mosquitoes (*Tripteroides* spp., *Culex* spp., and *Aedes* spp.) and the condition of "hairy" and "nonhairy" larvae may occur within a single species as evidenced by the studies of Rosen and Rozeboom (1954) on *Aedes polynesiensis* Marks. This attribute is usually considered to be environmentally induced and is most commonly encountered in larvae inhabiting tree holes, plant axils, or artificial containers with considerable debris. Colless (1956) postulates that the factors producing hairiness reside in some nonliving particle, commonly found in tree-hole water. In the Pandani Group, this attribute has become genetically fixed and appears to indicate a common origin for the constituent species.

Aedes guamensis, the fourth endemic *Stegomyia* species, is distributed on the southern Marianas including Guam, Rota, Saipan, and Tinian. It is a member of the Scutellaris Subgroup of the previously mentioned Scutellaris Group. Several species closely related to *A. guamensis* occur on other Micronesian islands. These include: *A. dybasi* Bohart–Palau; *A. hakanssoni* Knight and Hurlbut–Ponape; *A. hensilli* Farner–widespread in the Carolines, including several atolls; *A. marshallensis* Stone and Bohart–Marshall Islands and Kiribati; *A. palauensis* Bohart–Palau; and *A. scutoscriptus* Bohart and Ingram–Truk. At least two of these species were reported from Guam during the early 1970s (Reisen et al. 1971), but as later indicated, their presence cannot be substantiated.

The two remaining endemic species are both members of the subgenus *Culex* of the genus *Culex;* both higher taxa are cosmopolitan. These two species, *C. litoralis* and *C. annulirostris marianae,* are both within the Sitiens Subgroup of Belkin (1962) and Sirivanakarn (1976). The subgroup is divided into three complexes: Sitiens, Whitmorei, and Annulirostris. *Culex litoralis,* a species of the Sitiens Complex, is restricted to the northern and southern Marianas. Its immature stages commonly occur during the rainy season in nearly fresh to saline water in coral rock holes and other containers along the coasts. Its closest relatives in the Pacific area appear to be *C. roseni* Belkin from the Society Islands and *C. whittingtoni* Belkin from the Solomons (Belkin 1962). The nominate member of the complex, *C. sitiens* Wied., closely associated with brackish water habitats, is found almost worldwide in the Old World tropics, including many of the Pacific islands. Another species of the complex, *C. alis,* has a wide Asian distribution extending into Indonesia and islands of the PNG area.

Culex annulirostris marianae and *C. a. annulirostris* Skuse are the sole members of the Annulirostris Complex. Subspecies *marianae,* which is restricted to the northern and southern Marianas, was separated from the nominate subspecies by the presence of a narrow line of dull yellowish scales along the apices of abdominal tergites I-IV and sometimes on V and VI. Other characters have not been analyzed in sufficient detail to determine the true status of subspecies *marianae,* which in the future may be elevated to specific status or reduced to synonomy with *annulirostris*. However, some differentiation of the species does occur within Micronesia. As a whole, *C. annulirostris* has a broad distribution in the Pacific and occurs on many islands plus the Australian and Papuan areas. It is of interest that *C. annulirostris marianae* is the only endemic taxon which has been incriminated as a disease vector on Guam; for instance, it was the vector of Japanese B encephalitis virus during the 1947 epidemic.

MOSQUITOES INTRODUCED INTO GUAM

The introduced faunal component may be separated into four elements: a cosmotropical or worldwide group of three species (13%), four species (16%) present only in the Oriental area, one species (4%) only present in Micronesia, and a group of nine species (38%) occurring in the Oriental and one to four other faunal areas.

Cosmotropical Introductions

Aedes (*Stegomyia*) *aegypti* (L.), *A.* (*Aedimorphus*) *vexans* (Meigen), and *Culex* (*Culex*) *quinquefasciatus* Say are in the first group of widely dispersed species. These three species have been known from Guam since the early 1900s, primarily on the basis of reference to reports on medical conditions and economic entomology (Esaki 1939; Fullaway 1912; Leys 1905). The only museum specimen preserved from these early studies was one female *A. vexans* collected by Fullaway in 1911 (Bohart 1957). Other mosquito pest species had undoubtedly been introduced onto Guam many hundreds of years earlier; however, there is no historical record. The earliest reference to mosquitoes bothering humans appears in a paper by Safford (1912), who was assigned to Guam as a U.S. naval officer in 1899. He refers to an incident during 1899 as follows: "Before going to bed the lights were extinguished and a smudge was kindled to drive out the mosquitoes." During World War II, *A. aegypti* was responsible for widespread outbreaks of dengue. Extensive control campaigns eradicated this species from the island and the last larval collection was made during 1948 (Yamaguti and LaCasse 1950). In the interim, there have been a few intercepts of single adults, but no indication of new breeding populations.

Oriental Introductions

The four species footnoted* represent various introductions from the Oriental area during the period 1948–75. Due to the large numbers of specimens recovered, including adults and larvae from various locations, it is clear that these species are now established on Guam.

Anopheles indefinitus was first collected during March 1948 at four locations near the coast from a wide range of freshwater habitats, including lowland marshes, buffalo wallows, various ground pools, and brackish waterside pools in coastal tidewaters (Reeves and Rudnick 1951; Yamaguti and LaCasse 1950). From this dispersal pattern, it evidently had been introduced several years earlier, either through Japanese or U.S. troop movements. This species extends from Malaya and Java to Taiwan and the Philippines. There is no evidence that it is a vector of human disease in this area.

Culex fuscocephalus, a widespread Asian species, was recorded during a 1969 Public Health survey (Hayes and Whitworth 1969). Its presence in light trap surveys at Andersen Air Force Base (AFB) from 1971–79 indicates that it is well established. It is a common pest of domestic animals in rural communities of Southeast Asia and has been found to be naturally infected with two strains of Japanese encephalitis virus in Thailand (Gould et al. 1974).

In May 1975, mosquito collections were made by U.S. Army personnel during surveillance activities at the onset of "Operation New Life"—the program for use of Guam as a staging area for Vietnamese refugees prior to their entry to the United States. This survey produced two female specimens referable to the *Anopheles barbirostris* group (Ward et al. 1976). Specific identification could not be made at that time due to the absence of associated males and immature stages. Later that year, U.S. Navy Environmental Health Service entomologists disclosed larvae of another unrecorded species, *Anopheles litoralis,* from artificial containers at Orote Point and the Navy Beach. Identification of *A. litoralis* was confirmed through study of reared specimens. During 1976 further collections were made on the naval station grounds and larvae were collected, subse-

---

Anopheles (Anopheles) barbirostris Van der Wulp; *Anopheles (Cellia) indefinitus* (Ludlow); *Anopheles (Cellia) litoralis* King; *Culex (Culex) fuscocephalus* Theobald.

quently reared to adults and identified as *A. barbirostris* (Ward and Jordan 1979).

These two anophelines assume greater importance as potential vectors as compared with *A. indefinitus*. *A. litoralis* is also known from the Philippines and possibly Sabah. It has been incriminated as a malaria vector on Pangutaran Island, Sula Archipelago, Philippine Islands, and may be a vector on other Philippine islands where malaria is present, but *A. (Cellia) flavirostris* (Ludlow) is absent. The Asian distribution of *A. barbirostris* is considerably broader; from Pakistan in the west to Hainan Island, China, in the east and south through Indochina through portions of Indonesia. It does not appear to be a vector of malaria and filariasis except perhaps in Sulawesi (Reid 1968). Based upon the above distribution patterns, it appears likely that *A. litoralis* was introduced from the Philippines and *A. barbirostris* probably from Vietnam sometime prior to 1976, probably by aircraft.

Micronesian Introduction

Aedes neopandani, a member of the Pandani Group of the subgenus *Stegomyia,* represents an interisland introduction of an endemic Marianas species. Originally described from Saipan and Tinian (Bohart 1957), it has subsequently been found on Guam and Rota Islands by U.S. Air Force surveys during 1976 (Nowell 1980). Its continued presence in light trap collections at Andersen AFB from 1977 to 1979 indicates that *A. neopandani* is now established (United States Air Force [USAF] unpublished collection records).

Other Introductions

The remaining nine species comprise introductions from either the Oriental area or one or more additional areas.* Since some of these species also occur on other Pacific islands, the possibility of interisland transfer through human agency or air currents is highly possible. These

---

Anopheles (Cellia) vagus Dọnitz; *Anopheles (Cellia) subpictus* Grassi; *Mansonia (Mansonioides) uniformis* (Theobald); *Aedeomyia catasticta* Knab; *Aedes (Stegomyia) albopictus* (Skuse); *Armigeres (Armigeres) subalbatus* (Coq.); *Culex (Lutzia) fuscanus* Wied.; *Culex (Culex) sitiens* Wied.; *Culex (Culex) tritaeniorhynchus* Giles.

species will be treated in chronological sequence relating to date of discovery on Guam.

Aedes albopictus is one of the two most important vectors on Guam due to its role in the transmission of dengue and DHF. This species occurs in the Old World tropics, with the exclusion of the Afrotropical region, and is abundant on many Pacific islands. It was unknown on Guam until A. B. Weathersby found several larvae at Ylig Bay and Yona during 1944-45 (Hull 1952). Since then it has filled all the artificial niches previously occupied by *A. aegypti,* and now is also found in *Pandanus* axils and tree holes. The most recent epidemics of dengue on Guam have been attributed to *A. albopictus* (Haddock et al. 1979). *Aedes albopictus* was extremely abundant on Tinian and Saipan during the occupation of these islands by American forces during the fall of 1944, and it may have been carried to Guam shortly thereafter.

Culex sitiens was initially recorded by Bohart and Ingram (1946), although 1945-collected specimens are mentioned by Bohart in 1957. It has an extremely wide distribution through the South Pacific islands, Oriental, Papuan, Australian, Afrotropical, and some Palearctic areas; and it is never found far from the coast, where it inhabits brackish water pools, coral holes, and artificial containers. Larval surveys made during the early 1970s indicated that *C. sitiens* was widespread on Guam (Reisen et al. 1972). It is of no medical importance, although it may become a pest on some islands.

Aedeomyia catasticta was first found on Guam in 1958 and has subsequently been found in larval and adult surveys. The species is widely distributed from India and the Philippines to Fiji and northern Australia. Larvae are usually associated with thick, weedy vegetation, and adults are primarily bird feeders. In recent years, this species has been encountered occasionally in light trap surveys on Andersen AFB.

Culex tritaeniorhynchus was considered abundant during a May 1962 survey by Joyce (1963a). He indicates that it was there earlier, but probably unrecognized and possibly misidentified with *C. annulirostris marianae.* This is difficult to understand as *C. tritaeniorhynchus* was not found during either the 1948 survey covering 88 larval collections (Yamaguti and LaCasse 1950) or the 1951 survey of 194 larval collections (Hull 1952). Furthermore, Yamaguti and LaCasse were both very familiar with the Japanese fauna and there would be no reason for them not to correctly identify *C. tritaeniorhynchus* from Guam. This species is widely distributed in the Oriental, Afrotropical, and Asian areas of the Palearctic. It is the most important vector of Japanese B encephalitis virus in the Oriental Region.

Mansonia uniformis was initially recorded by Joyce (1963b) during a light-trap survey in May 1962. Its presence on Guam would have been considered dubious until it was again encountered in biting collections by U.S. Navy personnel during April 1964 (Holway 1964). This species occurs in the Old World tropics extending down to Australia and the Bismarck Islands. The larvae are intimately associated with aquatic plants, especially Water Lettuce (*Pistia stratiotes*), and it is reasonable that the mosquito was transferred to Guam on the roots of an aquatic plant.

Armigeres subalbatus was collected by Hayes and Whitworth (1969) both as adults and larvae. It is widely distributed throughout the Oriental Region, including the Philippines and the Ryukyus, and also the Asian Palearctic. To date it is not known from other islands in the Pacific.

Culex fuscanus was first encountered on Guam in 1968 (Bishop Museum Collection Records) and subsequently has appeared in most surveys. Larvae are particularly abundant in a variety of natural and artificial fresh water habitats, including sluggish streams. The larvae are predaceous upon other mosquito larvae and may effect some degree of natural control. This species is widely distributed in the Oriental region, Asian Palearctic, and several Pacific island groups, including the Carolines and Palau. There are recent records of its occurrence on Saipan and Rota (Nowell 1980).

Immature mosquito collections of Darsie and Reisen made in 1970 and 1971 disclosed two hitherto unreported anophelines (Darsie and Ramos 1971). The first, *Anopheles vagus,* was present in extremely large numbers and formed 92% of the anophelines collected from pools in Apra Heights. The second species from the same habitat, *A. subpictus,* represented 4% of the specimens. There was a third species, *A. indefinitus,* previously known from Guam in the same collection. This accounted for the remaining 4% of the specimens. *Anopheles vagus* is found from India through China and extends to Indonesia east to the Moluccas and northward into Borneo and the Philippines. It is not considered a vector of human disease. The distribution of *A. subpictus* is from the Middle East to India. From Malaysia eastwards it appears to be a coastal species and is present in Java, Sulawesi, New Guinea, and the Philippines (Reid 1968). Of all the introduced anophelines on Guam, *A. subpictus* poses the greatest potential as a malaria vector. It is a vector of some importance in Sulawesi and other parts of Indonesia and Timor. In parts of southern

India, it (or a closely related taxon) is apparently a secondary vector of malaria.

PREVIOUSLY PRESUMED MOSQUITO INTRODUCTIONS, NOW DELETED (also see Appendix)

The following 17 species or subspecies have been reported from Guam at various times:

Anopheles (*Anopheles*) *baezai* Gater
Anopheles (*Anopheles*) *lesteri* Baisas and Hu
Anopheles (*Anopheles*) *sinensis* Wiedemann
Anopheles (*Cellia*) *tesselatus* Theobald

Toxorhynchites (*Toxorhynchites*) *amboinensis* (Doleschall)
Toxorhynchites (*Toxorhynchites*) *brevipalpis* Theobald

Aedes (*Stegomyia*) *burnsi* Basio and Reisen
Aedes (*Stegomyia*) *dybasi* Bohart
Aedes (*Stegomyia*) *hensilli* Farner
Aedes (*Stegomyia*) *marshallensis* Stone and Bohart
Aedes (*Stegomyia*) *scutellaris* (Walker)
Aedes (*Aedimorphus*) *vexans nipponi* (Theobald)

Culex (*Culiciomyia*) *papuensis* Taylor
Culex (*Culex*) *hutchinsoni* Barraud
Culex (*Culex*) *pseudovishnui* Colless
Culex (*Culex*) *sinensis* Theobald
Culex (*Culex*) *vagans* Wiedemann

These have been deleted as faunal elements due to the following factors: (1) the original reports were based upon one or two specimens that were not saved for verification by a museum specialist; (2) the life history stage reported was inadequate for accurate species identification; (3) although the original material was preserved, its condition was too poor for taxonomic study (typical of much light-trap-collected material of *Aedes* and *Culex* spp.); and (4) the species had been introduced for biological control, but had not been subsequently recovered (for example, this is the situation for the two species of *Toxorhynchites* that were introduced in 1954).

Due to the thoroughness of the collecting of the late Henry Dybas, we have an excellent knowledge of the species actually on Guam in the year 1945. Dr. Dybas made extensive mosquito surveys in the Pacific during World War II, and at the end of the war, he returned to Micronesia to make insect collections for the Pacific Science Board during 1945. This material formed the basis for the *Insects of Micronesia* series sponsored by the Bernice P. Bishop Museum.

On the basis of the wartime records of *Aedes aegypti* and *Culex quinquefasciatus* and the Dybas collections, we know the fauna consisted of 10 species in 1945: *Aedes pandani, A. guamensis, A. aegypti, A. albopictus, A. vexans, A. oakleyi, Culex litoralis, C. sitiens, C. annulirostris marianae,* and *C. quinquefasciatus.*

After reviewing the dates when the other mosquito species were first reported from Guam (it should be remembered that a species may be undetected for many years either due to a lack of collecting effort or very low incidence in restricted habitats), it is concluded that the greatest increase in the number of newly established species has occurred within the past two decades as follows:

1940-49 (2 species)
Anopheles indefinitus
Aedes albopictus

1950-59 (1 species)
Aedeomyia catasticta

1960-69 (5 species)
Mansonia uniformis
Armigeres subalbatus
Culex fuscanus
Culex fuscocephala
Culex tritaeniorhynchus

1970-79 (7 species)
Anopheles barbirostris
Anopheles litoralis
Anopheles subpictus
Anopheles vagus
Aedes neopandani
Aedes rotanus
Aedes saipanensis

During the last 40 years, there has been a great increase in the amount of international air traffic between Guam and other areas, particularly in the Pacific. Typical of this is the route of Air Nauru, which can provide ready access to many hitherto remote areas. A 1979 Air Nauru advertisement in *South Pacific Bulletin,* vol. 29, no. 2, page 23 (Figure 8.1), emphasizes this point in demonstrating the airline's so-far unique Asian/Micronesian/Melanesian/Polynesian links. Thus it is not unexpected that introduced species can become established on an island situation with a multitude of aquatic habitats and a favorable climate.

Figure 8-1. Air Nauru advertisement from *South Pacific Bulletin,* 1979.

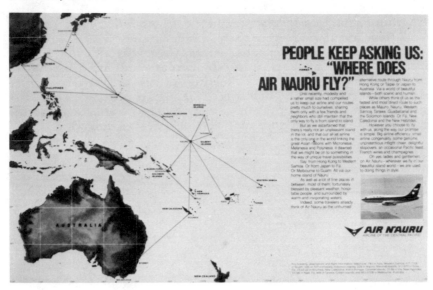

As a consequence of these introductions, there have been small and large epidemics of dengue fever on Guam. Between 1933 and 1937, 17 cases of dengue were reported on the island by the Guam Department of Health. These cases undoubtedly were transmitted by *Aedes aegypti,* which likewise was responsible for the large dengue outbreak in 1944. With the eradication of *A. aegypti* by 1945, any further dengue epidemics were apparently transmitted by *A. albopictus,* which filled the old *aegypti* habitats. Although strong potential was present during the period of "Operation New Life" for the transmission of dengue viruses and various malarial parasites from Vietnamese nationals to the citizens of Guam, no disease transmission occurred. (Six cases of dengue fever, including one death, and 55 cases of malaria were identified among the evacuees.) Due to intensive vector control measures that were applied on the island at this time, transmission was blocked and the island remained clear of these diseases (Haddock et al. 1979).

It is interesting that the only recorded epidemic of Japanese B encephalitis virus (JE) occurred prior to the introduction of its main vector, *Culex tritaeniorhynchus*. The 1947-48 outbreak was associated with *C. annulirostris marianae* on epidemiological grounds (Reeves and Rudnick 1951). This disease had apparently recently invaded the island through an infected person, who then served as a reservoir of infection. Hammon et al. (1958) indicated that JE virus was probably present on Guam for a few years before the outbreak occurred. They concluded that after the widespread epidemic, the virus then disappeared, apparently due to the absence of some factor necessary to maintain it at an endemic level.

The history of malaria on Guam has been documented by W. R. Nowell (unpublished manuscript 1980). In 1947 and 1948, there were reports of relapsing infections in military and civilian patients who had been infected in other countries; however, there was no indication of new transmission. Malaria was again reported during 1966 while the U.S. military used Guam as a treatment center for malaria cases from Southeast Asia. Although malaria patients were housed in screened quarters, five cases of *P. falciparum* malaria were reported, apparently contracted on Guam during the fall of 1966. Three of these cases occurred among civilians living in Dededo village at the time two wounded Guamanian U.S. Army veterans had malarial relapses while they were home on medical leave. At this time the only anopheline present on the island was *Anopheles indefinitus*. After a lapse of three years, one further *P. falciparum* malaria infection appeared in another local resident in Dededo village. Like the previous cases, this individual could have become infected by the bite of an anopheline that had fed upon a malaria patient at Andersen AFB or through transport of an infected anopheline from an airplane.

CONCLUSIONS

This review demonstrates that a critical faunal analysis is still dependent upon a strong taxonomic base, especially in situations concerning insects of medical and economic importance. Unfortunately, after routine identifications have been made on these insects, specimens are often discarded and verification of distributions cannot be confirmed. For Guam, such an analysis could not be made until each species had been critically reviewed. After this process, a species list of 41 was reduced to 24 species.

With the exclusion of seven species restricted to Guam and other islands of the Marianas, all species with the exception of the almost cosmopolitan *Aedes aegypti, A. vexans,* and *Culex quinquefasciatus* have been found on Guam since the end of World War II. Some species such as *Aedes albopictus* and *Anopheles indefinitus* represent wartime introductions from the Pacific islands or the Oriental Region. The remaining 14 species were introduced with increasing frequency in the three decades beginning with 1950. These species were introduced from the Philippines and various Southeast Asian countries through increased civilian and military air traffic. The latter increased dramatically during the period of U.S. military activity in Southeast Asia.

The absence of New World mosquito species on Guam, excluding the cosmotropical species, is probably indicative of the greater use and success of aircraft disinsection procedures for airplanes in transit at the Honolulu, Hawaii, airport. The efficiency of disinsection and quarantine measures is documented by the known mosquito fauna of the Hawaiian Islands. This fauna contains six species, only one of which—*Aedes vexans*—may have been introduced by aircraft during the early 1960s. It is evident that some Asian nations do not have such rigid quarantine procedures as the state of Hawaii, and the probability of an airplane from Asia carrying live mosquitoes to Guam would be much higher than one from the United States.

During the postwar era, the epidemics and outbreaks of mosquito-borne diseases were quickly brought under control, largely through concerted vector control programs. A retrospective review of these diseases and their vectors (dengue—*Aedes albopictus;* JE—*Culex annulirostris marianae, P. falciparum;* malaria—*Anopheles indefinitus*), indicates that in each of these episodes, an abnormal vector-pathogen relationship was involved, primarily due to the absence of primary vectors on the island. These examples may serve to indicate future patterns of vector-borne diseases in many areas of the world where an active pathogen-host involvement producing human disease can occur with hitherto unsuspected vectors.

APPENDIX

The following species or subspecies have been reported from Guam. For the reasons indicated below, they should not be considered as established or introduced faunal elements.

1. *Anopheles baezai.* Six larvae were collected from two carabao wallows, 7-15 February 1971 (Reisen et al. 1972). Alan Stone (in litt., 1971) stated: "I think you are correct in determining . . . *Anopheles baezai* Gater although the distal fraying of the inner clypeal hairs is less than usually found in that species." These specimens were not placed in a collection nor has *A. baezai* subsequently been collected on Guam. The usual distribution includes many nations of Southeast Asia, including the Philippines.

2. *Anopheles lesteri.* Four larvae were collected from a buffalo wallow on 10 February 1971 (Reisen et al. 1971). The single specimen examined by Stone was in poor condition and he recommended that further material be collected for verification. Further collections assignable to *A. lesteri* have not been made. The nominate subspecies, *A. lesteri lesteri,* occurs in the Philippines and southern China while *A. lesteri paraliae* Sandosham is known from Thailand, Peninsular Malaysia, Singapore, and southern Vietnam.

3. *Anopheles sinensis.* One damaged adult from Andersen AFB and two larvae from a carabao wallow were identified by Reisen et al. (1971). Like the two former mentioned anophelines, these are the only specimens reported. Species of the Hyrcanus Group, which include *A. sinensis, A. lesteri,* and at least 11 other Oriental species, are often difficult to determine unless accompanied by the associated immature larval and pupal skins.

4. *Anopheles tesselatus.* One collection of 12 larvae was made from a carabao wallow in 9 February 1971 (Reisen et al. 1972). This identification was verified by Alan Stone (in litt., 1971) who cautioned: ". . . we, including Botha deMeillon, both feel that it is dangerous to record new records for the island of Guam . . . based upon larvae alone." *Anopheles tesselatus* occurs throughout the Oriental Region and is also reported from the Moluccas and New Guinea.

5. *Aedes vexans nipponi.* One larva was found in a carabao wallow during February 1971 (Reisen et al. 1972). Additional material has not been collected. This subspecies occurs in China, Japan, South Korea, the Ryukyus, and the Baikal area of the USSR.

6. *Aedes burnsi* is known only from the type-series of six males (and associated skins) reared from a larval collection in *Pandanus* leaf axils at Andersen AFB on 9 February 1971 (Basio and Reisen 1971). According to the description, it is a member of Bohart's Group C

(Maehleri Group) of *Stegomyia*. Previously, this contained only *A. (Stegomyia) maehleri* Bohart from Yap Island. Unfortunately, the status of *A. burnsi* is in doubt as the authors did not compare their material with *A. maehleri*, none of the material was saved for subsequent research, their description was inadequate, and no material of the Maehleri Group has subsequently been found on Guam.

7. *Aedes scutellaris.* Fifteen specimens (sexes unknown) were collected on Andersen AFB during 1970 (Reisen et al. 1971). This is a highly variable species and can only be determined upon examination of the male genitalia. *Aedes scutellaris* is apparently restricted to the Papuan area and is quite similar to *A. hensilli.* The material of Reisen et al. (1971) may have been this latter species.

The next eight species are known from only one or two adults collected at Andersen AFB during 1970-71 (Reisen et al. 1972). As they did not appear in subsequent surveys at the air base, they may be considered as misidentified species, unsuccessful introductions, or introductions that were present in such low numbers that they failed to appear in the samples collected.

8. *Aedes dybasi* was described from *Nepenthes* sp. pitcher plants on the Palau Islands and has not been subsequently collected.

9. *Aedes hensilli* has a wide distribution throughout the Caroline Islands and, due to its peridomestic habitats, could be introduced onto Guam. Huang (1972) indicates *A. hensilli* can best be identified by the male genitalia, a point not noted by Reisen et al. (1972).

10. *Aedes marshallensis* occurs in the Caroline, Marshall, and Kiribati groups. Belkin (1962) believes this species originated on an eastern Caroline island, such as Kusai, and has been spread to other coral atolls by the Micronesians.

11. *Culex hutchinsoni* is a rural, inland species of the Oriental Region occurring in India, Pakistan, and the mainland of Southeast Asia. Sirivanakarn (1976) does not consider the Philippine record of Basio (1972) as valid. *Culex hutchinsoni* is very similar to *C. quinquefasciatus* in general adult habitus and the Guam report is apparently another misidentification by Basio.

12. *Culex pseudovishnui* is difficult to separate from

C. vishnui Theobald and *C. tritaeniorhynchus,* so this may be another incorrect record.

13. *Culex sinensis.* Although uncommon, this is one of the most widespread of the Oriental species with the range extending north and northeast into the Palearctic Region. Several specimens have been found on Luzon, Philippine Islands (Sirivanakarn 1976).

14. *Culex vagans* occurs in the Oriental and Palearctic Regions from Siberia south to Hong Kong and west to India and Pakistan. It appears to be restricted to higher elevations on hills or mountainous areas. There are no records of this species from the Philippines or other Pacific islands.

15. *Culex papuensis.* Species of the subgenus *Culiciomyia* are readily distinguished from the subgenus *Culex.* However, with only one record, it is not possible to establish the presence of this species on Guam. *Culex papuensis* is found in the Papuan and Oriental regions and also on several of the Solomon Islands.

16 and 17. *Toxorhynchites amboinensis* and *T. brevipalpis.* Larvae of these two predaceous mosquitoes were sent to Guam by Hu (1955) during February 1954, where laboratory colonies were established by G. D. Peterson. Adults were released in densely vegetated areas of Guam where *Aedes pandani* and *A. albopictus* occurred. This project was unsuccessful as these species were not encountered by future surveys.

REFERENCES

Basio, R. G. 1972. On Philippine Mosquitoes, IX. Notes and descriptions of *Culex (Culex) hutchinsoni* Barraud (Diptera, Culicidae). *Philippine Entomol.* 2:205-8.

Basio, R. G., and W. K. Reisen. 1971. On some mosquitoes of Guam, Marianas Islands (Diptera: Culicidae). *Philippine Entomol.* 2:57-61.

Belkin, J. N. 1962. *The Mosquitoes of the South Pacific (Diptera: Culicidae).* 2 vols. Berkeley and Los Angeles: University of California.

Bohart, R. M. 1957. Diptera: Culicidae. *Insects of Micronesia* 12(1):1-85.

Bohart, R. M., and R. L. Ingram. 1946. *Mosquitoes of Okinawa and islands in the Central Pacific.* NAVMED 1055. Washington: Bureau of Medicine and Surgery, Navy Department.

Colless, D. H. 1956. Environmental factors affecting hairiness in mosquitoe larvae. *Nature* 177:229-30.

—————. 1957. Records of two Pacific island species of mosquito from Singapore harbour. *Med. J. Malaya* 12:464-67.

Darsie, R. F., Jr., and A. Cagampang-Ramos. 1971. Additional species of *Anopheles* on Guam. *Mosquito Systematics Newsletter* 3:28-30.

Esaki, T. 1939. Injurious Arthropoda to man in mandated South Sea islands of Japan (First Report). In *Osaka Hakubutsu Gakkai, Volumen Tubilare pro Professore Sadao Yoshida,* pp. 230-52. Osaka: Osaka Imperial University.

Fullaway, D. T. 1912. Entomological notes. *Ann. Rpt Guam Agr. Expt Sta.* 1911:26-35.

Gould, D. J., R. Edelman, R. A. Grossman, A. Nisalak, and M. F. Sullivan. 1974. Studies of Japanese encephalitis virus in Chiangmai Valley, Thailand. IV. Vector studies. *Amer. J. Epidemiol.* 100:49-56.

Haddock, R. L., R. A. Mackie, and K. Cruz. 1979. Dengue control in Guam. *South Pacific Bull.* 29(2):16-21.

Hammon, W. McD., W. D. Tigertt, and G. E. Sather. 1958. Epidemiological studies of concurrent "virgin" epidemics of Japanese B encephalitis and of mumps on Guam 1947-1948, with subsequent observations including dengue, through 1957. *Amer. J. trop. Med. Hyg.* 7:441-67.

Hayes, G. R., Jr., and B. T. Whitworth. 1969. Survey of vector problems, Guam, U.S.A. Atlanta: Publ. Hlth Serv., US Dept Hlth Educ. Welfare. Mimeographed.

Holway, R. T. 1964. Disease vector and pest control technology; report of training and assistance. USN Preventive Medicine Unit No. 6. Mimeographed.

Hu, S. M. K. 1955. Progress report on biological control of *Aedes albopictus* Skuse in Hawaii. *Proc. Pprs. 23rd Ann. Conf. Calif. Mosq. Contr. Assn.* p. 23.

Huang, Y-M. 1972. Contributions to the mosquito fauna of southeast Asia. XIV. The Subgenus *Stegomyia* of *Aedes* in Southeast Asia. I–The Scutellaris group of species. *Contr. Amer. Ent. Inst.* 9(1):1-109.

Hull, W. B. 1952. Mosquito survey of Guam. *U.S. Armed Forces med. J.* 3:1287-1295.

Joyce, C. R. 1963a. June 13, 1962 notes and exhibitions. *Culex tritaeniorhynchus* Giles on Guam. *Proc. Hawaii. ent. Soc.* 18:207-8.

—————. 1963b. July 9, 1962 notes and exhibitions.

Mansonia (*Mansonioides*) *uniformis* (Theobald). *Proc. Hawaii. Ent. Soc.* 18:210.

Knight, K. L., and H. S. Hurlbut. 1949. The mosquitoes of Ponape Island, eastern Carolines. *J. Wash. Acad. Sci.* 39:20-34.

Leys, J. F. 1905. Report on the United States Naval Station, island of Guam, (1904). *Rpt of the Surgeon General, USN* pp. 91-96.

Nowell, W. R. 1980. Comparative mosquito collection data from the southern Mariana Islands (Diptera: Culicidae). *Proc. Pprs. Ann. Conf. Calif. Mosq. Vector Contr. Assn.* 48:112-16.

Nowell, W. R., and D. R. Sutton. 1977. The mosquito fauna of Rota Island, Mariana Islands (Diptera: Culicidae). *J. med. Ent.* 14:411-16.

Reeves, W. C., and A. Rudnick. 1951. A survey of the mosquitoes of Guam in two periods in 1948 and 1949 and its epidemiological implications. *Amer. J. trop. Med.* 31:633-58.

Reid, J. A. 1968. *Anopheline Mosquitoes of Malaya and Borneo.* Kuala Lumpur: Studies from the Institute for Medical Research No. 31.

Reisen, W. K., J. P. Burns, and R. G. Basio. 1971. A mosquito survey of Guam, Marianas Islands. 1st Medical Service Wing (PACAF), APO San Francisco. Mimeographed.

————. 1972. A mosquito survey of Guam, Marianas Islands with notes on the vector borne disease potential. *J. med. Ent.* 9:319-24.

Rosen, L., and L. E. Rozeboom. 1954. Morphological variations of larvae of the Scutellaris group of *Aedes* (Diptera, Culicidae) in Polynesia. *Amer. J. trop. Med. Hyg.* 3:529-38.

Safford, W. E. 1912. Guam. An account of its discovery and reduction, physical geography and natural history, and the social and economic conditions on the island during the first year of the American occupation. Washington, D. C.: reprint of a lecture, District of Columbia Society Sons of the American Revolution. April 19, 1911. 32 pp.

Sirivanakarn, S. 1976. Medical entomology studies–III. A revision of the subgenus *Culex* in the Oriental Region (Diptera: Culicidae). *Contr. Amer. Ent. Inst.* 12(2):1-272.

Ward, R. A., and B. Jordan. 1979. *Anopheles barbirostris*– confirmation of introduction on island of Guam. *Mosquito News* 39:802-3.

Ward, R. A., B. Jordan, A. R. Gillogly, and F. J. Harrison. 1976. *Anopheles litoralis* King and *A. barbirostris* group on the island of Guam. *Mosquito News* 36:99–100.

Yamaguti, S., and W. J. LaCasse. 1950. *Mosquito Fauna of Guam*. Tokyo: Office of the Surgeon, Headquarters US 8th Army.

Chapter 9

Preventive Measures against Importing Malaria Vectors into Pacific Islands

L. S. Self and A. Smith

GROWTH OF INTERNATIONAL TRAVEL

There is a growing concern that vectors of malaria may be introduced and established in nonmalarious areas of the Pacific islands where *Anopheles* spp. are now absent. Factors accounting for the greater risks of anopheline vector importation are the great increase in international travel and the large numbers of insects of medical impor- tance being found on international aircraft in Australia, Japan, Philippines, and New Zealand (Anonymous 1979b; Ogata et al. 1974; Basio et al. 1970; Laird 1951). Random to routine checks of aircraft arriving at international airports in the above countries have revealed the transport of exotic mosquito species, including malaria vectors, from one country to another. Guam, with a heavy influx of international travel by air and sea, has had post-World War II introductions and establishment of several anopheline species *Anopheles barbirostris, A. indefinitus, A. litoralis, A. subpictus,* and *A. vagus* (Reisen et al. 1972; Ward et al. 1976; Chapter 8).

The development of wide-bodied jet planes, capable of carrying large numbers of passengers rapidly and safely to distant destinations at budget prices, revolutionized travel and gave rise to the phenomena of mass tourism. The volume of passengers recorded in some countries of WHO's Western Pacific Region has increased tenfold within the past decade. While the vast improvement in transport has its advantages from the standpoint of tourism, trade, employment, and study, it also represents dangers of public health significance. Locally acquired malaria infections in at least six patients of metropolitan France, who had never been in an endemic area but had lived and worked in the vicinity of aircraft returning from Africa, indicates that transmission of malaria might have taken place at a French international airport, the vectors being anophelines imported via aviation from an endemic zone (Saliou et al. 1978). This example from Europe further supports the need for early and rapid detection of cases, the destruction of vectors responsible for infection, and measures to prevent malaria vectors from being transported from one place to another. The ease of travel has increased the demand for visits to picturesque Pacific islands where the danger of establishing imported malaria vectors is real.

CURRENT PROBLEMS

There are some pressing problems that need to be faced now if further anopheline introductions are to be prevented. The disinsection of aircraft has been one of the major lines of defense against importing anophelines into the Pacific islands. Many countries and areas in the high-risk regions still use this technique. However, the dichlorvos vapor disinsection method earlier anticipated by WHO (1961) never became operational and will never be used as a routine. The "blocks-away" technique (WHO 1961), which requires the spraying of aircraft after the doors are closed and before take off, has seldom been used. Because this procedure normally must be implemented by flight crews in the absence of quarantine officials, it has been abandoned by most countries in favor of spraying on arrival by quarantine staff, in spite of some inconvenience to passengers. In the United States, which has indigenous anopheline species, procedures for disinsecting aircraft were revised in 1979, permitting the passenger areas to be treated after passengers and crew deplane (Anonymous 1979a).

It has also been difficult for some countries and areas to comply with the International Health Regulations (IHR) in respect of Articles 19 and 20 on vector control (WHO 1974; Appendix). The first national priority to reduce risks of importing and establishing malaria vectors should be the maintenance of effective antimosquito measures within and around international airports.

ISLANDS WITH OR WITHOUT ANOPHELINES

Malaria transmission has not been recorded in the South Pacific east of 170°E longitude and south of 20° latitude, namely Buxton's Line (Buxton and Hopkins 1927). This anopheline-free area includes New Zealand and the Polynesian island groups of Samoa, Tonga, Cook, Tokelau, Tuvalu, Niue, and Society. There is also a large area extending over 120° longitude by 80° latitude which is malaria free (Bruce-Chwatt 1969). Anophelines have not been found in the Micronesian islands of Kiribati, Nauru, and the Caroline and Marshall Islands. They are also absent from New Caledonia and Fiji in Melanesia.

Anopheles and malaria occur in Melanesia in the South Pacific in the northwestern islands of Vanuatu, the Solomon Islands, and Papua New Guinea (PNG). Malaria also occurs in the adjacent Molucca group of Indonesia to the west. Geologists consider that there is a continental border, at least a part of which formerly edged an extensive continental mass (Melanesian Continent). Extensive sedimentary rocks (old land masses) occur in New Zealand, New Caledonia, and Fiji. However, the remaining Pacific islands are primarily volcanic or a combination of both volcanic and sedimentary. They are therefore relatively young. Tuvalu, Kiribati, Samoa, and Niue all lie east and north of southern Melanesia, pertaining to the ocean basin beyond the continental border area. In the greater part of the South Pacific, the surface waters of the ocean move in a generally westerly direction.

Lambert (1949) presented convincing evidence that malaria is a recent arrival in Melanesia and that anopheline species gradually filtered across from Indonesia, eventually reaching Australia via PNG. Although Fiji and New Caledonia are still anopheline-free, Buxton and Hopkins (1927) considered that *Anopheles punctulatus* was not a specialist in its breeding places and could easily establish itself in Fiji and Samoa. Laird (1954, 1956) believed that no ecological barrier existed to prevent the eastward extension of *A. farauti* and suggested that suitable environments are available in much of the central and eastern parts of the South Pacific. Belkin (1962), however, considered that the possibility of this eastward extension happening seemed unlikely.

The present distribution of *A. farauti* suggests that this species is not capable of crossing extensive ocean barriers by natural means in sufficient numbers to become established in marginal environments. It is possible that it has been spread as larval populations by Melanesians in canoes over relatively short distances to attain its present distribution, but a successful introduction of this malaria vector by ship or natural means into the central and eastern part of the South Pacific would seem very unlikely.

Peters (1965) has discussed ways in which mosquitoes could be transported into virgin areas of the South Pacific. With the ever-increasing speed and volume of air travel, Bruce-Chwatt (1969) submitted that the danger of anophelines and malaria invading Fiji and the islands of Micronesia and Polynesia is always present. *Culex annulirostris* (a common associate of *A. farauti* in larval habitats) occurs in Fiji and other island groups, hence the possibility of other surface-water breeding mosquitoes such as *Anopheles farauti* arriving aboard aircraft and establishing themselves must be entertained.

RISKS OF ANOPHELINE INTRODUCTIONS

Visits have been made during the past several years to malarious and nonmalarious countries of the Pacific islands to assess the risk of anopheline species being accidentally introduced and established in areas where they are now absent.

It is understandable that preventing the importation of malaria vectors into Indonesia is not considered to be a high priority inasmuch as the country has numerous malaria vectors already present. The three principal international airports are Djakarta in Java, Denpasar in Bali, and Medan in Sumatra. Those flights that depart at night pose a risk for transporting anophelines to other countries. Big jets with wide doorways can act as giant light traps to attract local insect populations. The "blocks-away" aircraft disinsection method is considered to be impractical because flight crews might not carry out the spraying conscientiously. If an emergency arose, aircraft would be disinsected on arrival by airport quarantine staff. More attention is now being given to vector control in international transport in Indonesia.

Aircraft disinsection is currently not carried out in Singapore. A unit responsible for vector control is assigned to the international airport to maintain the airport premises in a sanitary condition. Neither is routine aircraft disinsection carried out at the international airport of Kuala Lumpur, Malaysia, although good vector control services are maintained, as in Singapore.

Malaria is endemic in PNG, but vector control in international transport is principally motivated by fear of introducing into the country new strains of dengue viruses leading to potential outbreaks of DHF. A good plan of operations exists there for urban vector mosquito control. This includes emergency quarantine measures at international and domestic airports, and seaports too. Significant anopheline breeding has not been observed around the immediate seaport areas of Port Moresby, Kieta, and Arawa Bay. The risk of transporting *Anopheles* spp. through international aircraft entering or leaving PNG would appear to be low, as aircraft disinsection is practiced by the airlines.

The international airport in Honiara, Solomon Islands, is almost surrounded by swamp lands that are breeding places for *Anopheles farauti*. During the wet season (October-March), the many depressions in the land within the airport area become flooded and provide breeding places for mosquitoes, including *Anopheles* spp. The airport does not have facilities for night landing. Nearly all international aircraft leave the airfield before 1630 hours, generally taking less than one hour to turn around and depart. Under present conditions, the risk of anophelines being transported by aircraft from Honiara would seem negligible. Some flights departing from Kieta to Honiara are disinsected by the "blocks-away" method or by in-flight disinsection; otherwise passenger compartments are disinsected on aircraft arrival and before passenger deplaning.

The risk of introducing exotic *Anopheles* spp. into Vanuatu would seem to be low, the nearest source being the Solomon Islands where *A. farauti* has undergone many years of insecticide selection and is now refractory to DDT. The dominant strain there may thus be a different one from that found in Vanuatu. Disinsection of flights arriving in Port Vila from Honiara should continue.

With the *Anopheles*-free islands of Fiji to the east and New Caledonia to the southwest, Vanuatu occupies a crucial position with regard to the possible extension of *A. farauti* beyond its present boundary. This important malaria vector, the sole anopheline of Vanuatu, occurs in all islands except Futuna (Laird 1956). Its absence there may be attributed to a combination of the following factors: geographical isolation (Futuna lies 75 km from the nearest *Anopheles*-infested island [Tanna] and thus beyond the flight range [4 km] of *A. farauti*), infrequent shipping and no aircraft transport, and permeable volcanic soil with few potential breeding sites.

Climatic conditions and ocean currents also may be important factors contributing to the historic failure of *A. farauti* to spread to small oceanic islands to the south and west of Vanuatu. Ocean currents run strongly from east to west, inhibiting small craft as potential carriers of anophelines traveling eastward. Moreover, tradewinds blow strongly from the southeast throughout most of the year. Therefore, any adult mosquitoes being carried long distances by the wind would travel in a northwesterly direction. The generally low night temperatures in Noumea (which in the cool season [May–November] reach 12–13°C) would be expected to inhibit the exit of tropical mosquitoes from any night-landing aircraft.

Fiji's Nadi International Airport occupies a large area and is well-drained, but during the rainy season (October–April) a great deal of standing water accumulates in and around the airport. Temperatures are also high (75–95°F) and provide conditions conducive to mosquito breeding. In addition, there are sugarcane fields, rice fields, ponds, and mangrove swamps within 2 km of the airport area. Night-biting culicines (including C. annulirostris) capable of flying several kilometers are abundant in the airport area during the hot, rainy season. While no anophelines occur in Fiji, the conditions around Nadi airport are judged very suitable for A. farauti breeding. Great emphasis is placed on thorough disinsection of aircraft on arrival since effective mosquito control around Nadi (and Nausori airport near Suva, as well) is difficult due to availability of extensive larval habitats adjacent to the airport areas. Moreover, portions of the passenger lounge of Nadi International Airport are not screened to prevent mosquito bites. Passengers incubating dengue or RRV infections could thus precipitate local epidemics.

The risks of Anopheles spp. entering Australia through international aircraft and establishing themselves there exists. However, they would appear to be low, except with respect to aircraft arriving in Darwin from Denpasar (Bali, Indonesia), aircraft from which have reached Darwin with A. subpictus and A. sundaicus aboard (Chapter 7). Some risks also exist for aircraft departing from Kuala Lumpur, Manila, and Port Moresby. Particular attention is required where arrivals take place in Darwin, Cairns, and Townsville. On the basis of their geographical position in relation to the distribution of Anopheles species within Australia, the international airports of Sydney, Melbourne, Perth, and Hobart present a negligible risk of malaria vectors being accidentally exported by international aircraft departing from Australia. While A. farauti and A. hilli are present in the vicinity of the northern international airports, these "good" malaria vectors are absent from the southern half of Australia.

Flights from Cairns to Port Moresby, and Brisbane to Tokyo, pose some risks. While there is vigorous aircraft disinsection in Australia, regular surveillance and vector control in and around international airports may require strengthening in Darwin, Cairns, Townsville, and possibly Brisbane. The present risk of *Anopheles* spp. being introduced into Nadi from Sydney International Airport is virtually nil.

Although many flights entering Australia depart from the last foreign airport at night, many of them leave from international airports where anophelines do not occur, such as Honolulu, Nadi, Noumea, Auckland, or Christchurch, or from Singapore where vigorous vector control is practiced. Furthermore, nearly all international aircraft arrive in Australia during the day, thereby reducing the risk of any anophelines leaving the aircraft. The risk of *Anopheles* spp. entering Australia and establishing themselves through international aircraft arriving from the above places would appear to be low.

In Fiji and Australia, the routes and flights presenting the most risks of importing *Anopheles* spp. have been identified, and administrative steps have been taken to reduce the risks. In Fiji, flights from countries that are malarious are directed to Nadi International Airport, and flights from those that are nonmalarious into Nausori Airport. As far as practicable, flights departing from malarious countries and arriving in Australia are directed to the cooler, southern airports of Sydney and Melbourne.

There is good provision at Guam International Airport for plant quarantine inspection, but the health services do not have enough trained staff to carry out either mosquito control and surveillance either there or in the seaport areas, or inspection and disinsection of arriving aircraft. While it is not believed that malaria transmission takes place in Guam, two recent malaria cases might have been of indigenous origin. There is a present-day risk of malaria vectors being transferred (in both directions) between Guam International Airport and Manila International Airport, Philippines. Although Manila's runway is relatively close to rice fields, incoming and departing flights are not disinsected. Moreover, it is likely that flights from southern Vietnam constituted a risk for transporting malaria and other vectors into Guam via U.S. military aircraft during the 1960s and 1970s (Chapter 8).

By comparison with aircraft, cargo and passenger ships (being so much slower than aircraft) appear to present little risk of transporting *Anopheles* spp. into anopheline-free areas. Moreover, ports and wharfs are frequently too built up to provide significant larval habitats for anophe-lines. Fishing vessels, yachts, and small boats may, however, play a part in transporting *Anopheles* spp. across the Torres Strait, since many small vessels travel between Australia and PNG without port control.

The present flight timetables indicate that the principal risk to Nauru is the possible introduction of malaria vectors from Guam (Chapter 8). Each month, Nauru's seaport receives about ten cargo vessels to take on phosphate. However, all come from distant countries such as Australia, New Zealand, Japan, and Singapore.

From the above, it may be concluded that suitable aquatic environments for *Anopheles* spp. exist in the anopheline-free areas of the Pacific islands. It would thus be prudent to assume that any *Anopheles* spp. introduced would breed and become established. Nevertheless, the present-day risk of anophelines being introduced and established in areas from which they are now absent is judged to be low; nearly all international flights from countries infested with these vectors at present arrive and depart during the day.

FUTURE NEEDS TO CONTAIN ANOPHELINE SPREAD

There are plans for the expansion of present airports and the construction of new ones. Some of this construction and upgrading of airport facilities is expected to be com-pleted within the next few years. Thereafter, any sub-stantial increase in nighttime departures, especially from the malarious Melanesian countries, will increase the risks of anopheline importations unless the problem is anticipated by implementation of better mosquito surveillance and con-trol methods in and around international airports. The first step in overcoming this problem is greater recognition by WHO and Member States of the importance of mosquito surveillance in international transport in the nonmalarious, as well as malarious, countries.

Certain airline routes present a greater risk of anophe-lines being transported by international aircraft than others. In Melanesia, all flights from malarious to non-malarious countries require close surveillance and quaran-tine attention. The routes presenting the greatest risks to the countries concerned should be identified by health authorities. Pacific countries should be made aware of the greater risk of anophelines being transported in interna-tional aircraft, through nighttime arrivals and departures, than daytime ones. They should also be discouraged from increasing the number of nighttime arrivals and departures.

A serious constraint in evaluating present mosquito control methods to reduce risks of anopheline introductions is the deficiency of technical data on *Anopheles* spp. breeding in and around international airports. Weekly larval surveys and adult mosquito collections by light traps and other methods should be implemented or strengthened. Surveillance should be extended to the examination of aircraft for the presence and identification of mosquitoes, with particular attention being given to their condition, including whether they are alive or dead, male or female, unfed, fed or gravid. Appointment and training of new staff may be necessary to implement these activities at some airports. More information is needed on detailed descriptions of methods used to recover mosquitoes from aircraft.

In general, the present methods used to minimize the risk of new vector *Anopheles* spp. establishing themselves in and around international airports are largely based on aircraft disinsection, supplemented by varying degrees of source reduction. Space spraying, with ULV cold or thermal fogging for control of mosquito adults, is generally not practiced, or these methods are kept in reserve for emergency vector control situations. Greater country compliance with the IHR in respect of Article 20 on airport vector control (WHO 1974; Appendix) is needed. This involves active antimosquito measures extending for a distance of at least 400 m beyond the airport perimeter and the establishment of mosquito-proof passenger terminals.

As far as possible, the antimosquito measures should be of a permanent nature, such as land reclamation and drainage, supported by any insecticidal measures considered necessary. Larvicides may be applied to breeding places and residual insecticides to buildings. Countries considering the construction of new international airports should seek the advice of a sanitary engineer and entomologist experienced in mosquito control before planning reaches an advanced stage. Appropriate sanitary engineering in the design and maintenance of international airports to minimize both vector breeding and vector entry into buildings should be ensured.

A synthetic pyrethroid insecticide, d-phenothrin, has been widely used (at 2% concentration) as an aerosol for aircraft disinsection. It has been found to be effective in tests against mosquitoes confined in cages under the seats of aircraft (Sullivan et al. 1979). Dosages based on those indicated in Annex VI of the IHR (WHO 1974) have proved effective. The holding time of at least five minutes, based on earlier trials with other pyrethroids, is still widely used for "on arrival" disinsection. It would be prudent to continue using a five-minute holding period until there is more evidence that a shorter holding period is sufficient.

The disinsection of aircraft by the "blocks-away" method is recognized technically as the most effective means of aircraft disinsection. However, it has not been used as a routine, partly because the health authority of the country of arrival has not been provided with satisfactory evidence that disinsection has been properly carried out. An objection frequently made to "blocks-away" disinsection and in-flight aerosol disinsection applied shortly before descent is that it is done less effectively by the aircrews than by government and quarantine officials on arrival at the airports. The reasoning is that the government officials have a national commitment whereas the cabin crew are trained to care for their passengers—thus disinsection presents a conflict of interest, leading to only nominal disinsection of the passenger cabin and flight deck. Where the above shortcomings can be corrected, and where quarantine officers at airports of departure and arrival reach the required agreements to avoid spraying the aircraft a second time on arrival, the "blocks-away" technique should be encouraged and implemented. It is important also to consider taking other appropriate measures with respect to aircraft departing from *Anopheles*-infested countries bound for *Anopheles*-free areas. One of these measures could involve spraying the aircraft shortly before passengers board, even though it might be repeated by quarantine staff on arrival.

Development of new methods of aircraft disinsection, which do not disturb passengers, should be encouraged by the governments concerned and by WHO. Disinsection of aircraft on arrival, by quarantine staff, is the most widely-used procedure. It is also probably the best method of aircraft disinsection in use at present. However, there are some technical aspects of "on arrival" disinsection that merit attention. The addition of an inside split curtain in the doorway of the aircraft would reduce the risk of mosquitoes escaping as the door is opened for entry of the quarantine inspectors. With the increased use of an air bridge (or "jet-away") to facilitate passenger arrival and departure, tests should be made in which the air bridge is treated with residual or aerosol formulations to determine whether it might be practical to allow passengers and crew to deplane before the aircraft is disinsected.

Since international flights and shipping within the Pacific involve many countries, the problem of international anopheline transportation requires technical cooperation among the countries concerned. The means of strengthening consultations and cooperation among Member States should be promoted and the action required of them clearly identified. In principle, the overall health structure, and not just the Port Health or Quarantine Services, should be involved. For that matter, from an international standpoint, the prevention of the spread of *Anopheles* spp. also requires the cooperation of agencies dealing with tourism, trade, and transport.

The WHO Regional Office for the Western Pacific has directed its efforts toward strengthening epidemiological services, surveillance, and vector control through the organization of training programs, seminars, and the provision of technical staff. These activities have helped to remind Member States of their responsibilities with regard to the danger of the international spread of disease and anophelines. However, more effort needs to be exerted by all concerned to achieve the implementation of truly effective preventive measures.

APPENDIX*

Article 19

1. Depending upon the volume of its international traffic, each health administration shall designate as sanitary airports a number of the airports in its territory, provided they meet the conditions laid down in paragraph 2 of this Article, and the provisions of Article 14.
2. Every sanitary airport shall have at its disposal:
    (a) an organized medical service with adequate staff, equipment and premises;
    (b) facilities for the transport, isolation, and care of infected persons or suspects;
    (c) facilities for efficient disinsection and disinsecting, for the control of vectors and rodents, and for any other appropriate measure provided for by these Regulations;
    (d) a bacteriological laboratory, or facilities for dispatching suspected material to such a laboratory;

---

*Extracted from Part III—HEALTH ORGANIZATION, International Health Regulations (1969). Second annotated edition, 1974, p. 17. [See editorial footnote, p. 175—Ed.]

(e) facilities within the airport for vaccination against smallpox, and facilities within the airport or available to it for vaccination against cholera and yellow fever.

Article 20

1. Every port and the area within the perimeter of every airport shall be kept free from *Aedes aegypti* in its immature and adult stages and the mosquito vectors of malaria and other diseases of epidemiological significance in international traffic. For this purpose active anti-mosquito measures shall be maintained within a protective area extending for a distance of at least 400 metres around the perimeter.
2. Within a direct transit area provided at any airport situated in or adjacent to an area where the vectors referred to in paragraph 1 of this Article exist, any building used as accommodation for persons or animals shall be kept mosquito-proof.
3. For the purposes of this Article, the perimeter of an airport means a line enclosing the area containing the airport buildings and any land or water used or intended to be used for the parking of aircraft.
4. Each health administration shall furnish data to the Organization once a year on the extent to which its ports and airports are kept free from vectors of epidemiological significance in international traffic.

REFERENCES

Anonymous. 1979a. *United States of America Federal Register*. Foreign Quarantine, Disinsection of Aircraft 44: No. 199.
——————. 1979b. Arthropod-borne vectors of human disease discovered on aircraft. *Communicable Dis. Intell.* Commonwealth Dept Hlth, Australia. Bull. 79/20.
Basio, R. G., M. J. Prudencio, and I. E. Chanco. 1970. Notes on the aerial transportation of mosquitoes and other insects at the Manila International Airport. *The Philippine Entomologist* 1:407-8.
Belkin, J. N. 1962. *The Mosquitoes of the South Pacific (Diptera: Culicidae)*. 2 vols. Berkeley and Los Angeles: University of California.
Bruce-Chwatt, L. J. 1969. Global review of malaria control and eradication by attack on the vector. *Misc.*

Pub. ent. Soc. Amer. 7:7-27.

Buxton, P. A., and G. H. E. Hopkins. 1927. Researches in Polynesia and Melanesia. Parts I to IV. London: No. 1 Men. Ser. Lond. Schl. Hyg. Trop. Med.

Laird, M. 1951. Insects collected from aircraft arriving in New Zealand from abroad. *Zool. Publ. Vict. Univ. Coll.,* Wellington, 11:1-30.

————. 1954. A mosquito survey in New Caledonia and the Belep Islands, with new locality records for two species of *Culex. Bull. ent. Res.* 45:285-93.

————. 1956. Studies of mosquitoes and freshwater ecology in the South Pacific. *Roy. Soc. N. Z. Bull.* 6.

Lambert, S. M. 1949. Malaria incidence in Australia and the South Pacific. *Boyd's Malariology,* 1949, *vol. II:* 820-30.

Ogata, K., I. Tanaka, Y. Ito, and S. Morii. 1974. Survey of the medically important insects carried by the international aircraft to Tokyo International Airport. *Jap. J. Sanit. Zool.* 25:177-84.

Peters, W. 1965. Ecological factors limiting the extension of malaria in the southwest Pacific—their bearing on malaria control or eradication programmes. *Acta Tropica* 22:62-68.

Reisen, W. K., J. P. Burns, and R. G. Basio. 1972. A mosquito survey of Guam, Marianas Islands with notes on the vector borne disease potential. *J. med. Ent.* 9:319-24.

Saliou, P., et al. 1978. Deux nouveaux cas de paludisme autochtone dans la région parisienne illustrante deux modes de contamination differents. *Bull. Soc. Path. exot.* 71:342-47.

Sullivan, W. N., B. M. Cawley, M. S. Schechter, N. O. Morgan, and R. Pal. 1979. Aircraft disinsecting: the effectiveness of freon-based and water-based phenothrin and permethrin aerosols. *Bull. Wld Hlth Org.* 57:619-23.

Ward, R. A., B. Jordan, A. R. Gillogly, and F. J. Harrison. 1976. *Anopheles litoralis* King and *A. barbirostris* group on the island of Guam. *Mosquito News* 36:99-100.

WHO. 1961. Aircraft disinsection. Eleventh Report of the Expert Committee on Insecticides. *WHO Tech. Rep. Ser.* 206.

————. 1974. International Health Regulations (1969). Second annotated edition. Geneva: WHO. [The third annotated edition, 1983, renumbers Article 20 to 19 and 19 to 18, but this information was received too late for textual amendment—Ed.]

The Introduction of Vectors and Disease into Australia: An Historical Perspective and Present-day Threat

J. M. Goldsmid

INTRODUCTION

The present volume is concerned primarily with the introduction of *insects* from one area to another. From the medical standpoint, though, this is only the tip of the iceberg as regards the overall problem of the spread of disease from country to country and its importation and introduction into new geographical areas. The aim of this contribution, therefore, is to provide an overview of the whole problem of the international spread of disease—especially as it relates to Australia, a country that offers a unique opportunity for such a study.

PRE-HUMAN AUSTRALIA

Australia has always tended to be rather isolated (Figure 10-1)* and her fauna and flora evolved highly distinctively after the continents drifted apart from the single land mass of Pangea and the southern land mass of Gondwanaland, 150-200 million years ago (Figure 10-2) (Cockburn 1980; Haegi 1981). It is estimated that man colonized Australia and New Guinea about 40,000 years ago, presumably from

---

*I should like to thank my wife, Hilary, for drawing Figures 1-3.

the northern Southeast Asian islands, possibly Melanesia (Bellwood 1979; Murray 1980). Humans then spread slowly southwards until even the extreme south of the continent was settled. The Aborigines of Tasmania were then finally further isolated when they were cut off from the mainland by rising sea levels and the flooding of the Bass Strait approximately 10,000-13,000 years ago (Murray 1980; Cockburn 1980).

Australian wildlife consequently evolved its own diseases, probably sharing some with the related animals below Weber's Line (Figure 10-3), a hypothetical line dividing the Pacific fauna and flora into Asian and Australian segments, especially after the severing of the land-bridge link some 12,000 years or so ago. With the arrival of the first aboriginal settlers, their diseases must have come with them, supplemented by zoonotic diseases already in the local faunal population and perhaps diseases introduced by migrating birds and transmitted by transported arthropods (for example, ixodid ticks) that were not averse to attacking man.

HUMAN DISEASE IN PRE-EUROPEAN
AUSTRALIA

In Australia prior to the arrival of the whites, population densities were low. This, together with the nomadic habits of the Aborigines, in all likelihood precluded the persistence of many of the acute human infectious diseases (for example, measles) that require a large population (probably well in excess of 1.25 million people) for maintenance in any given community (Cockburn 1977). A further factor against the survival of diseases of pollution (for instance, soil-transmitted parasites) in these early days of human occupation was the fact that the small nomadic groups of Aborigines seldom returned within a short time to previously occupied locations (Baldwin 1938).

The Australian Aborigines were thus probably left with only the more chronic infections—about which we have few records—perhaps supplemented from time to time by enzootic zoonotic infections that may have been relatively chronic (for example, zoophilic dermatophyte infections [Basedow 1932d]) or acute (for example, infection with Ross River Virus [RRV] or Australian Encephalitis). In 1772, Labillardière on board the vessel *Recherche,* remarked that the Tasmanian Aborigines seemed generally free of disease (West 1852; Ryan 1981), although they were full of "vermin" (Ryan 1981).

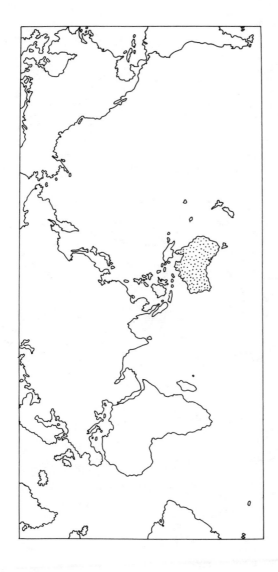

Figure 10-1. Australia in relation to the rest of the world, showing its relative isolation.

Figure 10-2. Evolution of the world's land masses by the Theory of Continental Drift.

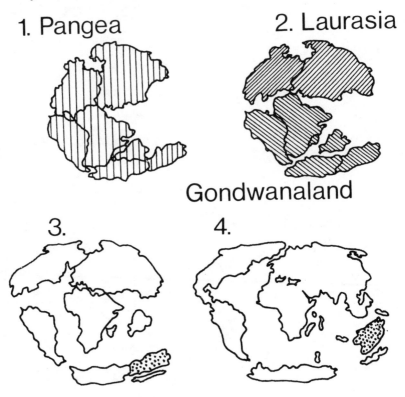

1. Pangea

2. Laurasia

Gondwanaland

3.

4.

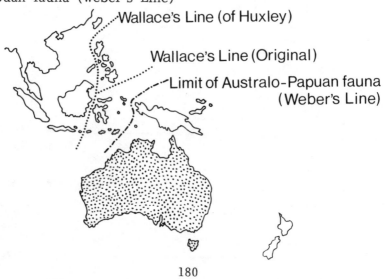

Figure 10-3. Australia and the limits of the Australo-Papuan fauna (Weber's Line)

Wallace's Line (of Huxley)

Wallace's Line (Original)

Limit of Australo-Papuan fauna (Weber's Line)

Despite the fact that one-third of Australia is tropical to subtropical (Baldwin 1938), early medical observers in northern Australia were of the opinion that no tropical diseases, with the possible exception of malaria, were endemic there prior to the arrival of nonaboriginal settlers between 1788 and the early 1800s. In fact, even up to 1845 tropical and other infectious diseases were noticeably absent even in the northern parts of Australia (Basedow 1932a; Cilento 1932).

Malaria is more problematical. Although Cleland (1914) and Cilento (1932) considered it as most probably absent, Black (1956) felt that "benign tertian malaria has probably been endemic since before European times," possibly being brought in with traders, whether Malayan (Black 1956; Cleland 1928a) or Sumatran; it is known that the latter had traveled widely, even as far westward as India and Madagascar, for at least the last 2,000 years (Lewis 1980).

A long-lasting relapsing and chronic malaria such as that caused by *Plasmodium vivax* could probably survive with low-level transmission by effective indigenous *Anopheles* spp. (for example, *A. farauti*). However, the acute form of the disease due to *P. falciparum,* causal agent of malignant tertian malaria, was probably not endemic at that time, although outbreaks could conceivably have occurred sporadically along Australia's northern coastline through contact with Papua New Guinea (PNG) via Malayan and other traders prior to the European era. Such outbreaks would probably have had disastrous results for the isolated, nonimmune aboriginal communities, among whom it could have continued to be transmitted for a time by susceptible and efficient local mosquito vectors before again dying out due to the small numbers of the human population and their nomadic habit (Cleland 1928a). Further evidence against the endemicity of *P. falciparum* infections is the lack of genetic markers (for example, sickle cell and perhaps less proven glucose-6-phosphate-dehydrogenase-deficiency) in the aboriginal population (Budtz-Olsen and Kidson 1961; Martin et al. 1979). For it is an accepted fact that such genetic markers are of survival value in hyperendemic *P. falciparum* areas (Elsdon-Dew 1962; Tobias 1974) and may persist in a population for some time even after the removal of the selecting agent.

Cleland (1914) quotes numerous historic records suggesting the absence of endemic malaria from tropical Australia prior to post-European introduction from elsewhere. He does, however, record a number of malaria deaths in newly arrived passengers (for instance, from the *Amity* which arrived from Coupang), and he also remarks that malaria was present among soldiers of the 17th Regiment in 1833 and suggests some local transmission by indigenous *Anopheles*.*

He felt however, that "the thinly scattered aboriginal population of these parts and the fact that the various voyagers and travellers can seldom have been for long in the neighbourhood of natives may account for this original absence of malaria in Australia." He further believed that in southern parts of Australia "though anopheline mosquitoes do occur, their generally small numbers indicate that little or no danger exists of an introduction of malaria, or of a spread southwards."

Possibly the first endemic records of malaria in northern Australia were in 1849, when Dr. Leichenhardt's expedition failed due to "ague" and in 1867 for which good clinical records of malaria are available (Cleland 1914).

By 1879 malaria seems to have become well established, but in 1912 Dr. Elkington recorded the introduction from New Guinea of a "severe and fatal form of malaria" that was being spread by a "potentially dangerous anopheline" existing in the northern parts. On the Einasleigh Gold Fields in 1910, in a population of 400, there were 120 cases and 24 deaths following the infecting of local mosquito vectors by two parasitized miners from New Guinea (Cleland 1914).

A disease of uncertain aetiology referred to as "Mossman Fever" is described by Clarke (1913) as possibly being found in Aborigines prior to white settlement in the Mossman district of Queensland. The identity of this disease was never established. It seemed to have clinical features of a number of febrile illnesses, including leptospirosis and scrub typhus, and could have been an endemic zoonotic disease—especially as many of these febrile illnesses were rural (Cilento 1942).

Mudge (1982), in a discussion of the arbovirus diseases of Australia, stated that the earliest accounts of aboriginal illnesses did not seem to fit closely any of the clinical features of diseases such as that caused by Ross River

---

*There was a similar situation in Ontario, Canada, in the same period, when a reservoir of malaria infection for local anophelines was introduced into the Ottawa Valley by soldiers who had been stationed in the West Indies and other then-endemic areas (Ffrench, G. 1957. The wider view—possibilities in the Canadian pattern of disease. *Can. Med. Assoc. J.* 76:198-205)—Ed.

Virus (RRV), transmitted by *Culex annulirostris* and *Aedes vigilax*. He pointed out, however, that recent serological studies in Queensland and Western Australia have shown that many Aborigines have antibodies to Alphavirus, suggesting that such infections may have been ones of long-standing in these people. He went on to suggest that RRV may have reached Australia via the land-bridge linking the continent to PNG and other northern land areas at least 12,000 years ago.

It is interesting to speculate on the possible endemicity in Australia of yaws due to *Treponema pertenue*. The disease was reported in the first half of this century to be widespread and endemic throughout Asia, Polynesia and New Guinea (Cilento 1942). It proved to be common among aboriginal children on the northern coast of tropical Australia, but less so, or even absent, inland (Cilento 1932). This might suggest its introduction from the north and/or the Pacific at some stage, but its absence as an endemic disease elsewhere. Certainly the disease was widespread and well-recognized by many aboriginal tribes, being known as "larrikincha" or "errekincha" (Basedow 1932a, 1932c). It could well be that where syphilis was reported to be an endemic disease among the Aborigines (for example, that of Sturt in 1830 as reported by Basedow 1932b), confusion with yaws might be the correct answer; for syphilis is not usually recorded in areas where yaws is highly endemic, especially among the children, the latter disease conferring a cross-immunity to the former (Duguid et al. 1978).

Sandison (1980) asserts that venereal syphilis was introduced into Australia by white explorers and settlers and that prior to this, the Aborigines had suffered from yaws in many of the tropical regions and from endemic syphilis or treponarid (irkinja) in the drier areas. He suggested that climatic change, with an increase in arid areas, resulted in the evolution of treponarid from yaws. Basedow (1932a, 1932b) considered it likely that syphilis was introduced by whites and Chinese, although he admitted that earlier sporadic introductions may have been effected on the north coast of Australia by Macassan fishermen.

While there are comparatively few records regarding the infections of Aborigines in pre-European times, we have, in contrast, at least speculative evidence of the ectoparasitic and endoparasitic infections of the New Zealand Maori, based upon medical writings and observations of the early European explorers, Maori folklore, and so on. Thus Andrews (1976) lists the following as possible parasites of the Maori even prior to the arrival of whites in New Zealand:

Pediculus humanus capitis
Pediculus humanus corporis
Phthirus pubis
Sarcoptes scabiei
Demodex folliculorum
Ascaris lumbricoides
Enterobius vermicularis

Although the Australian Aborigine has a profoundly different ethnic origin from the Maori, can anything be deduced from Andrews' results relating to diseases of the former?

While long ago Labillardière commented on the Tasmanian Aborigines as being full of "vermin," the nature of these ectoparasites is open to speculation. The body louse seems unlikely, as most Aborigines in the north of Australia (the area from which they originally migrated across the continent) wore few clothes in the hot climate; body lice, living on and laying their eggs on clothing—*not* the body—tend to be absent from such people (Grundy 1979). Even the Tasmanian Aborigines, living in a colder climate, seem to have worn few clothes according to early observers (West 1852; Ryan 1981). By 1932, however, body lice had become a scourge, infesting blankets, and so on, of the Aborigines (Basedow 1932a).

Although head lice do not commonly infest Africans or Negroes (Juranek 1977), they infect Aborigines readily (Basedow 1932c). Thus, these ectoparasites may have been harbored by pre-European Aborigines, as suggested by observations on tribes who had never been in contact with whites (Basedow 1932c).

Sarcoptes scabiei and *Demodex folliculorum* could also possibly have occurred, both being widespread among human populations everywhere. Although it would be purely hypothetical to postulate the early presence of *Ascaris lumbricoides* and *Enterobius vermicularis,* the former worm would seem an unlikely parasite in such small and nomadic groups; and although direct transmission of *E. vermicularis* is possible, pinworms have been shown to be less common in tropical regions (from which the Aborigine originated) than in temperate ones.

Using Andrews' deductions regarding the parasites of the Maori and the writings of early Australian observers, some educated guesses may be ventured, as follows.

Thus in a detailed unpublished document, Daisy Bates,

by close questioning of Aborigines and studies of their folklore and of historic documents, concluded that few communicable diseases were found before the coming of the whites—a conclusion endorsed by West (1852), Ryan (1981), and Basedow (1932a, 1932b, 1932c, 1932d). Aboriginal folklore indicated the presence of "itch" (?scabies), which was known variously as "jip-jip," "Iyari dala" or "Inyari dauari," "Gumbar-gumbar" or "Goom-boor Goom-boor," and a skin disease or itch known as "Nyeerang" or "Nyeering."

Ophthalmia, reported to be associated with flies, was widespread and was described as a cause of blindness—suggesting trachoma (Cleland 1928b). The fly referred to must have been the native bush fly (*Musca vetustissima*), which does feed on sores and exudates, for the common housefly (*Musca domestica*) was only introduced after white settlement (Waterhouse 1982). Evidence given by one informant that a venereal disease called "koo-ar'-roo" was common in the coastal tribes, and afflicted newborns as well, could have been related to the occurrence of yaws in the pre-European era. Both syphilis and gonorrhea are more likely to have been introduced by white and other settlers (Basedow 1932b).

Most skin diseases described from the Aborigines were believed to be due to dietary imbalance. Records of tuberculosis in the Aborigine as evidenced by the "spitting of blood" are unconvincing as regards the period before the whites arrived. So, on the contrary, is the claim by one Aborigine that neither toothache nor headache existed before the coming of the whites, unless one relates it to tooth decay due to sugar consumption and hangovers due to alcohol!

Chickenpox has a rather more difficult history to trace in Australia, and it may well have been one of the few childhood diseases present before the coming of the whites (Gandevia 1978). The reason for this could well have been the ability of the Herpes zoster virus to remain latent in the body after an attack of chickenpox and then to become reactivated—often many years later—to give rise to an attack of zoster (shingles), which can be infectious to a susceptible subject (often a child of the next generation).

The Aboriginal importation of the dingo into Australia, possibly via New Guinea between 3,000 and 10,000 years ago (Harden 1981; Newsome 1982), probably saw the introduction of some zoonotic dog parasites such as *Toxocara canis* and perhaps the mosquito-borne *Dirofilaria immitis*. Both of these are widespread in Australia today. The latter species at least is commoner in the Aborigine than in the white in the northern part of the country

(Moodie 1977). *D. immitis* could, however, have been a later import (for example, with dog breeds from the United States or Caribbean), which again adapted to susceptible local mosquito vectors.

Hydatid may have come into the country at this stage and survived as a sylvatic cycle in wallabies and dingoes, as is still the case today over much of mainland Australia. However, it seems more probable that it was imported later with dogs and sheep of European origin (Basedow 1932c)—a theory held also for hydatid in New Zealand (Andrews 1976). Recent studies have shown, though, that there seem to be three distinct strains of hydatid in Australia. Thompson and Kumaratilake (1982) have postulated that these strains may have been introduced independently: first by Aborigines and their dingoes, and again at a later stage by whites with their domestic dogs and sheep. However, even by 1879, hydatid of the liver was said to be known by Aborigines (Cleland 1928a).

EARLY SETTLEMENT AND DISEASE

The disease situation in Australia at this stage probably remained fairly static, with the Aborigines harboring a few diseases and being occasionally afflicted by endemic zoonotic infections, as well as occasional outbreaks of infection resulting from contact with Malay or other traders calling at Australia.

However, due to small population numbers and nomadic habits, imported diseases probably never became established to any degree. It was really only after the arrival of increasing numbers of white settlers that the disease picture in Australia began to change. The first white settlers arrived in the late 1700s and early 1800s. Even then, in fact, the new settlements (the tropical northern parts included) were relatively free from disease until the great period of colonial expansion between 1850 and 1860.

Of the southern settlements, Tasmania seemed free from epidemics for the first 15 years or so of white settlement, although an outbreak of influenza almost decimated the Aborigines at Port Phillip (Ryan 1981). There were disease problems in the convict transports, especially typhus, cholera, and smallpox. In the Sydney settlements, smallpox was probably first introduced as early as 1788, when the disease spread rapidly through the Aboriginal population of New South Wales and continued to flourish epidemically among them for a further 50 years, finally dying out in about 1845 (Cilento 1942; Cleland 1967; Kiss 1967). In 1865-66 smallpox was again introduced possibly this time by

Malays, again with tragic results for the Ngoorla and Ngallooma tribes (Bates n.d.; Gandevia 1978).

Another early introduction was typhus, especially in the convict settlements, arriving in the overcrowded convict ships from England. It caused problems in some of the penal settlements, where it was known as "spotted fever" or "gaol fever" and was at times confused with typhoid (Cumpston 1927). In 1799 Smyth, as quoted by Ford (1950), was already advocating nitrous vapor to prevent and destroy "contagion" in ships, prisons, and hospitals to prevent typhus. This must be one of the earliest references to disinsection (albeit unwittingly!) by fumigation on record. It was a direct reference to the *Hillsborough,* which arrived at the convict station of Botany Bay near Sydney in 1798 after a voyage in which 95 of the 300 convicts on board died of typhus and six more died subsequently on shore.

It is interesting that despite the frequency of typhus on ships from England, and especially on the prison ships, the disease did not really become established on the Australian mainland. Thus McCrea in 1864-66, noted (when defending the necessity of maintaining quarantine stations after an outbreak of typhus in the *Golden Empire* had caused much alarm in Melbourne) that despite frequent records of the importation of this infection in ships over the preceding 13 years—including the *Ticonderonga* in which of 795 people on board, 98 died of typhus en route and 75 died after arrival in Melbourne—only 4 cases had occurred among people nursing the sick, while the disease never extended beyond these nor established itself (Ford 1950). This could have been due to disease recognition on the voyage and efficient quarantine on arrival. However, it might also be that while overcrowding on these ships facilitated louse transfer—and hence disease transmission—the less crowded, low density population settlements of early Australia (except in the prisons and convict stations) were not conducive to louse transmission.

The situation was slightly different though in Tasmania, where in 1839-40 there was a serious outbreak of typhus in Hobarton (now Hobart). This was directly traced to the arrival of the prison ship *Marquis of Hastings* with 240 male convicts. Very little fever had existed in Hobarton to that date; the final tally was 914 cases and 78 deaths. Fresh cases were added to the outbreak in 1839 and 1840 with the arrival of the convict transport *Layton* and the French exploration ship *La Zelée.* The outbreak was mostly limited to the confined convicts, who were in all probability heavily infested with body lice; but it soon spread to convicts in private service and then presumably to some free settlers. In the outbreak, two prison medical officers, one medical apprentice, and one apothecary also died.

The last record of imported typhus in Australia occurred in Melbourne in 1869 (Cumpston 1927), although there is a record of "low malignant fever"—believed to be typhus—among the overcrowded and poorly housed mutton-birders in the Bass Strait Islands in 1879 (according to Vines, as quoted by Ford 1950).

Typhoid was introduced in ships from time to time and had become a scourge in all the main Australian cities by 1850 (Gandevia 1978). It became endemic in Tasmania (Cumpston 1927) and had a high mortality rate in New South Wales between 1876 and 1878, and then again from 1882-87 and 1895-1904. With the influx of immigrants after the discovery of gold in Australia, further large outbreaks occurred. Eventually, with the overall improvement in hygiene and sanitation, it receded to become at most a sporadic infection in parts of the country.

Measles is often recorded as having been introduced into Australia in 1850; but it seems more likely that it appeared about 1830 with soldiers and missionaries, after which it spread from Sydney to Tasmania and then to New Zealand. The 1850 epidemic probably resulted from a reintroduction at Melbourne, measles thereafter becoming endemic due to the population increasing to a level able to support it, although it did die out in Western Australia between 1860 and 1883. There were subsequent explosive epidemics in the gold rush days with a high mortality (Bates n.d.; Gandevia 1978).

Of the other "childhood diseases," pertussis (whooping cough) seemed best able to survive the long sea voyage from England, probably because of its overall inherent chronic nature (Gandevia 1978). The first recorded epidemic occurred in 1828 in Sydney (and was only preceded among epidemic disease introductions by outbreaks of influenza, smallpox, and mumps). The disease had reached Tasmania by 1833 and all states by 1850, after which it readily became endemic (Gandevia 1978). Its introduction into Western Australia is of particular interest, as it appeared to have arrived with the families of soldiers of the 21st Regiment in the 1840s. It caused many deaths among the susceptible local Aborigines in the area around Perth. The Aborigines blamed the infection on the army bugles, associating the harsh notes of the bugle with the characteristic "whoop" of the infected people (Bates n.d.).

As it is also true for typhoid, the history of diphtheria

is difficult to unravel due to diagnostic confusion with such other infections as croup. However, diptheria was first specifically diagnosed in Australia in Victoria in 1858 and then spread rapidly to South Australia and Tasmania, reaching Queensland and Western Australia by 1860. It declined after the introduction of specific antitoxin in 1892-95 (Gandevia 1978).

Influenza was introduced repeatedly and was the first serious epidemic disease to afflict the newly founded colony in Sydney, where it killed large numbers of the very young and the very old in 1820. It recurred in 1826. It is interesting that these epidemics were not part of any world pandemic. However, in 1836-37 and 1847-48 the influenza pandemics sweeping the world also struck Australia; and then in 1860 a further Australian epidemic occurred (Gandevia 1978), foreshadowing the 1919 disaster during the global Spanish influenza pandemic (Basedow 1932a, 1932b).

Tuberculosis probably did not occur in Australia prior to white settlement (Basedow 1932c), despite a disease termed "spitting of blood" by the Aborigines (Bates n.d.). It may nevertheless have been an early introduction into Tasmania (Cleland 1928c). In Australia the disease seems to have been uncommon—at least as a cause of death—before the middle of the nineteenth century. What is fascinating is that in the latter 1800s many people knowingly introduced tuberculosis into Australia by traveling there to "take the cure" in a hot, dry climate. There must thus have existed a large reservoir of infection (further reinforced by new arrivals during the gold rush period) from which a new generation—the Australian-born descendents of recent immigrant stock as well as susceptible Aborigines—became infected. This resulted in a general period of increasing mortality from tuberculosis between 1860 and 1885 that, strangely enough, Western Australia seems to have been spared (Gandevia 1978).

We see, therefore, that in the early colonial days following the arrival of the first three fleets in 1788 and in the years immediately thereafter, infectious diseases were comparatively rare. Most deaths were due to dietary deficiency and, in the young children, to congenital disorders (including, however, syphilis). Even as late as 1852-54 syphilis accounted for 10% of childhood deaths in Hobart. Some deaths in the early period were caused by typhoid, typhus, influenza, diarrhea, and measles, but as more people arrived, more diseases were introduced and more became endemic in the increasing population.

DISEASE IN THE LATER PERIOD
OF SETTLEMENT (AFTER 1850)

Although initially in the early years of settlement, most infectious diseases were uncommon or absent, the period 1788 to 1850 saw the importation, probably repeatedly, in convict and migrant ships of all the prevalent human infections of those times, including all the common childhood diseases. By the late 1800s the population had stabilized to some extent and had grown in all the young Australian colonies to a sufficiently large level to support these diseases on an endemic basis. In many cases, the effects of these diseases on the local indigenous aboriginal people had been disastrous, with high morbidity and mortality.

The situation after 1860 deteriorated rapidly in the previously relatively healthy tropical areas of Australia, associated with contemporary population growth due to the gold rush and the "colonial expansionist" era between 1860 and 1900. During this period, the European powers of Britain, France, and Germany, together with the United States, were looking towards the Pacific. A direct result of this in Australia was an expansion into the vast, undeveloped tropical areas of the continent. Coinciding with this territorial extension and development was the importation of cheap Asian and Oceanic labor, which had serious implications from a medical standpoint (Cilento 1932).

Both species of hookworm (*Ancylostoma duodenale* and *Necator americanus*) occur in Australia, having been first recorded from Queensland in 1889. Cilento (1932, 1942) believed that the former was introduced from Chinese and southern European sources, while the latter came from the Melanesian archipelagoes with the imported "Kanaka" labor. The worms readily became established in the warmer areas of Australia. Severe hookworm disease is recorded even today as an important cause of ill health, especially anaemia, in Aboriginal children (Walker and Bellmaine 1975).

Diarrhea in the early days of settlement in both Tasmania and Sydney was often termed "cholera," but there is little direct evidence to confirm the presence of Asiatic cholera during this period (Ford 1976). In 1886, however, Asiatic cholera from Batavia resulted in 17 deaths, 6 of them in quarantine at Peel Island. In all, up to 1942 cholera was introduced at least six times by ship into Australia. However, it never succeeded in becoming established. Ships on the Australia-England route are also recorded as being afflicted (for example, the *S.S. Dorunda* from Bombay) (Ford 1976). Cilento (1942) recorded the most important ports for possible introduction of cholera into Australia as China (all ports); India (Calcutta, Madras, Chittagong); and Burma (Bassein, Moulmein, Rangoon).

With the emergence of the El Tor biotype of *Vibrio cholerae,* the disease spread even more widely throughout the world, to extend to the previously cholera-free areas of southern Africa (Cruickshank et al. 1975). Outbreaks of endemic cholera were recorded along Queensland river valleys (Anonymous 1980), where the disease seems to have developed a reservoir in the rivers themselves (Feachem 1982).

Dengue was introduced into Australia a number of times: 8 cases on the *Charles Auguste* from Mauritius in 1873 and 5 cases on the *Gungas* from Fiji and Noumea in 1885 (Cleland 1914). Subsequently, the disease was diagnosed in Victoria (1886), Thursday Island (1894), Townsville (1898), Queensland generally (1897), and in 1898 in New South Wales (Cleland 1914). It eventually reached Western Australia (Cilento 1942). These epidemics usually spread from north to south, suggesting introduction in the north and carriage southwards by internal population movements or epidemic spread from area to area with transmission by local mosquito vectors. At one stage it was established that 75% of school children in Queensland suffered from dengue (Gandevia 1978). According to Cilento (1942), the vector in Queensland, where sporadic epidemics occurred, was *Aedes aegypti.*

Leprosy also seemed to have been introduced during this period of colonial expansion. In a detailed study of the problem, Cook (1927) concluded that "[l]eprosy was unknown amongst the Aborigines and early European settlers. It was introduced from China and the Pacific Islands during the last century by the importation of colored labour from those countries," a view supported by Basedow (1932e).

Malaria, as mentioned previously, probably became established during this general period. Ford (1950) wrote that "[w]hile malaria is not present in the major part of the Australian mainland, foci are found in the northern parts of the continent and conditions of potential danger from its introduction exist over a wide area." The malarial areas of Australia at that time were defined as lying north of latitude 19°S in Queensland and Western Australia and north of latitude 17°S in the Northern Territory (NT) (Goldsmid 1980a). Especially in the NT up to 1929-34, endemic malaria—mostly due to *Plasmodium vivax* but with some *P. falciparum*—persisted in Australia, with occasional flare-ups until eradication of the disease was finally achieved about 20 years ago, although the vector mosquitoes (for example, *Anopheles farauti* and *A. hilli*) still occur (Goldsmid 1980a; Black 1980). There was a particular awareness of the dangers of spreading malaria after both World Wars, when returning soldiers with gametocytes in their blood posed a potential threat for wide dissemination of the disease among susceptible indigenous mosquito vectors, although contemporary workers doubted that malaria would ever really become established on a large scale in Australia "unless a reservoir of infection comparable to that present in the natives of tropical countries is allowed to develop in the Australian population" (Anonymous 1943). The first definite clinical record of malaria is probably the epidemic of "black fever" that in 1864 almost wiped out the inhabitants of Burketown. It is believed this was *P. falciparum* brought in by Malays coming across in prahus; as a result of the infection, three-quarters of the community died. From this time, malaria seemed to have been increasingly frequently introduced. It eventually became endemic, although the overall sparseness of the population at that time probably prevented it assuming severely epidemic proportions (Cilento 1932).

The development and recent rapid spread of drug resistant *P. falciparum* through Southeast Asia and PNG has heightened concern as regards the reintroduction of malaria (Goldsmid 1980), although the problem remains essentially one of diagnosis and treatment of cases recently arrived or returned to the country after overseas travel (Goldsmid 1979a, 1979b, 1980a). A recent mini-epidemic of imported cases in the Torres Strait Islands (Black 1980), however, serves to emphasize that such small outbreaks could occur via indigenous vectors. If this happened in an isolated community, a number of deaths could result before appropriate measures could be undertaken to eradicate it.

The problem of filariasis due to *Wuchereria bancrofti* in Australia was quite different. This infection was first diagnosed in Brisbane in 1876 and described in the *Lancet* by Cobbold (Ford 1976). It was probably introduced into northern Australia in the late 1800s with imported "Kanaka" laborers who infected susceptible local mosquitoes with parasites that they had acquired in their Pacific island homes. As a result, the disease became endemic along the coastal areas of Queensland; while it possibly spread to northern NSW too, it is less likely that the NT became involved (Goldsmid 1980a). In 1900-10 the prevalence of *W. bancrofti* in Brisbane reached 15% in the surgical wards, with clinical cases of severe elephantiasis being recorded (Cilento 1932). However, with the repatriation of the Pacific islanders between 1900-10, the disease rapidly disappeared. Its prevalence had fallen to 1-3% by the 1920s, and it was only rarely encountered by 1949-56 (Mackerras 1958; Goldsmid 1980a).

The reason for the disappearance of filariasis from Queensland remains an intriguing one, the solution to which is still unclear. Mackerras (1958) felt that the infection may have died out due to changes in mosquito populations, perhaps due to "a gradual replacement in some localities of *C. quinquefasciatus* by an allied mosquito, *C. pipiens australicus,* which breeds away from houses." It may also have been, however, that changes in the mosquito environment—such as drainage of water and clearance of domestic breeding sites—played some role (Mackerras 1958).

An alternative suggestion was put forward by Cilento (1942), who felt that the disappearance of filariasis might have been related to the departure of the Pacific islanders, thus depriving the vectors of their source of infection. If this is so, however, an inexplicable feature of the situation would seem to be the fact that filariasis as seen in Queensland at that time was essentially an urban disease, developing and spreading from areas of white settlement (Mackerras 1958).

One might well ask why the Pacific islanders were necessary, if indeed they were, to maintain transmission. Why could not the whites or Aborigines have maintained the infection?

The answer might lie in the fact that the mosquito is a relatively inefficient vector of *Wuchereria bancrofti* (Hairston and de Meillon 1968) and that, in addition, relatively heavy parasitaemias are necessary to infect biting mosquitoes. Thus, it has been calculated that microfilarial rates of 3 microfilariae per mm^3 of blood are optimal for infection of the mosquito, while microfilarial rates of 0.5 mm^3 of blood or less will fail to infect. These weaknesses at both points of worm transfer between vector and final host would indicate that heavy human parasitaemias and plentiful bite contacts were necessary to maintain infection. The position is even more complicated by the fact that recent work by Ottesen (1980) and Weller et al. (1982) indicate that only a proportion of infected people show a significant microfilaraemia and that this might be associated with some form of immunological deficiency (Forsyth, personal communication).

The white population in Queensland would thus not suffice as a reservoir, as they probably mostly used mosquito nets, so cutting down on biting contacts, resulting in low parasitaemias in general, while the Aborigines were few in number and nomadic of habit, thus also reducing their effectiveness in the role of reservoirs for the maintenance of filariasis.

Filariasis, therefore, serves as an example of a disease that was in all probability imported to Australia, became well established and clinically significant by the importation into receptive areas of a large number of heavily parasitized people, and then disappeared, possibly when the reservoir was subsequently removed (Goldsmid 1980a).

Another insect-borne disease, bubonic plague (caused by *Yersinia pestis*) was introduced a number of times from ships into Australian ports. The oriental rat flea (*Xenopsylla cheopis*), one of the main vectors of this disease, is now present in all Australia's main east coast ports from Sydney northwards (Cilento 1942; Dunnett 1973). Despite this, and the fact that plague has been introduced at various times from Java, China, India, and New Caledonia (Cilento 1942), it has never become established, while sylvatic plague does not occur in Australia (Dunnett 1973). The last epidemic in this country occurred about 40-50 years ago (Cilento 1942; Dunnett 1973). Earlier, the outbreak of 1900-09 had affected many of Australia's coastal ports, including Melbourne and Adelaide (Armstrong; Caro; Gresswell; Thompson; Neale: all quoted by Ford 1976). The 1921-22 appearance of plague on the Queensland and NSW seaboards comprised part of a general world pandemic at the time (Cilento 1942).

Schistosomiasis, a snail-borne disease caused by blood-flukes of the genus *Schistosoma,* has caused concern at various times over the last 80 years. The problems of the introduction of, and the dangers of the establishment of, schistosomiasis into Australia, have been reviewed by Goldsmid (1979a, 1980a). There was great concern regarding the possibility of introducing schistosomiasis into Australia through infection of local freshwater snails by returning soldiers at the end of the Boer War in 1902 and of World War I in 1918. At that time, one report even claimed that the ability of local snail species to transmit the infection had been established (Anonymous 1919), and there were sporadic reports of the disease having been contracted from water bodies in Australia (McWhee and Jagger 1921; Holland and Woodward 1924). It was certainly wise that such dangers should be taken seriously. Thus, in South America schistosomiasis had become rife after the introduction of *Schistosoma mansoni* with imported slaves from Africa resulted in the infection of a highly susceptible local snail vector, *Biomphalaria glabrata*.

In a recent review, however, Goldsmid (1980a) expressed doubts as regards the dangers of the disease becoming established to any extent due to lack of recent scientific evidence of the susceptibility of local snails to act as vectors, and the relative sparseness of the population over most rural areas in tropical Australia.

CURRENT PROBLEMS OF DISEASE IMPORTATION INTO AUSTRALIA

The most important factor involved in the spread of disease is human population movements. In recent years there has been a phenomenal increase in travel throughout the world, a trend seen also in Australia (Table 10-1) if we compare worldwide visitor-arrival figures and Australian figures for short-term visitors and total arrivals for the years 1956, 1966, 1977, and 1980.

Table 10-1. Visitor arrivals (worldwide) and visitor arrivals (Australia).

Visitor arrivals (worldwide)		Visitor arrivals (Australia)		
Year	No. of arrivals	Year	Visitor arrivals	Total arrivals
1966	139,000,000	1956	66,018	153,450
1976	221,000,000	1966	187,262	557,591
		1977	563,282	1,697,771
		1980	904,558	2,283,613

Of late years there has also been an increase in the number of travelers from tropical countries. Thus in the United Kingdom, it has been calculated that one in every 600 of the world's population makes an air journey each year, and one in every 750 (200 million people) makes an intercontinental journey. In London alone, at least 4 million people arrive from the tropics and subtropics each year (Woodruff 1978).

The same trend can be observed in Australia, where increasing numbers of people are coming from tropical embarkation points (Table 10-2).

Table 10-2. Origins of visitor arrivals in Australia.

Origin	1967	1977	1980
C. & S. America	1,533	3,046	6,129
Africa	4,028	8,915	13,885
Oceania (excl. NZ)	29,762	46,390	52,333
Asia	25,513	127,403	138,699

However, not only has there been an increase in the number of people traveling and a change in their origins and destinations, with increasing numbers traveling to and from disease-ridden Third World countries, but there has also been an important change in their mode of travel. Originally, man had to walk or travel by ox-cart, horse, or camel. This limited his travel distance and took long periods of time. International travel was mostly by sea, initially by sail, with voyages taking months or even years. Then steam replaced sail, and voyage times were reduced to weeks or days. Now, however, people travel by air. With the advent of the jumbo jet, groups of 400 or more people can be transported from one part of the globe to another in a matter of hours. What this means in terms of disease is that whereas previously diseases had time to incubate and be recognized en route, enabling efficient quarantine at the port of arrival, the advent of large aircraft has allowed extensive passenger dispersal in the country of destination before development of symptoms. This greatly complicates contact-tracing and quarantine regulation, where aircraft as large as jumbo jets are concerned.

Such a change has not passed unnoticed by medical workers. Fenner (1971) noted that "air travel is converting the World of Man into one ecological unit" and that while "in 1957 pandemic influenza spread around the World at the speed of ship and train travel, in 1968 the Hong Kong variant was distributed by aeroplane." Woodruff (1978) even coined the phrase of "airline imported disease."

This is particularly noticeable in Australia, where because of relative isolation over 98% of all arrivals were by 1976 being carried by air and less than 2% by sea (Goldsmid 1980a).

There has been considerable concern expressed recently regarding the disease hazards of increased travel both in

Europe (Maegraith 1971; Wright 1971; Bruce-Chwatt 1973; Zuidema 1975; Bell 1978; Woodruff 1978) and in Australia (Rutter 1977; Boughton 1978a, 1978b; Radford 1978; Goldsmid 1979a, 1980; Webb 1978; Grove 1981). Most of the concern has concentrated on the need to advise travelers on prevention of disease while abroad and on promoting an awareness in medical circles regarding the problems of diagnosis and treatment of so-called "exotic" diseases contracted overseas.

Imported diseases recorded in Australia include typhoid, cholera, dengue, amoebiasis, schistosomiasis, cysticercosis, filariasis, intestinal helminthiases, coccidiodomycosis, tinia, pityriasis versicolor, histoplasmosis, and leprosy. In addition, immigrants make up one-third of all tuberculosis notifications in Australia (Goldsmid 1980a). Table 10-3 shows that imported malaria has increased dramatically year by year in Australia.

Table 10-3. Imported malaria in Australia 1969-80.

Year	No. cases	Year	No. cases
1969	166	1975	255
1970	199	1976	265
1971	220	1977	291
1972	170	1978	325
1973	194	1979	473
1974	201	1980	628
		Total No. cases	3387

Source: Black 1981.

Of these cases, 82.3% were due to *Plasmodium vivax;* 14.8% to *P. falciparum;* 0.5% to *P. malariae;* and 0.3% to *P. ovale.* Mixed infections comprised 1.1%, and in a further 1.1% the species was unidentified (Black 1981). It is also of interest that in 1980, the 14,785 Southeast Asian refugees who came to Australia accounted for 36% of all malaria cases that year (Black 1981).

It is often implied that imported diseases occur only at the point of entry (Helliwell and Turner 1980). Such a view can be misleading, for imported infections in these days of rapid air travel can, and do, occur anywhere—a fact that can be well seen by examining figures for Tasmania (Goldsmid 1979a, 1979b, 1980a, 1981).

Tasmania has the lowest figures for initial point of entry into Australia for any state (Table 10-4), and yet a significant range of infections have been recorded as being imported (Table 10-5).

Table 10-4. Clearance of international passengers to Australia by state (1977).

State of clearance	N.S.W.	Vic.	Q'land.	W.A.	N.T.	A.C.T.	Tas.	Total
Arrivals (percent)	59.1	23	8.8	8.3	0.8	0.02	0.001	1,697,770

In addition to these imported parasitic infections, other imported diseases recently diagnosed in Tasmania include: shigellosis, typhoid, salmonellosis, cholera, leprosy, gonorrhea (including β-lactamase producing strains), lymphogranuloma venereum, and chancroid.

In early studies, Goldsmid (1980b) reported that most imported parasitic infections in Tasmania were recorded in Australians who had been holidaying or traveling overseas (77.8%), as opposed to immigrants who had brought their infections with them (22.2%). At that time, he concluded that in Tasmania parasitic diseases were diseases of affluence—only a danger to those who could afford to travel!

However, with the increase in Southeast Asian refugees into the state, the situation has changed. Of 190 refugees entering Tasmania from Southeast Asia, 93 (61.2%) were found to be infected with parasites, 70 (46.1%) by protozoa, and 40 (26.3%) by helminths. Of those infected, 40.8% were infected with 1 species and 20.4% by 2 or more species. Table 10-6 lists the species recorded.

In addition, 32 (51.4%) of 72 Indochinese refugee children were found to be infested with head lice.

As well as these recent imports into Australia, 2 cases of introduced malaria contracted endemically have been recorded (Black 1981); and an outbreak of imported malaria has been recently reported in the Torres Strait Islands, emphasizing the potential threat in receptive areas (Black 1980).

Table 10-5. Parasitic infections imported into Tasmania.

Species	Origin	No. cases
Giardia lamblia	Asia; India	4
Chilomastix mesnili	Vietnam; India	2
Leishmania tropica	? Mediterranean/Middle East	1
Entamoeba histolytica	Asia; India, Nepal; Vietnam; Southeast Asia; PNG	8
Entamoeba coli	Vietnam; India	2
Iodamoeba butschlii	Vietnam	1
Endolimax nana	Vietnam; India; Bangladesh	3
Plasmodium vivax	PNG; Solomons; Kenya/Tanzania; Ghana; India; Southeast Asia	15
Plasmodium falciparum	Kenya/Tanzania; PNG	2
Schistosoma mansoni	Kenya; Zimbabwe	2
Schistosoma haematobium	Zimbabwe	1
Hymenolepis nana	Bangladesh	1
Taenia saginata	Lebanon	1
Hookworm	Vietnam; N. Africa	4
Cutaneous larva migrans	Pacific islands	1
Strongyloides stercoralis	Timor; PNG; Southeast Asia; India	15
Trichuris trichiura	India; Bangladesh; Asia; Maldives	7
Enterobius vermicularis	India	1
Ascaris lumbriocides	India; Bangladesh; Maldives; PNG; Fiji; Zimbabwe	8
Loa loa	W. Africa	1
Tropical eosinophilia	Maldives	1
Wuchereria bancrofti	India	1
Dermatobia hominis	S. America	1

Introduced cholera seems to have become established in certain rivers in Queensland with sporadic local cases being recorded, throwing doubt on the belief that an active human reservoir is necessary for the maintenance of this infection (Feachem 1982).

Imported cases of dengue were recorded in 1981-82 originating from Sri Lanka (Anonymous 1982). Local transmission resulted in the first outbreak in Australia for many years, with cases being diagnosed in Cairns, Townsville, Chillagoe, Mossman, and Thursday Island (Anonymous 1981; Anonymous 1982). Mosquitoes known to be capable of transmitting the diseases or that can be regarded as potential vectors in Australia include *Aedes aegypti,*

Table 10-6. Intestinal parasites and commensals recorded in 190 Southeast Asian refugees arriving in Tasmania.

Species	No. infected	
Giardia lamblia	30	(15.8%)
Chlilomastix mesnili	2	(1.1%)
Entamoeba histolytica	11	(5.8%)
Entamoeba hartmanni	12	(6.3%)
Entamoeba coli	24	(12.6%)
Endolimax nana	25	(13.2%)
Iodamoeba butschlii	5	(2.6%)
Blastocystis hominis	23	(12.1%)
Ascaris lumbricoides	19	(10.0%)
Trichuris trichiura	21	(11.1%)
Hookworm	4	(2.1%)
Strongyloides stercoralis	3	(1.6%)
Enterobius vermicularis	2	(1.1%)
Fasciolopsis buski	1	(0.5%)

A. tremulus, A. vigilax, A. katherinensis, A. scutellaris, Culex annulirostris, and *C. quinquefasciatus* (Walker et al. 1982).

An interesting reversal of the trend for diseases to be imported into Australia has been the spread of RRV from the traditionally endemic areas of northern Australia, not only southwards into South Australia and Tasmania (Mudge unpublished) but eastwards into the Pacific, to Fiji and the Cook Islands, for instance, Rarotonga (Kanamitsu et al. 1979; Aaskov et al. 1981; Rosen et al. 1981; Tesh et al. 1981; Chapter 11), where an important vector has been *Aedes polynesiensis* (Rosen et al. 1981).

POTENTIAL PROBLEMS REGARDING THE
FUTURE SPREAD OF DISEASE

A number of potential threats emerge from the study of the spread of disease in Australia and the Pacific:

1. Will RRV spread further and become endemic in the Western Pacific or even New Zealand? (Mudge unpublished; Chapter 11).

2. Could dengue spread further in Australia and will Chikungunya spread into Australia as it has into Southeast Asia—where it was introduced from Africa and where it has now become established in urban areas? (Grove 1981).

3. Will other diseases continue to be a diagnostic and therapeutic problem or even increase in importance with further increase in human population movements? This applies especially to refugees from politically unstable areas where (even though screening may take place for intestinal pathogens and blood parasites) monitoring of viraemia is impractical. Blood-borne viral infections and even low parasitaemias may thus escape detection, resulting in introduction into receptive areas with infection of local vectors, and in the case of many arbovirus infections, exposure of the local vertebrate reservoir.

MODE OF SPREAD AND ESTABLISHMENT

1. Imported diseases become established in a new area when brought in by travelers to a receptive area with poor hygiene (cholera, typhoid), susceptible vectors (malaria, filariasis, arbovirus) or reservoir hosts (RRV).

2. A disease may also become introduced by travelers *after* the prior introduction of a susceptible vector. This threat exists in Hong Kong where snail vectors of schistosomiasis have become established in local water bodies (Meier-Brook 1975). A similar recent threat to Australia was averted when water plants with the *Schistosoma* vector, *Australarlis straminea,* were intercepted at Sydney's international airport in a batch of tropical fish (Walker 1978).

3. A disease could be introduced by the importation (in a ship or aircraft) of an infected vector that infects a local person or susceptible reservoir animal and then breeds or leads to infection of susceptible local vectors, resulting in establishment of the disease. Again, a potential threat of this kind is recorded in the United Kingdom, where Woodruff and Ansdell (1977) detected a case of Le Dantec virus infection in a docker who was bitten by an insect while unloading a ship from Nigeria and West Africa. They concluded that "the case is notable in focussing attention on the need for vigilance in containing viral infections that could be transmitted by insects carried on transport

arriving from Africa." Similarly, we have *assumed* that RRV and dengue have spread due to the movement of viraemic humans or animals. Can we, though, altogether rule out the movement of infected mosquitoes by aircraft or ship or even on wind currents?

OVERALL CONCLUSIONS

What can be learned from this study of the history of imported disease in Australia?

1. Australia lies in a very vulnerable position as regards disease importation. There is increasing travel to and from the tropics; and even to get to Europe and the United States, it is necessary to travel via tropical areas. This trend towards international travel is likely to increase in the coming years, intensifying the problem of imported disease.

2. Australia is a very receptive area for vector-borne diseases with many effective local vectors and potential vectors, a fact that makes constant vigilance essential if we are to prevent the introduction of a range of presently nonendemic diseases.

3. Australia is ecologically receptive to introduced snail and arthropod vectors, which must be denied entry. As Mudge (unpublished) has warned: "More stringent barriers and vector surveillance at airports must be a top priority for Public Health authorities in the coming decades." In fact, the airplane, in particular, is proving an efficient counter to the previously effective water barrier surrounding this formerly isolated continent.

4. Australia has abundant animal life to serve as a reservoir for introduced zoonoses (for instance, rabies could spread rapidly among dingoes and introduced foxes if allowed to penetrate our disease defenses).

5. Increased travel, in particular, the increased influx of refugees from war-torn tropical countries, presents a serious potential disease importation threat unless strict precautions are enforced.

6. The movement and importation of vectors, while undeniably important, is only a small part of the overall problem of the importation of disease.

REFERENCES

Aaskov, J. G., J. U. Mataika, G. W. Lawrence, V. Rubukawaqu, M. M. Tucker, J. A. R. Miles, and D. A. Daglish. 1981. An epidemic of Ross River virus infection in Fiji. *Amer. J. trop. Med. Hyg.* 30:1053–59.

Andrews, J. R. H. 1976. The parasitology of the Maori in pre-European times. *N.Z. med. J.* 84:62–65.

Anonymous. 1919. Antimony in bilharziosis. *Med. J. Aust.* (2):269–70.

——————. 1943. The malaria problem in Australia. *Med. J. Aust.* (1):539–40.

——————. 1980. Cholera in Queensland. *Communicable Dis. Intell.* 80/3. Woden: Aust. Dept Hlth.

——————. 1981. Virus reporting scheme. *Communicable Dis. Intell.* 81/22. Woden: Aust. Dept Hlth.

——————. 1982. Virus reporting scheme. *Communicable Dis. Intell.* 82/5. Woden: Aust. Dept Hlth.

Baldwin, A. H. 1938. Observations on morbidity in tropical and subtropical Queensland. *Med. J. Aust.* (1):733–38.

Basedow, H. 1932a. Diseases of the Australian Aborigines. *J. trop. Med. Hyg.* 35:177–85.

——————. 1932b. Diseases of the Australian Aborigines. *J. trop. Med. Hyg.* 35:193–98.

——————. 1932c. Diseases of the Australian Aborigines. *J. trop. Med. Hyg.* 35:209–13.

——————. 1932d. Diseases of the Australian Aborigines. *J. trop. Med. Hyg.* 35:273–77.

Bates, D. n.d. Diseases, remedies, death (burial). Typescript from unpublished ms. Section 10:1a, 2a, 2c (ANL-MS. 365-32/2-95; 33/2-57; 72-80) 2a–diseases of natives before White contact–names for diseases.

Bell, D. R. 1978. Emergency situations–is it tropical? *Brit. J. hosp. Med.* 19:213–17.

Bellwood, P. 1979. The real pioneers. *Hemisphere* 23:370–74.

Black, R. H. 1956. The epidemiology of malaria in the southwest Pacific: Changes associated with increasing European contact. *Oceania* 27:136–42.

——————. 1980. Malaria in Australia, 1979. *Trop. Med. Techn. Pap.* No. 5. Sydney: Commonwealth Inst. Hlth.

——————. 1981. Malaria in Australia, 1980. *Trop. Med. Techn. Pap.* No. 7. Sydney: Commonwealth Inst. Hlth.

Boughton, C. R. 1978a. Travelling overseas? I Immunisation requirements and recommendations. *Aust. Prescriber* 2:64–67.

————. 1978b. Travelling overseas? II Precautions against infectious diseases. *Aust. Prescriber* 2:93-94.

Bruce-Chwatt, L. J. 1973. Global problems of imported disease. *Adv. Parasitol.* 11:75-114.

Budtz-Olsen, O. E. D., and C. Kidson. 1961. Absence of red cell enzyme deficiency in Australian aboriginal natives. *Nature* 192:765.

Cilento, R. W. 1932. Australia's problems in the tropics. *Rpt. 21st Mtg. Aust. N.Z. Assoc. Advncmnt Sci.*:216-33.

————. 1942. *Tropical diseases in Australasia* 2nd Ed. Brisbane: Smith and Paterson.

Clarke, P. S. 1913. Report on Mossman fever. *Wld Hlth med. Serv. Brnch Ann. Rpt:*32-35.

Cleland, J. B. 1914. Contributions to the history of disease of man in Australia. *Third Rpt Govt Bur. Microbiol.*:226-32.

————. 1928a. Disease amongst the Australian Aborigines. *J. trop. med. Hyg.* 31:157-60.

————. 1928b. Disease amongst the Australian Aborigines. *J. trop. med. Hyg.* 31:216-20.

————. 1928c. Disease amongst the Australian Aborigines. *J. trop. med. Hyg.* 31:232-35.

————. 1967. Mystery at Port Hacking—the smallpox. *Mankind* 6:432-33.

Cockburn, A. 1977. Where did our infectious diseases come from? In *Health and Disease in Tribal Societies.* Hugh-Jones, P. (Chairman) 103-13. Amsterdam: Elsevier.

————. 1980. Palaeopathology and the parasites. *Aust. Microbiol.* 1:3-6.

Cook, C. 1927. The epidemiology of leprosy in Australia. Aust. Dept. Health. *Serv. Publ.* No. 38.

Cruickshank, J. G., H. B. McD. Farrell, and B. P. B. Ellis. 1975. Cholera in the Manicaland Province of Rhodesia, February to May, 1974. *Centr. Afr. J. Med.* 21:1-10.

Cumpston, J. H. L. 1927. *The History of the Intestinal Infections (and Typhus Fever) in Australia,* 1799-1923. Melbourne: Commonwealth of Australia.

Duguid, J. P., B. P. Marmion, and R. H. A. Swain. 1978. *Mackie and McCartney's Medical Microbiology.* 13th ed. Vol. I. Edinburgh: Churchill-Livingstone.

Dunnett, G. M. 1973. Siphonaptera. In *The Insects of Australia* CSIRO, 647-55 Melbourne: Melbourne Univ. Press.

Elsdon-Dew, R. 1962. Protective and lethal genes. *S. Afr. J. Sci.* 58:387-88.

Feachem, R. G. 1982. Environmental aspects of cholera epidemiology. III Transmission and control. *Trop. Dis. Bull.* 79:1-47.

Fenner, F. 1971. Infectious disease and social change. *Med. J. Aust.* (1):1043-47, 1099-1102.

Ford, E. 1950. The malaria problem in Australia and the Australian Pacific territories. *Med. J. Aust.* (1):749-60.

————. 1976. *Bibliography of Australian Medicine 1790-1900.* Paramatta: Macarthur Press.

Gandevia, B. 1978. *Tears Often Shed.* Gordon: Charter Books.

Goldsmid, J. M. 1979a. The travel bug. *Occ. Ppr No. 17, Univ. Tasmania.* Hobart: Univ. Tasmania.

————. 1979b. Imported parasitic infections in Tasmania. *Med. J. Aust.* 2:338-39.

————. 1980a. Imported disease: A continuing and increasing threat to Australia. *Soc. Sci. Med.* 14D:101-9.

————. 1980b. Imported parasitic infections in Tasmania. *Communicable Dis. Intell.* 80/18. Woden: Aust. Dept Hlth.

Grove, D. I. 1981. Diseases of overseas travel: Recognition and treatment. *Curr. Therapeut.* 22:51-56.

Grundy, J. H. 1979. *Medical Zoology for Travellers.* 3rd ed. Chilbolton: Noble.

Haegi, L. 1981. Caught in the drift. *Aust. Nat. Hist.* 20:211-15.

Hairston, N. G., and B. De Meillon. 1968. On the inefficiency of transmission of *Wuchereria bancrofti* from mosquito to human host. *Bull. Wld Hlth Org.* 38:935-41.

Harden, B. 1981. A look at the dingo. *Aust. Nat. Hist.* 20:191-94.

Helliwell, C. J. V., and A. C. Turner. 1980. Imported disease at point of entry. *Practitioner.* 224:793-96.

Holland, E. P., and E. A. Woodward. 1924. A case of bilharziasis endemic in Australia. *Med. J. Aust.* (2):606.

Juranek, D. D. 1977. Epidemiologic investigations of pediculosis capitis in school children. In *Scabies and Pediculosis,* ed. M. Orkin, H. I. Maibach, L. C. Parish, and R. M. Schwartzman, 168-73. Philadelphia: Lippincott.

Kanamitsu, M., K. Taniguchi, S. Urasawa, T. Ogata, Y. Wada, and J. S. Saroso. 1979. Geographic distribution of arbovirus antibodies in indigenous human populations in the Indo-Australian archipelago. *Amer. J. trop. med. Hyg.* 28:351-63.

Kiss, C. 1967. Mystery at Port Hacking—more on smallpox.

Mankind 6:432-33.

Lewis, D. 1980. Navigators of the narrow seas. *Hemisphere* 24:122-27.

Mackerras, M. J. 1958. The decline of filariasis in Queensland. *Med. J. Aust.* (1):702-4.

Maegraith, B. 1971. *Imported Diseases in Europe.* Basle: CIBA-GEIGY.

Martin, S. K., L. H. Miller, D. Alling, V. C. Okoye, G. J. F. Esan, B. O. Osumkoyo, and M. Deane. 1979. Severe malaria and glucose-6-phosphate-dehydrogenase deficiency: A reappraisal of the malaria/G-6-P.D. hypothesis. *Lancet* (1):524-26.

McWhee, D. J., and T. R. Jagger. 1921. Bilharziosis in Western Australia. *Med. J. Aust.* (2):217-19.

Meier-Brook, C. 1975. A snail intermediate host of *Schistosoma mansoni* introduced to Hong Kong. *WHO/SCHISTO/75.37.* Mimeographed.

Moddie, P. M. 1977. Medical aspects of aboriginal health. *Aust. Fam. Physician* 6:1309-1317.

Mudge, P. 1982. Clinical and epidemiological features of epidemic polyarthritis in Australia. Unpublished monograph.

Murray, P. 1980. A vigorous and agreeable people. *Aust. Nat. Hist.* 20:35-38.

Newsome, A. E. 1982. The dingo. *Australia's Wildlife Heritage* 4, Part 31:1953-1961.

Ottesen, E. A. 1980. The clinical spectrum of lymphatic filariasis and its immunological determinants. *WHO/FIL/80.160.* Mimeographed.

Radford, A. 1978. Protection against infectious diseases—advice to travellers. *Med. Aust.* 2:141-44.

Rosen, L., D. J. Gubler, and P. H. Bennett. 1981. Epidemic polyarthritis (Ross River) virus infection in the Cook Islands. *Amer. J. trop. Med. Hyg.* 30:1294-1302.

Rutter, J. F. 1977. Travelling. *Aust. Fam. Physician* 6:1596-1601.

Ryan, L. 1981. *The Aboriginal Tasmanians.* St. Lucia: Univ. Queensland Press.

Sandison, T. 1980. Treponemal infections in pre-European contact exhumed Australian Aboriginal skeletons. *3rd Europ. Mtg. Palaeopathol. Assoc.*, Caen, France.

Tesh, R. B., R. G. McLean, D. A. Shroyer, C. H. Calisher, and L. Rosen. 1981. Ross River virus (Togaviridae: *Alphavirus*) infection (epidemic polyarthritis) in American Samoa. *Trans. roy. Soc. trop. Med. Hyg.* 75:426-31.

Thompson, R. C. A., and L. M. Kumaratilake. 1982. Intraspecific variation in *Echinococcus granulosus*: The

Australian situation and perspectives for the future. *Trans. roy. Soc. trop. Med. Hyg.* 76:13-16.

Tobias, P. V. 1974. An anthropologist looks at malaria. *S. Afr. Med. J.* 48:1124-27.

Walker, J. 1978. The finding of *Biomphalaria straminea* amongst fish imported into Australia. *WHO/SCHISTO/ 78.46.* Mimeographed.

Walker, A. C., and S. P. Bellmaine. 1975. Severe alimentary bleeding associated with hookworm infestation in aboriginal infants. *Med. J. Aust.* (1):751-52.

Walker, P. J., J. F. Douglas, J. R. Murray, I. D. Fanning, and P. Mottram. 1982. Dengue outbreak, Thursday Island. *Communicable Dis. Intell.* 82/4. Woden: Aust. Dept Hlth.

Waterhouse, D. F. 1982. Bushflies. *Australia's Wildlife Heritage* 4. Part 30:1906-1911.

Webb, R. C. 1978. Problems of infections relating to international travel. *Aust. Fam. Physician* 7:1370-84.

Weller, P. F., E. A. Ottesen, L. Heck, T. Tere, and F. Neva. 1982. Endemic filariasis on a Pacific Island. I. Clinical, epidemiological and parasitologic aspects. *Amer. J. trop. Med. Hyg.* 31:942-52.

West, J. 1852. *The History of Tasmania.* [Ed. A. Shaw, London: Angus and Robertson. 1981 Reprint.]

Woodruff, A. W. 1978. Airline imported diseases: A new community hazard. *J. roy. Coll. Physicians* 12:323-28.

Woodruff, A. W., and V. E. Ansdell. 1977. Le Dantec virus infection in a patient who had not been to West Africa. *Brit. Med. J.* (2):1632-1633.

Wright, F. J. 1971. Tropical disease and general medicine. *Scot. Med. J.* 16:209-14.

Zuidema, P. J. 1975. Tropical diseases in Europe. *J. roy. Coll. Physicians* 10:67-71.

Chapter 11

On the Spread of Ross River Virus in the Islands of the South Pacific

J. A. R. Miles

INTRODUCTION*

In 1928 Nimmo, doctor to the small town and rural community of Narrandera (34.45°S 146.33°E) in southern New
South Wales (NSW), Australia, described an epidemic of
polyarthritis in which some of the patients had a characteristic rash. He noted that there were many relapses in
an epidemic with over 100 cases. He suggested that this
might be due to bites of "stinging flies" but thought that
mosquitoes could be ruled out as vectors. Edwards (1928)
reported seeing six similar cases in Hay, NSW (34.30°S
144.51°E) and suggested that they were dengue, although
he failed to find *Aedes aegypti* in the area. Nimmo re-
futed this, pointing out that E. W. Ferguson had not found
A. aegypti so far south as latitude 34°S and that the
1926-27 dengue epidemic had stopped at 32°S. Nimmo's was
the first clear account of the syndrome of epidemic polyarthritis and rash, which, until very recently, had only
been recognized in Australia.

During World War II Australia moved substantial numbers
of troops to the far north of the country at the time when
the Japanese were advancing rapidly southwards. It was in
this period that the classical description of the above

*This work was supported by the Medical Research
Council of New Zealand and the Wellcome Trust.

disease was given (Halliday and Horan 1943) from an epidemic in soldiers stationed in the Northern Territory (NT). In the following year Harris (1944) reported another epidemic in the same area. From that time on, numerous small epidemics were recorded, and it has become clear that the disease occurs in all states of Australia and that, in that country, it is mainly a rural disease.

Shope and Anderson (1960) studied an unusually large epidemic occurring in the Murray Valley region of southeastern Australia in the late summer of 1956. They found that 6 of 16 paired sera from cases had rising titres of antibody against certain alphaviruses, particularly Bebaru (MM 2354). In 1959 a further alphavirus belonging to the same subgroup as Bebaru was isolated from *Aedes* (*Ochlerotatus*) *vigilax* near Townsville in northern Queensland and was named Ross River virus (RRV) (Doherty et al. 1963). They also showed that six patients who had had an attack of polyarthritis and rash had much higher titres of antibody against RRV than against Bebaru, Getah, or Sindbis. Although the virus could not be isolated from typical cases, accumulated evidence made it clear that RRV was the causative virus of epidemic polyarthritis and rash (Doherty et al. 1964, 1966). The only isolation of RRV from human material in Australia was from the blood of a child with a nonspecific fever (Doherty et al. 1972).

Tesh et al. (1975) studied the distribution and prevalence of alphavirus neutralizing antibodies in Southeast Asia and the Pacific. Apart from one serum from Vietnam that had a higher titre against Bebaru, the only areas where RRV antibodies were detected were the Moluccas in Indonesia, where 3 of 121 sera were positive; New Guinea, where 222 of 647 in West Irian and 204 of 604 in PNG were positive; and the western and central Solomon Islands. They only found 1 of 68 sera from Guadalcanal positive (our unpublished data showed a higher positive rate from there). Their data and our own study failed to record antibody in sera from the eastern Solomons or from Vanuatu. At that time, they found no positive sera in collections from New Caledonia, Samoa, or Palau; and our collections of Rarotonga sera were all negative. Weber, Appel, and Raymond (1946) reported two small outbreaks of a disease characterized by fever, rash, and arthritis in American troops in Biak, West Irian, and on Bougainville during World War II. Except for their emphasis on fever (which is not usual in RRV infections), these could well have been due to this virus rather than Chikungunya, which has not been found so far east. Thus, although there was no unequivocal evidence of clinical disease outside Australia, there was evidence that the virus had been in the Moluccas and Solomon Islands and that it was endemic throughout the island of New Guinea, but none of it having been present in Pacific islands further to the east.

RESERVOIR HOSTS AND VECTORS IN AUSTRALIA

Doherty and his colleagues in Queensland (1966, 1971) studied sera from man and other animals for antibodies to alphaviruses. The 1966 paper showed that there was an interesting contrast between RRV and Sindbis viruses. Only 1 out of 145 native birds had RRV antibodies, while 12 of 152 had antibodies to Sindbis. Among mammals, 54 of 97 Macropodidae (55.7%) and 63 of 148 domestic mammals (42.6%) had RRV antibodies, while only 4% of Macropodidae and 10.5% of domestic mammals had Sindbis antibodies. Rodents and small marsupials had little antibody against either virus. The 1971 paper added to the evidence that Macropodidae might be important reservoir hosts of RRV and reported isolation of virus from *Wallabia agilis* and from a second species of mosquito, *Culex (C.) annulirostris*. Whitehead (1969) studied viraemia produced by RRV in a variety of animals in the laboratory. He found viraemia in rabbits, rats, bandicoots, marsupial mice, and day old chicks, but not in adult fowls or pigeons, thus adding to the evidence that mammals are more important hosts of RRV than birds.

Aedes vigilax and *C. annulirostris* are, from epidemiological considerations, regarded as the most important vectors in Australia. The virus has also been isolated in that country from *Aedes normanensis, A. theobaldi, Anopheles amictus, Mansonia (Mansonioides) uniformis,* and *Mansonia (Coquillettidia) linealis* (Doherty 1977; Gard, Marshall, and Woodroofe 1973; Marshall 1979).

Most of the earlier work on RRV had been done in Queensland on material from that state, although epidemics of polyarthritis and rash had been reported from all states except Tasmania. In 1965 cases were found on the Port Stephens peninsula. These were shown to occur regularly every year and it was found that antibodies were common in man in the central coastal region of NSW (Clarke, Marshall, and Gard 1973). Woodroofe, Marshall, and Taylor (1977) showed that these strains differed immunologically from Queensland strains. Recently Munday (1981) has shown that a high proportion of Tasmanian marsupials, including small carnivorous species, have RRV antibodies; and three human cases of disease due to the virus have been proven in that state.

Thus Australian data indicate that RRV is a virus of mammals whose reservoir may be in marsupials; that in that country the main vectors are *Aedes vigilax* and *Culex annulirostris,* but that a variety of both culicine and anopheline mosquitoes can be infected in nature; and that the virus is endemic from New Guinea in the north to Tasmania in the south.

FIJI EPIDEMIC

Late in April 1979, a doctor in Nadi on the west side of the main Fiji island—Viti Levu—reported eight cases of a syndrome with polyarthritis and rash occurring in his area close to Nadi International Airport. Cases were not reported elsewhere for about ten days, when they began to appear more widely around the western side of Viti Levu and rapidly spread throughout the main islands of the group to give an estimated 50,000 clinical cases; and judging from serological studies, there were more than 300,000 human infections in an island group with a population of 630,000 (Aaskov et al. 1981).

Two isolations of virus were made early in the epidemic by intracerebral inoculation into suckling mice of human blood taken in the first twenty-four hours of the disease. With the help of antisera supplied by the Queensland Institute of Medical Research (QIMR), we were able to identify them rapidly as identical with or very closely related to RRV. More thorough later studies showed them to be indistinguishable from Queensland strains.

At the time of the epidemic, all of nine dog sera from Suva and all of fourteen goat sera from Bua in Western Vanua Levu contained antibodies. In August 1979, in southeastern Viti Levu, 8 of 17 pigs, 6 of 10 bovine, and 1 of 3 feline sera were positive above 1 : 10 by haemagglutination inhibition and were confirmed by a neutralization test. None of 10 fowl sera from a location where human infections were numerous was positive. Over 100 animal sera from before the epidemic were tested at QIMR, and the only positive was one cow giving a titre 1 : 80 by H.I. (Aaskov, personal communication). A further 25 sera collected in March 1978 were tested in Suva, including 12 more cattle from the same herd as the positive. All were negative.

Pig sera from the Suva area continued to be tested by neutralization test in Fiji and New Zealand, and all batches contained positives up to February 1981, when 10 of 33 were positive. Ninety sera from young pigs collected in late March were all negative, as were pig sera collected later in 1981 (Table 11-1).

Table 11-1. RRV Neutralization by Pig Bloods early in 1981 (Suva area).

Blood collected	Locality	No. tested	No. positive
January 1981	Colo-i-Suva	14	2
January 1981	Naboro	13	3
February 1981	Naboro	9	3
February 1981	Sawani	24	7
March 1981	All localities	90	0

Several rat and mongoose sera collected early in 1980 gave a positive complement fixation test against RRV, but none neutralized the virus. It is likely that this was due to a nonspecific complement fixing substance.

The epidemic on Viti Levu reached its peak in late May and early June and then spread to Vanua Levu and other of the larger islands. By September 1979, few cases were being reported. No clinical cases were reported from the Lau Islands to eastward, but while our library of pre-epidemic sera all proved negative, 90% of over 700 sera collected in December 1980 had neutralizing antibodies (Austin and Maguire 1982). Laboratory-proven human cases continued in the Suva area until September 1980, and virus was isolated from two cases from Labasa on Vanua Levu that had been diagnosed as dengue in January 1981 (Table 11-2).

FURTHER SPREAD

In August 1979 the disease spread to American Samoa, where Dr. Tesh (Tesh et al. 1981) isolated virus from human blood and estimated that about half the population had been affected. No virological investigations were

Table 11-2. Tests on human material 1980-81.

Date	No. sera*	H.I.	Neutralization	Isolation	Location origin of sera
1980					
January	9	5	--**	--	SE Viti Levu
February	29	5	--	--	SE Viti Levu
March	92	2	--	--	SE Viti Levu
April	53	2	19	--	SE Viti Levu
May	123	--	15	--	SE Viti Levu
June	1	1	--	--	SE Viti Levu
July	9	1	--	--	SE Viti Levu
August	4	1	--	--	SE Viti Levu
September	17	1	--	--	SE Viti Levu
October	31	0	--	--	SE Viti Levu
November	24	0	--	--	SE Viti Levu
December	13	0	--	--	SE Viti Levu
1981					
January	45	0	--	2	Serology⁻ SE Viti Levu Isolation⁻ Labasa, Vanua Levu
February	17	0	--	--	--

*All serology on paired sera, positive showing a four-fold or greater rising titre.
 **Test not performed.

214

carried out in Western Samoa until April 1980, when only evidence of current dengue was obtained. However, sera did contain antibody against RRV, and some patients described two painful attacks within a few months, one with and one without small-joint involvement. It appears likely that a relatively small RRV outbreak did occur there concurrently with dengue.

In February 1980 a brisk epidemic of polyarthritis and rash due to RRV occurred on Rarotonga in the Cook Islands, where a large number of isolations from human blood were made using C6/36 mosquito cells (Rosen, Gubler, and Bennett 1981).

In November 1979 the disease spread to Wallis and Futuna Islands and then to New Caledonia. Dr. Fauran made isolations from human blood from all these islands. Dr. Fauran's strains were indistinguishable from the 1979 Fiji strains.

Human pre-epidemic sera from Fiji were tested by two groups. At QIMR 225 sera were tested by H.I., and thirty gave a titre of 1 : 20 or higher. Some were confirmed by neutralization. In Dunedin, using the neutralization test, two positives were found among 703 sera. The Queensland results did not show any increase in antibody rate with age and suggested the possibility of a single small invasion by a virus related to RRV within the previous three to four years (Aaskov et al. 1981). The Dunedin results indicated that if this was due to RRV, the outbreak did not spread widely.

VECTORS

When the Fiji epidemic started, there were unusually large numbers of *Aedes vigilax* in the western coastal regions of Viti Levu and they may well have been responsible for early high infection rate. *Culex annulirostris* is widespread in Fiji but is not usually present in very large numbers. In most of the other island groups affected, *A. vigilax* is absent. Even in Fiji, numerous infections occurred in areas where both are absent. Therefore, other vectors must be involved. *Aedes aegypti* has always been known to be susceptible and could be important in Fiji. However, the most likely candidate to be important in all the island groups involved except New Caledonia is *A. polynesiensis* (Tables 11-3 and 11-4).

The Fiji strain of this member of the subgenus *Stegomyia* can be infected with a rather smaller dose of virus than Fiji strains of either *A. aegypti* or *C. annulirostris* and is an

Table 11-3. Infection of mosquito species with RRV.

Species	Infected in field	By feeding	Experimental transmission	Efficiency
Aedes vexans	-	+	+	low
Aedes australis	-	+	+	?
Aedes oceanicus	-	+	NT	?
Aedes notoscriptus	-	+	NT	?
Aedes vigilax	+	+	+	high
Aedes aegypti	-	+	+	fair to high
Aedes albopictus	-	+	+	high
Aedes polynesiensis	+	+	+	high
Aedes pseudoscutellaris	-	+	+	low
Aedes tongae tabu	-	+	+	low
Aedes funereus	-	+	NT	?
Aedes normanensis	+	NT	NT	?
Aedes theobaldi	+	NT	NT	?
Anopheles amictus	+	NT	NT	?
Culex annulirostris	+	+	+	fair to high
Culex quinquefasciatus	-	±		negligible
Culex sitiens	-	+	NT	?
Mansonia linealis	+	+	NT	?
Mansonia uniformis	+	+	NT	?

Data from Kay et al. 1982   NT = not tested

Table 11-4. Distribution of main vectors of RRV in the affected South Pacific island groups.

Vector	Island groups
Aedes aegypti	Fiji, New Caledonia, Samoa, Wallis
Aedes polynesiensis	Cook Islands, Fiji, Samoa, Wallis
Aedes vigilax	Fiji, New Caledonia
Culex annulirostris	Cook Islands, Fiji, New Caledonia, Samoa, Wallis

effective transmitter. On Rarotonga where *A. aegypti* is not present, it was almost certainly the main vector. In Fiji another Scutellaris Subgroup *Stegomyia, A. pseudoscutellaris,* is endemic, but this is, in the laboratory, a relatively poor vector.

EXPERIMENTAL VECTOR STUDIES

The large number of species of mosquito from which the virus has been isolated in Australia indicates that it has a wide range of potential vectors, and this may well have increased its ability to spread through the islands of the South Pacific. The available evidence has recently been summarized (Kay, Miles, Gubler, and Mitchell 1982). Sixteen species of mosquito have been tested in the laboratory and all of them have proved to be able to be infected in some experiments, and 3 species that have not been tested experimentally have been found infected in the field. Among 8 strains of *C. quinquefasciatus* tested, 3 proved refractory and a low proportion of individuals in the others were infected. The remaining species could all be infected by biting (Table 11-3).

In Australia epidemiological data suggest that the important vectors are *A. vigilax* and *C. annulirostris,* whose efficiency is rated in the laboratory as high and fair to high. Among the Pacific islands infected in 1979-80, *A. vigilax* is only found in New Caledonia and Fiji. It may have been important in establishing the infection on the west side of Viti Levu where the numbers of this mosquito were unusually large at the time when the epidemic started, but it is not present in the islands further to the east. *C. annulirostris* is present in all the infected island groups, but it is not as numerous there as in Australia and is unlikely to have been very important (Table 11-4). *A. aegypti* has fair to high vector efficiency; it is present in the urban centers where infection occurred except for the Cook Islands where, although it was present in 1954, it has completely disappeared. Three thorough recent studies have failed to locate it. Three studies have found *A. polynesiensis* to be an efficient vector, and both Gubler (1981) and I found it more susceptible than *A. aegypti*. It is present on all infected islands except New Caledonia. It was almost certainly the main vector on Rarotonga in the Cook Islands and on many of the smaller islands in the Fiji group. *A. albopictus* is an efficient vector in the laboratory, but it is not present in any of the South Pacific islands E of the Solomons (p. 93). Thus, it cannot have been involved. *A. vexans, A. oceanicus, A. pseudoscutellaris,* and *A. tongae tabu* have not been found to be efficient vectors and could only have played a minor role in the epidemic on the islands where they are present.

The situation in New Zealand presents an interesting contrast. Many cases of the disease occurred in people returning from Fiji. Two introduced species of mosquito in New Zealand have been shown to be susceptible to infection by feeding. *A. australis* is a strictly coastal mosquito breeding in brackish water and is unlikely to be important. *A. notoscriptus* is a peridomestic species present in large numbers in parts of the north of the country. If this were an efficient vector, we would have expected indigenous cases, but, despite wide publicity and requests in the medical press for specimens from possible cases, no indigenous infections were detected. It is probable that no common New Zealand mosquito is an efficient vector of RRV.

REASONS FOR THE SPREAD TO THE SOUTH PACIFIC

Arrival in Fiji

The evidence presented suggests that the virus had reached Fiji on at least one occasion before 1979. It seems likely that on the earlier occasion, which serological data indicate to have been 1975 or 1976, the virus infected a limited number of people and died out, although it is possible that it had survived either in man or other mammals until suitable conditions arose for an epidemic in 1979. However, the evidence that it has now failed to survive beyond the beginning of 1981, the location of the early cases in the tourist area around the Nadi International Airport, the identity of the virus strains with the classical Queensland strains, and the fact that large numbers of cases were occurring in Australia at the time, make it more likely that the virus arrived either in a human incubating the disease or in a mosquito that had escaped aircraft disinsection. The unusually large population of an efficient vector, *A. vigilax,* in the locality at that time assisted the establishment of the virus.

Were There Changes in the Virus?

The spectacular spread of the virus in the South Pacific islands and the very high morbidity were certainly partly due to the lack of past experience of the virus in the populations exposed, but a change in the virus giving enhanced transmissibility would have caused it to spread more quickly.

There are two important differences between the usual picture in Australia and that recently seen in the South Pacific. In Australia the virus has only once been isolated from human blood. This was from a child with a nonspecific fever (Doherty, Carley, and Best 1972). No isolations have been made in Australia from typical cases of polyarthritis and rash, but in the Pacific isolating virus from the blood of typical cases has proved easy. Secondly, in Australia this has been predominantly a rural disease in which man is likely to have been infected casually through involvement in a cycle between other mammals and vector mosquitoes. In the islands there have been large urban outbreaks with the character of a man-mosquito-man cycle. Such a cycle would be likely to be established if there were a change in the virus giving a higher titre and/or more prolonged viraemia.

These probable changes may have been present in the virus when it arrived from Australia, but it is at least equally likely that rapid passage in a highly susceptible population allowed the development of a strain giving increased viraemia and consequently increased transmissibility. It is also possible that the new vectors that were important in Fiji and most, if not all, the other island groups affected, were two members of the subgenus *Stegomyia, Aedes aegypti,* and *A. polynesiensis;* selected strains of virus giving high blood titres and long-lasting viraemia.

Fraser and Cunningham (1980) in Australia reported a minimum incubation period of 7-9 days and suggested that an incubation of less than 5 days indicated a different diagnosis. Rosen, Gubler, and Bennett (1981) found a maximum incubation of 3-4 days in recent arrivals in Rarotonga. This also suggests more rapid virus multiplication leading to early symptomatic illness.

Method of Spread Through the Islands

The most probable way in which RRV reached Fiji was in a human—incubating the disease—who infected local mosquitoes at a time in 1979 when *A. vigilax,* an efficient vector, was in unusually large numbers in the area of Viti Levu around Nadi International Airport. It is now generally believed that frequent rapid air transport is often responsible for the spread of human pathogens and that man himself is the most common carrier. However, other possibilities need to be considered and the arrival of an infected mosquito may have initiated the Fiji epidemic.

Mosquitoes can be transported by plane or on prevailing winds. Viable mosquitoes have been recovered from the upper atmosphere, but they do not survive actual freezing. The main RRV vector species are killed in less than five minutes at -10°C. However, it is theoretically possible that infected mosquitoes from Queensland could reach Fiji in this way. It is just possible that they could have spread from Fiji to Samoa and then on to the Cook Islands in the same way, although the chance of three such events occurring in a 10-month period is astronomically small. The reverse movement from Samoa to Wallis and then to New Caledonia during the same period is quite beyond credibility. The possibility of transfer of mosquitoes by plane remains, but the island governments generally attempt to exclude vectors by disinsecting incoming aircraft, and the chance of six such events occurring with infected mosquitoes in a single 10-month period is again astronomically small.

Migrating birds should be mentioned, although all the evidence indicates that RRV has a mammalian rather than an avian reservoir. However, since the migration routes of birds at the relevant times of year are incompatible with such a theory, it can be discarded. Spread by mammals other than man is impossible on such a scale in so short a time period.

The theory of human transportation is then by far the most likely. Many humans reached New Zealand from Fiji who were incubating the disease. More than 30 were definitely diagnosed serologically and at least as many more clinical cases were not investigated in the laboratory. Had efficient vectors been present, spread would inevitably have occurred. All the island groups involved have frequent air connections and most have scheduled air services with substantial movements of tourists. Evidence has been presented that the strains responsible for this spread were unusual in the ease with which they could be isolated from human blood, and it is highly probable that infection of mosquitoes from man could easily have occurred. The available evidence combines to give a high probability that rapid human transportation was responsible for this spread.

IS RRV NOW ENZOOTIC IN THE
SOUTH PACIFIC ISLANDS?

Investigation of the amount of infection in domestic mammals in Fiji at the time of the epidemic and shortly afterwards had shown that a high proportion were infected. It was thought that with a large population of rats of the genus *Rattus* and a substantial population of domestic pigs, most of which are slaughtered at about 6 months of age, Fiji, in spite of the very high level of human immunity, might be able to maintain RRV as an enzootic infection. It was thought that if the virus could not survive in Fiji, it was very unlikely that it would survive in smaller islands with smaller mammalian populations. No human cases have been diagnosed in Fiji since January 1981, and the last positive porcine sera were in the batch collected in February 1981. No cases have been reported from any other island group since 1980. It therefore appears that the virus has failed to establish.

It does then seem likely that, although RRV has a very broad range of potential vectors and can infect and produce viraemia in a wide range of mammals, it has more specific essential reservoir hosts that are present in Australia and New Guinea but not in the South Pacific islands. From Australian data, marsupials would seem the most likely group. In Tasmania, where only three human cases of RRV infection have been proven, Munday (1981) found antibodies in 56% of marsupial sera, and it is likely that the virus is highly enzootic. Much more work is needed to identify main reservoir hosts, but there are some indications. In Queensland Macropodidae seem the most likely, but in Tasmania small carnivorous marsupials appear to be infected equally often.

WHAT IS LIKELY TO BE THE FUTURE OF RRV IN THE SOUTH PACIFIC?

The high level of human immunity to RRV in the islands affected in the recent epidemics is such that no new introduction of virus in the next few years would be likely to lead to any substantial spread. Since children under the age of 10 years rarely develop typical symptoms, no characteristic epidemic is likely for at least 10 years; and a large epidemic is improbable for the next 25 years.

Notifications of RRV infection have increased in Australia over the last four years. If this is a true increase, and provided tourism between Australia and the South Pacific is maintained, it is probable that repeated introductions of the virus will occur. In this event future large epidemics in those islands affected in 1979-80 are improbable, but similar outbreaks may occur in Vanuatu, the eastern Solomon Islands, Tonga, French Polynesia, and other groups not yet involved.

REFERENCES

Aaskov, J. G., J. U. Mataika, G. W. Lawrence, V. Rabukawaqa, M. M. Tucker, J. A. R. Miles, and D. A. Daglish. 1981. An epidemic of Ross River virus infection in Fiji, 1979. *Amer. J. trop. Med. Hyg.* 30:1053-1059.

Austin, F. J., and T. Maguire. 1982. In *Viral Diseases in Southeast Asia and the Western Pacific.* (ed. J. MacKenzie) London and New York: Academic Press.

Clarke, J. A., I. D. Marshall, and G. Gard. 1973. Annually recurrent epidemic polyarthritis and Ross River activity in a coastal area of New South Wales: I. Occurrence of the disease. *Amer. J. trop. Med. Hyg.* 22:543-50.

Doherty, R. L. 1977. Arthropod-borne viruses in Australia, 1973-76. *Aust. J. exp. Biol. med. Sci.* 55:103-30.

Doherty, R. L., J. G. Carley, and J. C. Best. 1972. Isolation of Ross River virus from man. *Med. J. Aust.* 1:1083-1084.

Doherty, R. L., B. M. Gorman, R. H. Whitehead, and J. G. Carley. 1964. Studies of epidemic polyarthritis. The significance of three group A arboviruses isolated from mosquitoes in Queensland. *Aust. Ann. Med.* 13:322-37.

————. 1966. Studies of arthropod-borne virus infections in Queensland. V. Survey of antibodies to group A arboviruses in man and other animals. *Aust. J. exp. Biol. med. Sci.* 44:365-78.

Doherty, R. L., H. A. Standfast, R. Domrow, E. J. Wetters, R. J. Whitehead, and J. G. Carley. 1971. Studies of the epidemiology of arthropod-borne virus infestions at Mitchell River Mission, Cape York Peninsula, North Queensland: IV. Arbovirus infections of mosquitoes and mammals: 1967-69. *Trans roy. soc. trop. Med. Hyg.* 65:504-13.

Doherty, R. L., R. H. Whitehead, B. M. Gorman, and A. K. O'Gower. 1963. The isolation of a third group A arbovirus in Australia, with preliminary observations on its relationship to epidemic polyarthritis. *Aust. J. Sci.* 26:183-84.

Edwards, A. M. 1928. An unusual epidemic. *Med. J. Aust.* 1:664-65.

Fraser, J. R. E., and A. L. Cunningham. 1980. Incubation time of epidemic polyarthritis. *Med. J. Aust.* 1:550-51.

Gard, G., I. D. Marshall, and G. M. Woodroofe. 1973. Annually recurrent epidemic polyarthritis and Ross River virus activity in a coastal area of New South Wales. 2. Mosquitoes, viruses and wildlife. *Amer. J. trop. Med. Hyg.* 22:551-60.

Gubler, D. J. 1981. Transmission of Ross River virus by *Aedes polynesiensis* and *Aedes aegypti*. *Amer. J. trop. Med. Hyg.* 30:1303-1306.

Halliday, J. H., and J. P. Horan. 1943. An epidemic of polyarthritis in the Northern Territory. *Med. J. Aust.* 2:293-95.

Harris, L. 1944. Polyarthritis in the Northern Territory. *Med. J. Aust.* 1:546.

Kay, B. H., J. A. R. Miles, D. J. Gubler, and G. J. Mitchell. 1982. In *Viral Diseases in Southeast Asia and the Western Pacific* (ed. J. MacKenzie). London and New York: Academic Press.

Marshall, I. D. 1979. In *Arbovirus Research in Australia* (eds. T. D. St. George and E. L. French). Proc. Second Symp., CSIRQ-QIMR. p. 47.

Munday, B. 1981. Ross River virus in Tasmania. Canberra: *Communicable Dis. Intell.* Woden: Aust. Dept Hlth.

Nimmo, J. R. 1928. An unusual epidemic. *Med. J. Aust.* 1:549-50.

Rosen, L., D. J. Gubler, and P. H. Bennett. 1981. Epidemic polyarthritis (Ross River) virus infections in the Cook Islands. *Amer. J. trop. Med. Hyg.*

30:1294-1302.

Shope, R. E., and S. G. Anderson. 1960. The virus aetiology of epidemic exanthem and polyarthritis. *Med. J. Aust.* 1:156-58.

Tesh, R. B., D. C. Gajdusek, R. M. Garruto, J. H. Cross, and L. Rosen. 1975. The distribution and prevalence of group A arbovirus neutralising antibodies among human populations in Southeast Asia and the Pacific islands. *Amer. J. trop. Med. Hyg.* 24:664-75.

Tesh, R. B., R. G. McLean, D. A. Shroyer, C. H. Calisher, and L. Rosen. 1981. Ross River virus (Togaviridae: *Alphavirus*) infection (epidemic polyarthritis) in American Samoa. *Trans. roy. Soc. trop. Med. Hyg.* 75:426-31.

Weber, F. C., T. W. Appel, and R. W. Raymond. 1946. A mild exanthematous disease seen in the Schouten Islands. *Amer. J. trop. Med.* 26:489-95.

Whitehead, R. H. 1969. Experimental infection of vertebrates with Ross River and Sindbis viruses, two group A arboviruses isolated in Australia. *Aust. J. exp. Biol. med. Sci.* 47:11-15.

Woodroofe, G., I. D. Marshall, and W. P. Taylor. 1977. Antigenically distinct strains of Ross River virus from North Queensland and coastal New South Wales. *Aust. J. exp. Biol. med. Sci.* 55:79-88.

Chapter 12

Transport Services as an Aid to Insect Dispersal in the South Pacific

P. S. Dale and P. A. Maddison

INTRODUCTION

After more than two centuries of European exploration of the South Pacific, the written record of its insect fauna has remained fragmentary and the task of interpreting patterns of insect distribution beset with many hazards. Recently, however, a carefully planned survey of plant pests and diseases was conducted over much of the area by a team sponsored jointly by UNDP/FAO and the South Pacific Bureau for Economic Co-operation. For the islands and groups covered, it is unlikely that many of the more common plant pest species have gone unrecorded. Perhaps for the first time we are now in a position to look at the phytophagous insect fauna of the South Pacific with some degree of confidence. If we confine our attention to the more obvious and visible pests of the better-known crop plants, we may be able to draw conclusions that have some validity. It is still necessary, however, to tread warily and to resist the temptation to regard the absence of evidence as being evidence of a pest's absence.

In this chapter the known distribution of insect pests of some of the more ubiquitous food plants of the region is examined, unexpected presence or absence is noted, and an attempt is made to explain anomalous distribution.

METHODS OF DISPERSAL

The geographic range over which phytophagous insects can establish is, of course, related to their mobility and to the availability of suitable host plants. Insects that are capable of maintaining themselves aloft for long periods should be more widespread than those that cannot, and polyphagous insects will in general have a better chance of finding a host plant than those that are host-specific. Those whose host plants are ubiquitous should establish more widely than those whose hosts are restricted or scattered in their distribution.

The mobility of insects is achieved in various ways. Some Lepidoptera (particularly noctuids, sphingids, and nymphalids) are capable of long periods of sustained flight, and with favorable winds can cover transoceanic distances in excess of 2,000 km (Fox 1978; Wise 1968; Tindale 1981). Juvenile Coccoidea have the ability to float considerable distances on air currents with the aid of gossamer threads (Willard 1974), while small insects of many kinds are able to maintain themselves aloft in wind currents for long periods presumably by some combination of flying and floating. Numerous investigators have trapped such airborne insects, using nets attached to ships and aircraft (Gressitt and Nakata 1958; Gressitt et al. 1962; Gressitt and Yoshimoto 1964; Holzapfel and Perkins 1969; Johnston 1969; Wise 1971; Yoshimoto and Gressitt 1964), and although it has not always been possible to determine whether or not the insects were alive when captured, some at least have been known to survive journeys of several hundred kilometers. Lepidoptera, Homoptera, small Diptera, and Hymenoptera are among the insects most commonly captured over the Pacific.

Ocean currents and flotsam may account for the dispersal of certain kinds of insects (Wise 1971), though it is a means of transport better suited to xylophagous or saprophagous species than to recognized pests of food plants.

The dispersal of phytophagous insects can also be aided by man. Such aid may occasionally be intentional or even malicious, but is more often an inadvertent consequence of some other, unrelated human activity. Insects can be carried on or in produce that may be in transit as cargo, as luggage, or as food for consumption on the voyage. They can also be associated with plant material used as packing or packaging, or with seeds, tubers, and other plant parts intended for propagation. Some insects may be transported in conveyances or containers that they have entered casually, either as a result of being confused by bright light, seeking shelter from bright light, being attracted by odors from people or products, or being left behind from previous cargoes. Philanthropy has not infrequently provided the means of establishing insects in new locations when well-intentioned people have unwittingly introduced pest species along with soil, plants, or beneficial insects that they were bringing to those they believed to be in need of them.

Until the advent of steamship services, the spread of insects by human agency was limited by the infrequency of interisland travel, by the perishable nature of the host material carried, and by the slow speed and long duration of the voyage. Since then the establishment of regular steamship, motor vessel, and air services have done much to facilitate the movement of insect pests. It is only the establishment, in comparatively recent times, of effective quarantine systems that has enabled the problem to be brought under reasonable control. One way of assessing the effectiveness of routine quarantine practices is by considering some of the disasters that have occurred when routine procedures were not followed.

PLANT PESTS

The heterogeneity of the Pacific islands with respect to their topography and plant cover makes a comparison of their phytophagous insect faunas rather difficult. The following discussion is therefore confined to the pests of a few widely grown crops, and to some other insects whose host range is such as would give them an opportunity to establish on the majority of the islands under consideration.

Taro Pests

Taro—primarily *Colocasia esculenta* and *Cyrtosperma chamissonis*—is the most characteristic root crop in the South Pacific and occurs almost universally on those islands that have sufficient topsoil to support it. The edible tubers are commonly carried between islands as gifts or in commerce. Less commonly, the crown of the plant and surrounding leaf petioles, which serve as propagative material, are also transported, sometimes in large amounts as a disaster relief measure. The leaves, which are also used as food, are too perishable for journeys of long duration, but air transport has made the carriage of fresh leaves a practical proposition.

Insect pests of taro are shown in Table 12-1. Among the most widely distributed are the moths, *Spodoptera litura, Hippotion celerio,* and *Agrotis ipsilon aneituma.* All three have migratory habits and are capable of long transoceanic flights, under favorable conditions, in excess of 2,000 kilometers (Fox 1978). This ability may well have contributed to their wide distribution, but they are also attracted to lights, and they are not uncommonly found in cargo containers and the holds of ships and aircraft (Keall 1981). Larvae of *S. litura* may also burrow in leaf petioles of taro and could conceivably be carried with propagative material. This moth also has the habit of ovipositing on all manner of flat surfaces, including the exteriors of ships and aircraft, so this could provide it with yet another means of dispersal. Finally, all three moth species have alternative host plants with which they could conceivably be transported.

Aphis gossypii is also very widely distributed. Being parthenogenetic, it requires only a single individual to establish a new colony, so its dispersal by air currents and turbulence following cyclones is quite possible, though the fact that few other aphids have achieved such distribution would suggest other factors, such as its very wide host range, may be a contributing factor.

Tarophagus proserpina, a delphacid and a weak flier, oviposits in the petioles of taro and its eggs which take 8-9 days to hatch are probably often transported with propagative material on voyages of medium duration. The fact that it did not reach Hawaii until 1930 (Fullaway and Krauss 1945) suggests, however, that its spread through the South Pacific may well have had to wait for the advent of mechanized transport and regular shipping services before it could overcome the larger gaps between island groups.

At the other end of the scale, the coreid leaf-feeding bug *Brachylybas variegatus* shows how little distribution can be achieved by exclusively leaf-feeding species, even with human aid. The taro-whitefly *Bemisia tabaci* shows only a slightly broader distribution, much of it achieved in very recent times since air travel has made the carriage of fresh leaves in luggage a practicable possibility.

Of intermediate distribution are two species, *Adoretus versutus* and *Teleogryllus oceanicus,* which are not primarily pests of taro, but which are carried in commerce as casual passengers through their susceptibility to confusion by bright lights and their tendency to burrow in dark places when they alight. Ships and aircraft loading at night are likely to be invaded, and the insects can probably survive journeys of several days.

The root-burrowing weevil *Elytroteinus subtruncatus* must have achieved its spread by being transported with the tubers, but the scarab *Papuana hubneri,* whose adult tunnels in the tubers but which pupates in the soil, has not apparently been able to get much use from the tuber as a medium of transport. Its presence in Kiribati is said to result from an importation of soil for a mission garden.

The absence of specific taro pests from the Tokelau Islands is largely a reflection of the paucity of topsoil in which the crop can be grown. The few plants that are grown are cultivated in specially prepared compost pits (Hinckley 1969).

With the possible exception of the Lepidoptera, the pests of taro reveal, in their South Pacific distribution a good deal of evidence of human aid arising from man's close association with their host plant.

Pests of Sweet Potato

Sweet potato (*Ipomoea batatas*) is widely grown in the South Pacific, though it becomes less important as a food item east of Fiji. On the atolls its cultivation is limited by the lack of topsoil. However, a close relative, *Ipomoea pes-caprae,* is a common sand-binding plant of almost universal occurrence, so that even on those islands where sweet potato is not normally grown, there is suitable host material to support many of its pests. There is still some controversy about the means by which sweet potato came into the Pacific. Purseglove (1968, 79-81) and Yen (1974) present various aspects of the argument but do not consider that the aid of man need be invoked to account for its transfer from South America to Polynesia, preferring to believe that floating seed, possibly aided by driftwood, was the means by which it traveled. A consideration of the distribution of its insect pests would point in a different conclusion.

The tuber of the sweet potato differs as an article of commerce from the tuber of taro in two important ways. Properly cured, it has a much longer storage life and was probably a preferred article for victualing canoes for this reason. Secondly, it is not only the edible part of the plant but is also the source of propagative material or can itself be used as propagative material, so that unused victuals could, at the end of a voyage, be used to establish new crops. This method, rather than a purposeful attempt at plant introduction by transfer of rooted cuttings, seems more likely to be the manner in which sweet potato was first introduced into Polynesia. As the least edible tubers

Table 12-1. Insect Pests of Taro.

	Aust	PNG	Sol	Van	NC	Kir	Tuv	Fiji	Ton	Tok	Sam	Niue	Cook	Poly
COLEOPTERA														
Elytroteinus subtruncatus (Fairm.)								x	x		x	x	x	
Adoretus versutus Har.				x				x	x		x	x		
Papuana hubneri (Fairm.)	x	x				x								
HETEROPTERA														
Brachylybas variegatus Le Guill.								x	x					
HOMOPTERA														
Aphis gossypii Glover	x	x	x	x	x	x	x	x	x	x	x	x	x	x

230

Species	Aust	PNG	Sol	Van	NC	Kir	Tuv	Fiji	Ton	Tok	Sam	Niue	Cook	Poly
Bemisia tabaci (Genn.)	x	x		x	x	x	x	x			x		x	x
Tarophagus proserpina (Kirkaldy)	x	x	x					x	x		x	x	x	x
LEPIDOPTERA														
Agrotis ipsilon aneituma (Walk.)	x	x	x	x	x	x	x	x	x		x	x	x	x
Hippotion celerio (L.)	x	x	x	x	x	x	x	x	x	x	x	x	x	x
Spodoptera litura (Fab.)	x	x	x	x	x	x	x	x			x	x	x	x
ORTHOPTERA														
Teleogryllus oceanicus (Le Guill.)	x	x	x	x	x	x	x	x			x	x	x	x

231

Abbreviations: Aust/Australia; PNG/Papua New Guinea; Sol/Solomon Islands; Van/Vanuatu; NC/New Caledonia; Kir/Kiribati; Tuv/Tuvalu; Fiji/Fiji; Ton/Tonga; Tok/Tokelau Islands; Sam/Samoa; Niue/Niue; Cook/Cook Islands; Poly/French Polynesia.

would be the ones most likely to be available for propagation at the end of a long voyage, it is probably that this was also the method by which its most persistent pests were also transferred from their native environment.

Among the pests of sweet potato (Table 12-2), the polyphagous and migrant Lepidoptera show a similar ubiquity to that noticed when they were considered as pests of taro, except that there are now 6 species involved instead of only 3 species. Five of these species, *Agrius convolvuli, Hippotion celerio, Hymenia (Spoladea) recurvalis, Precis villida,* and *Spodoptera litura* have been recorded by Fox (1978) as more or less regular migrants from Australia to New Zealand. They are thus theoretically capable, given favorable winds, of crossing almost any of the ocean gaps that occur between Papua New Guinea and the Tuamotus. *Hippotion swinhoei* and *Aedia sericea* may be assumed to have a similar capability. Man may have contributed to their spread through transport of some of their alternative hosts, but his intervention does not seem necessary to explain current distribution.

Almost equally widespread, however, are the two weevils, *Cylas formicarius* and *Euscepes postfasciatus,* whose ability to cross oceans without human aid must be minimal. Capable of passing their complete life cycle within the confines of a single tuber, these inconspicuous burrowers are ideally adapted to occupy tubers during transit and to exploit the propagated plants when the tubers are set out in a new environment. Their apparent absence from parts of Melanesia probably reflects the paucity of collections from there, and their absence from New Zealand, where their host plant is an important commercial crop, is almost certainly due to their inability to survive temperate winter conditions. Their restricted range in South America reinforces this view (Kuschel personal communication).

The only other species with general distribution is *Nezara viridula.* With its limited flight capability, it could scarcely have achieved this spread without human aid, but its broad host range and its habit of depositing clusters of quite resistant eggs on them, give it many opportunities to exploit commercial transport. It was probably assisted by the trade in temperate-zone vegetables from Australia, for it did not reach New Zealand until 1944 (Cumber 1949).

Myzus persicae, which has a similarly broad host range, may well spread in a similar way. Its absence from Tonga and Samoa suggest that this aphid's ability to move on air currents is not great. Its actual distribution bears an interesting relation to shipping routes, mentioned again below.

The pyralid moth *Antiercta ornatalis* is another whose distribution seems to owe more to shipping services than to geographical proximity. Its absence from French Polynesia is perhaps more apparent than real.

The little bronze bug *Brachyplatys pacificus* has a similarly anomalous distribution, no doubt related to its abundance on weeds and to the readiness with which it attaches itself to anything that moves. It too will be considered again under "shipping services."

The leaf miners *Bedellia orchilella* (in Samoa and French Polynesia) and *B. somnulentella* (in Fiji)—the latter also occurs in New Zealand and Australia—have a distribution that is difficult to explain, but that is unlikely to have been achieved without human aid. The pupa (the resistant stage) is attached to the leaf and so there is an opportunity for transport on dead or wilted foliage.

In general, the widely distributed pests of sweet potato are the polyphagous migrant moths, the pests of the tuber, and the polyphagous foliar pests that have opportunities for transport on other products. The true foliar pests of sweet potato have the limited distribution one would expect to be associated with their limited opportunities for artificial transport.

Pests of Coconut

The coconut (*Cocos nucifera*) is one of the most characteristic plants of the South Pacific. There can scarcely be an island where it does not grow. For the insects that can survive on it, it provides an unparalleled opportunity for colonization. However, as it is invariably propagated from seed, and as the seed supports few of its pests (and these only for a limited time), traffic in seed nuts—whether by ocean currents or by artificial means—provides little assistance in transporting its insect fauna from one island to another. The commercially valuable kernel of the nut provides even less assistance, for it does not support any of the insect pests that attack the living palm. Though the coconut palm may have been taken originally by man to most of the places where we now find it, it would seem at first sight that most of the pests that now live on it must have made their own way there. However, the fronds of the coconut also have their uses to travelers, being used to make temporary baskets in which all manner of foodstuffs can be transported. They also form a ready conveyance for such associated insects as can withstand the rigors of the journey. Germinated nuts with young fronds are also

Table 12-2. Insect Pests of Sweet Potato.

	PNG	Sol	Van	NC	Kir	Tuv	Fiji	Wal	Tok	Sam	Ton	Niue	Cook	Poly
COLEOPTERA														
Cylas formicarius Fab.	x	x		x	x	x	x			x	x	x	x	x
Euscepes postfasciatus (Fairm.)	x			x	x	x	x	x		x	x	x	x	x
Metriona strigula (Montr.)										x				
DIPTERA														
Liriomyza sp. ? brassicae (Riley)							x							
HETEROPTERA														
Brachyplatys pacificus Dallas							x	x		x	x			
Nezara viridula (L.)	x			x	x		x			x	x	x	x	x

234

HOMOPTERA

Delphacodes
muirella Metcalf

Myzus persicae
(Sulz.)

THYSANOPTERA

Dendrothripoides
ipomoeae Bagn.

LEPIDOPTERA

Acrocercops
homalacta Meyr.

Acrocercops prosacta
Meyr.

Agrius convolvuli (L.)

Aedia sericea (Butl.)

Antiercta ornatalis
Duponchel

Table 12-2. Continued

	PNG	Sol	Van	NC	Kir	Tuv	Fiji	Wal	Tok	Sam	Ton	Niue	Cook	Poly
Bedellia orchilella Walshingham														x
Bedellia somnulentella (Zell.)							x			x				
Hippotion celerio (L.)	x	x	x	x	x	x	x			x	x	x	x	x
Hippotion swinhoei (Moore)	x	x	x	x		x	x		x	x	x	x	x	
Hymenia recurvalis (Fab.)	x	x	x	x	x	x	x	x	x	x	x	x	x	x
Myconita lipara Bradley							x							
Precis villida (Fab.)	x	x	x	x	x	x	x	x	x	x	x	x	x	x
Spodoptera litura (Fab.)	x	x	x	x	x	x	x	x		x	x	x	x	x

Abbreviations: PNG/Papua New Guinea; Sol/Solomon Islands; Van/Vanuatu; NC/New Caledonia; Kir/Kiribati; Tuv/Tuvalu; Fiji/Fiji; Wal/Wallis; Tok/Tokelau Islands; Sam/Samoa; Ton/Tonga; Niue/Niue; Cook/Cook Islands; Poly/French Polynesia.

236

sometimes carried from place to place as planting material, and occasionally potted palms are carried on ships as a form of decoration.

The distribution of pests of coconut is shown in Table 12-3. The flightless coconut stick insect *Graeffea crouanii* has a surprisingly widespread occurrence. Devoid of obvious aids to dispersal, it has, however, an egg that is remarkably resistant and that can remain viable for 2 to 3 months (Swaine 1971). These eggs often lodge in the bases of the palm leaflets, and it is presumably in this way that coconut-frond baskets have provided the means for their dispersal to almost every island group in the region (see Chapter 13).

The weevil *Diocalandra taitensis,* which breeds in dead and dying tissue at the frond bases, may have likewise survived in frond baskets: however, it is also associated with inflorescences and may have been carried with mature nuts. The other widespread weevil borer, *Rhabdoscelus obscurus,* probably achieved most of its dispersal within its more favored host—sugarcane (see Chapter 13).

The continuity of distribution of most of the other coconut pests is similarly related to their ability to survive in dead or dying fronds. Those with a resistant (pupal) form, such as *Agonoxena argaula* or *Tirathaba rufivena,* spread quite widely, while those more closely dependent on the living leaf tissue are more confined.

The coconut termite *Neotermes rainbowi* may well have attained its range without human aid, by utilizing drifting logs; but the fact that it does not infest coconuts on any of the major islands where it occurs seems to indicate that it drifted to the atolls of the Cook Islands and Tuvalu on some other kind of timber and adapted to coconut on arrival.

Nevertheless, the discontinuities in the distribution of coconut pests shown in Table 12-3 indicate that neither aids to artificial dispersal, nor the operation of natural forces, have succeeded in achieving for most pests of coconut the kind of ubiquity that the distribution of their host plant would allow.

Miscellaneous Plant Pests

Consideration of the distribution of pests of taro, sweet potato, and coconut has drawn attention to the importance of human agency in their dispersal, and also to the significance of a pest's ability to survive for considerable periods in or on the transportable portion of the host plant. Various other plant pests (Table 12-4) serve to emphasize these points.

Table 12-3. Insect Pests of Coconut.

	Aust	PNG	Sol	Van	NC	Kir	Tuv	Fiji	Wal	Tok	Sam	Ton	Niue	Cook	Poly	Haw
COLEOPTERA																
Brontispa longissima Gestro	x	x	x	x	x										x	
Diocalandra taitensis (Guér)		x		x	x	x		x	x	x	x	x	x	x	x	x
Oryctes rhinoceros (L.)*	x	x						x	x	x	x	x				
Promecotheca caeruleipennis Blanch.								x	x		x	x				
Promecotheca opacicollis Gestro			x	x												
Rhabdoscelus obscurus Bois.	x	x	x	x	x			x			x	x	x	x	x	x

Rhynchophorus
bilineatus (Montr.)

Scapanes
australis Bois.

HETEROPTERA

Amblypelta
cocophaga China§

Axiagastus
cambelli Dist.

HOMOPTERA

Aleurodicus
destructor Mackie

Stenaleyrodes
vinsoni Tak.¶

Aspidiotus
destructor Sign.

Dysmicoccus
cocotis (Mask.)

Table 12-3. Continued

	Aust	PNG	Sol	Van	NC	Kir	Tuv	Fiji	Wal	Tok	Sam	Ton	Niue	Cook	Poly	Haw
Chrysomphalus aonidum (L.)	x					x	x				x			x	x	
Ischnaspis longirostris (Sign.)	x	x	x		x			x				x			x	
Palmicultor palmarum Ehrh.					x	x			x		x			x	x	
Pinnaspis buxi (Bouché)	x	x	x	x				x						x	x	
ISOPTERA																
Neotermes rainbowi Hill#							x	x			x	x		x		
LEPIDOPTERA																
Agonoxena argaula Meyr.				x	x	x	x	x	x	x	x	x	x			x

240

Agonoxena
pyrogramma Meyr.

Decadarchis
psammaula Meyr.

Levuana
iridescens Beth.-Baker

Tirathaba
rufivena Walk.

ORTHOPTERA

Graeffea crouanii
(Le Guill.)

Locusta migratoria L.

Segestidea spp.

Sexava spp.

*Not on PNG or Australian mainland; §Only Bougainville in PNG; ¶Also from Reunion; #Not on coconut in Fiji, Samoa, Tonga

Abbreviations: Aust/Australia; PNG/Papua New Guinea; Sol/Solomon Islands; Van/Vanuatu; NC/New Caledonia; Kir/Kiribati; Tuv/Tuvalu; Fiji/Fiji; Wal/Wallis and Futuna; Tok/Tokelau Islands; Sam/Samoa; Ton/Tonga; Niue/Niue; Cook/Cook Islands; Poly/French Polynesia; Haw/Hawaii.

Table 12-4. Miscellaneous Plant Pests.

	Aust	PNG	Sol	Van	NC	Kir	Tuv	Fiji	Wal	Tok	Sam	Ton	Niue	Cook	Poly
Dacus kirki Frogg.*	x										x	x	x		x
Dacus passiflorae Frogg.*								x				x	x		
Dacus tryoni (Frogg.)*		x			x										
Dacus xanthodes (Broun)*								x			x	x			x
Cosmopolites sordidus (Germ.)§	x	x	x	x	x			x	x		x	x		x	x
Lamprosema octasema Meyr.§	x	x	x	x	x			x			x	x			
Pentalonia nigronervosa Coq.§	x	x	x	x			x	x		x	x	x	x	x	x
Icerya aegyptiaca (Dougl.)¶	x					x		x			x			x	x

	Aust	PNG	Sol	Van	NC	Kir	Tuv	Fiji	Wal	Tok	Sam	Ton	Niue	Cook	Poly
Hypothenemus hampei (Ferr.)#		x													x
Pieris rapae (L.)+		x		x											
Plutella xylostella (L.)+	x	x	x	x		x		x			x	x	x		x
Phthorimaea operculella (Zell.)=	x	x	x					x							x

*Various fruits; §Banana; ¶Breadfruit; #Coffee; +Brassicas; =Potato

Abbreviations: Aust/Australia; PNG/Papua New Guinea; Sol/Solomon Islands; Van/Vanuatu; NC/New Caledonia; Kir/Kiribati; Tuv/Tuvalu; Fiji/Fiji; Wal/Wallis and Futuna; Tok/Tokelau Islands; Sam/Samoa; Ton/Tonga; Niue/Niue; Cook/Cook Islands; Poly/French Polynesia.

Those pests that can continue their life cycle on or in the part of the plant used in vegetative propagation are readily transported and have become widespread. Examples are the weevil borer *Cosmopolites sordidus* and the aphid *Pentalonia nigronervosa* on bananas (*Musa* spp.), and the tuber moth *Phthorimaea operculella* of potatoes (*Solanum tuberosum*), which have spread to almost every place where their host plants are grown. Also widespread are those that feed and pupate on the transported produce. Thus, the banana scabmoth *Lamprosema octasema* and the diamond-back moth *Plutella xylostella* of cabbages (*Brassica oleracea*) are widespread, while the cabbage white butterfly *Pieris rapae* and the fruit flies *Dacus* spp., which do not pupate on the produce, have, in general, quite limited distribution. The advent of air travel has blunted somewhat the protective effect of this last characteristic and, unless, adequate precautions are taken, living insects can now be conveyed over great distances in association with quite perishable host material. Fortunately, the development of plant quarantine services has paralleled the development of air services in the South Pacific, though not in time to prevent the introduction of the Queensland fruit fly *Dacus tryoni* into New Caledonia, French Polynesia, and Easter Island in the last 15 years.

SHIPPING SERVICES

The extent to which the hand of man has contributed to the current distribution of plant pests has already become evident in the foregoing sections. Consideration will now be given to the extent to which shipping in its various forms may have contributed to the distribution pattern.

Ancient Voyagers

Pacific islanders already had a reputation as navigators and transocean travelers when Europeans first began Pacific exploration. The distribution of plant pests within island groups and between neighboring groups would indicate that canoe voyages may well have contributed to it, particularly in respect of the sweet potato weevils, the coconut stick insect (see Chapter 13), and the taro leaf-hopper. However, the comparative paucity of pests, and the absence of certain crops in pre-European times mean that their contribution to the overall pest distribution pattern must have been a minor one. The infrequency of their voyages and their tiny cargo capacity would not be much help to pest dispersal.

Early Europeans

To some extent, the same restrictions applied to the early Europeans. Interested as they were in exploration, colonization and "R and R," they took little interest in interisland trade in plant materials before the latter part of the nineteenth century.

The colonists no doubt introduced (with vegetatively propagated plants) the more intimately associated scales and burrowing insects, but interisland traffic in these was limited both by lack of regular shipping and by international rivalry.

Regular Commercial Services

The adoption of the triple-expansion steam engine about 1880 gave a measure of economic viability to long range steamship services and was followed by the French company "Messageries Maritimes" operating a regular service to New Caledonia via Réunion and Mauritius from 1881. (The coconut whitefly *Stenaleyrodes vinsoni,* known from Reunion—and in the Pacific, only from New Caledonia—may owe its Pacific presence to this service.) In 1910 a regular "banana run" operated between Fiji and Australian ports, and the Union Steamship Company began a regular service between New Zealand and San Francisco via Rarotonga (Cook Islands) and Tahiti (French Polynesia).

However, the real impetus to interisland shipping in the South Pacific came in 1914 with the opening of the Panama Canal and the annexation of German colonies in PNG by Australia and in Western Samoa by New Zealand. From the end of World War I until the mid-1960s, regular freight and passenger services operated (a) from France through the Panama Canal to Tahiti and New Caledonia (with connections to Fiji, Vanuatu, Wallis, and Futuna), (b) from Australia via Vanuatu and the Solomon Islands to PNG, and (c) from New Zealand through Tonga, Niue, Samoa, and Fiji. These were regular 2-4 weekly sailings, which with minor changes served the region for more than 40 years and which still form the framework of the surviving cargo connections. One of the features of these services on the shorter interisland runs was the practice of carrying "deck passengers." For a modest fare, these passengers received their passage only. They were sheltered on deck under some sort of awning and were required to provide their own rations, bedding, and so on. The rations consisted largely of precooked meat, fish, root crops, and fruit carried in coconut-frond baskets. The latter—along with the customary gifts of vegetables—carried as luggage, seem to have contributed significantly to the present distribution of plant pests.

Other shipping services carrying nonperishable cargoes, and some carrying passengers, have operated in the region during the period since World War I; but the three circuits mentioned above transported the vast bulk of perishable plant material. It appears from a consideration of the patterns of pest distribution that they also distributed many of the plant pests (Figures 12-1, 12-2, and 12-3).

The Coral Sea circuit (Figure 12-1) links many islands that also share quite a range of economically significant plant pests that are only occasionally found outside this area. Many of them were doubtless indigenous to one or other of the island groups before regular shipping services began to operate; but they are now spread quite widely through islands on the circuit, without having invaded nearby groups that are not on the circuit. Examples are the heteropteran pests of coconut: *Amblypelta cocophaga, Axiagastus cambelli,* and *Aleurodicus destructor;* and the cabbage white butterfly *Pieris rapae.* The taro pest *Papuana hubneri* has extended its range to Kiribati, probably with soil imports, and the migratory locust *Locusta migratoria* has reached Fiji.

Other pest species found in the Coral Sea area have extended their distribution to Fiji and French Polynesia, becoming established more or less exclusively along the route followed since 1923 by the shipping line "Messageries Maritimes" (Figure 12-2) and more recently by French air services. The green peach aphid *Myzus persicae,* the coconut scales and mealy bugs *Aspidiotus destructor* (see Chapter 13), *Chrysomphalus aonidum, Palmicultor palmarum,* and *Pinnaspis buxi,* the Queensland fruit fly *Dacus tryoni,* the potato tuber moth *Phthorimaea operculella,* the coffee bean borer *Hypothenemus hampei,* and the coconut leaf beetle *Brontispa longissima* (see Chapter 13), all show close associations with this transregional route, though some (*Brontispa longissima, Palmicultor palmarum*) have later reached back into the islands (those of Samoa and Tonga respectively) which they had previously bypassed.

A third grouping of pests is shared by Fiji, Tonga, Samoa, and Niue, and is more or less isolated from Melanesia on the one side and eastern Polynesia on the

Figure 12-1. The Coral Sea shipping circuit and insect plant pest distribution.

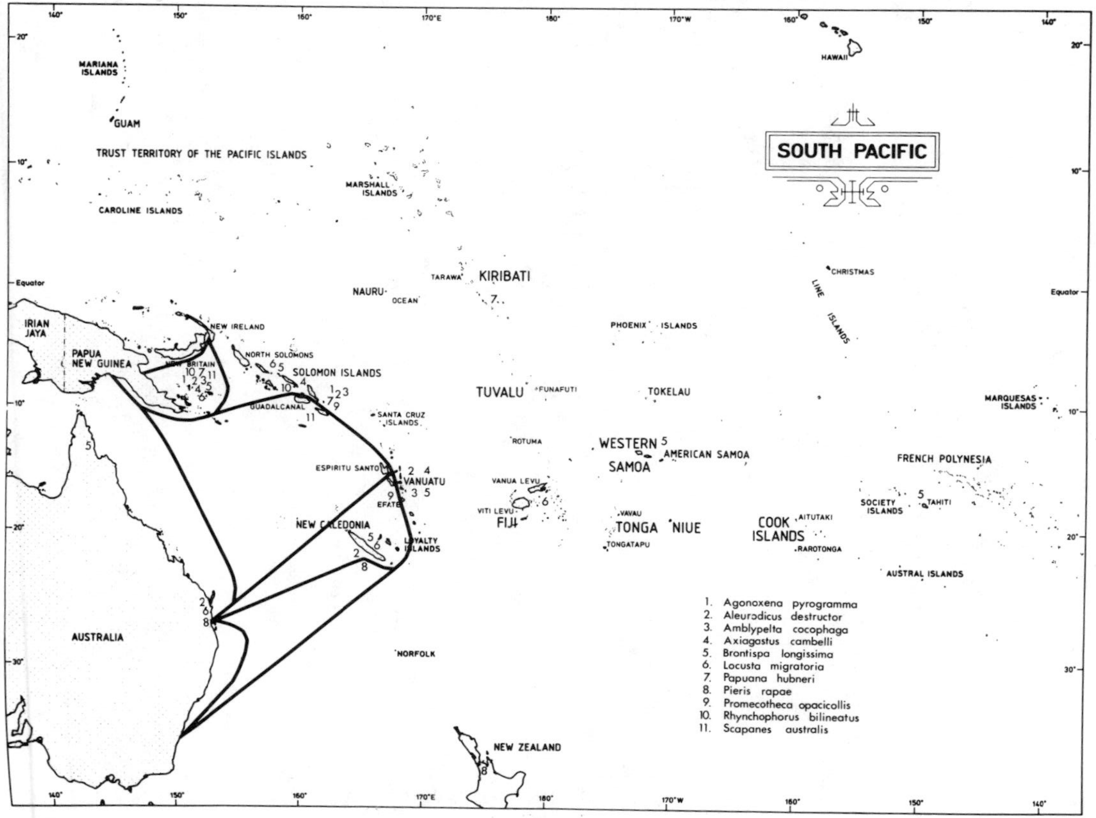

1.   Agonoxena pyrogramma
2.   Aleurodicus destructor
3.   Amblypelta cocophaga
4.   Axiagastus cambelli
5.   Brontispa longissima
6.   Locusta migratoria
7.   Papuana huebneri
8.   Pieris rapae
9.   Promecotheca opacicollis
10. Rhynchophorus bilineatus
11. Scapanes australis

Figure 12-2. The "Messageries Maritimes" shipping route and insect plant pest distribution.

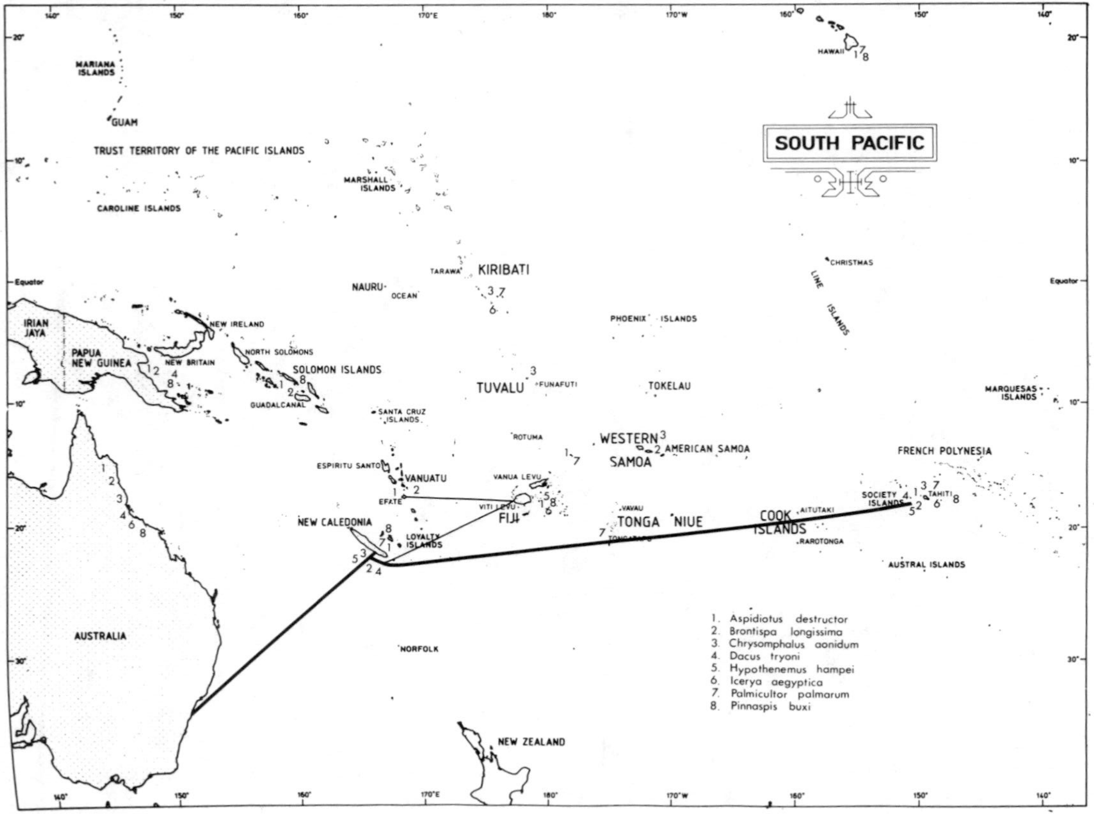

other. This grouping corresponds to the area served for more than forty years by the vessels "Tofua" and "Matua" of the Union Steamship Company of New Zealand (Figure 12-3). Pests characteristic of the grouping are the fruit flies *Dacus kirki, D. passiflorae,* and *D. xanthodes;* the leaf bugs *Brachyplatys pacificus* and *Brachylybas variegatus;* the taro weevil *Elytroteinus subtruncatus;* the sweet potato pyralid *Antiercta ornatalis;* the coconut leaf miner *Promecotheca caeruleipennis;* and the coconut mealy bug *Dysmicoccus cocotis.* The scarabs *Oryctes rhinoceros* and *Adoretus versutus,* though not associated with commercial produce, have also been distributed round this orbit.

Insects not Associated with Goods in Transit

Most of the insects mentioned above in connection with shipping services are more or less intimately associated with fresh plant material carried as luggage or cargo.

There are, however, other insects that are found in ships and cargo containers but are not associated with cargo items. According to New Zealand records (Manson and Ward 1968; Richardson 1979; Keall 1981) about 15-20% of these are in families that contain potential plant pests (Cerambycidae, Chrysomelidae, Curculionidae, Geometridae, Gryllidae, Noctuidae, Pieridae, Scarabaeidae, Sphingidae). Some, such as certain polyphagous weevils, may attach themselves to almost any item of cargo, but the majority seem to enter ships or containers when they are confused by bright lights and seek refuge in shadow after alighting. Many must subsequently die from desiccation. In fact, nearly all are picked up dead. Some, nevertheless (particularly scarabs, weevils, and noctuids), are able to survive long periods in such surroundings; and a few whose oviposition requirements are not too exacting may well extend their geographic range in this way. The rose-beetle *Adoretus versutus,* which oviposits in soil, appears to have done so; Keall (1981) records it 11 times from ships in New Zealand. *Oryctes rhinoceros,* which oviposits in rotting logs, may have reached Fiji and Tonga from Samoa in a similar manner. There are four New Zealand records of *O. rhinoceros* being taken from effects and from ships' holds (Richardson 1979; Keall 1981). The fact that it took 45 years to extend its range from Samoa to Fiji suggests, however, that dispersal by this means is not a very frequent occurrence. The dispersal of *O. rhinoceros* in the Pacific in general, and Polynesia in particular, is further

Figure 12-3. The former circuit of the Union Steam Ship Company of New Zealand and insect plant pest distribution.

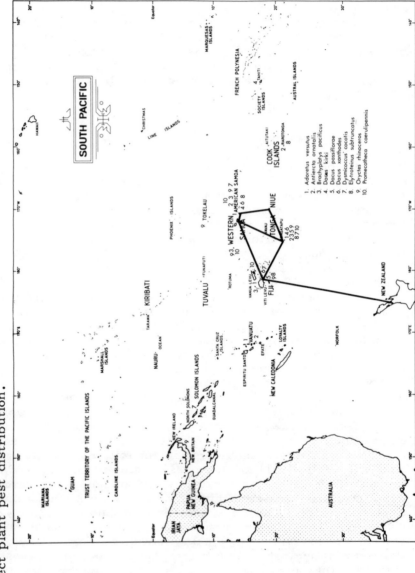

250

considered in Chapter 13. *Teleogryllus oceanicus,* which is readily attracted to lights and which oviposits in soil, could be another candidate for dispersal by shipping, but for most plant pests that have less resistance to desiccation, more specific oviposition requirements, or less inherent mobility, it can hardly be important.

AIR SERVICES

The development of interisland air services in the South Pacific since World War II has had a profound effect on travel and transport in the region. From the late 1950s they successively replaced the shipping services as carriers of passenger traffic and made steady increases in the carriage of perishable freight. To the extent that they could (a) link islands and island groups in a matter of hours rather than days, (b) provide daily rather than weekly services, and (c) carry plants and plant produce without recourse to refrigeration, it is rather surprising that aircraft have not had more impact than they have had on the distribution of phytophagous pests. No doubt the parallel development of quarantine services and of plant quarantine awareness has been a factor. Weight restrictions and fashion trends have also had their effect. Coconut frond baskets of uncooked taro and bananas are not such appropriate luggage as they were in the "deck passenger" days, while airfreight charges restrict the carriage of other fresh produce to small quantities of high value items that can be readily handled by routine quarantine procedures.

Yet there is need for continued vigilance. Fresh leaf material, fresh green beans, and fresh fruit can now be transferred from country to country and from plantation to plantation in a matter of hours, so the endurance that was once required of insects in transit is no longer necessary. Fruit flies, foliar feeders, and pod borers are readily spread by aircraft, as witness the spread of Queensland fruit fly, *Dacus tryoni, Liriomyza sativae,* and *Bemisia tabaci* in recent years.

There is plenty of evidence that insects dissociated from produce are carried in aircraft (Pemberton 1944; Laird 1951; Rainwater 1963; Manson and Ward 1968; Richardson 1979; Keall 1981). While these papers, with the exception of Laird (1951), make no attempt to distinguish between live and dead insects, unpublished studies by the Australian Department of Health and the New Zealand Ministry of Agriculture and Fisheries show that flies and mosquitoes, at least, readily can and do survive the desiccation of high-altitude jet flights and the low temperatures of their unheated cargo compartments. However, very few of the insects taken from passenger cabins are of economic or public health importance, and there is little evidence that insects carried in this way—as distinct from phytophagous insects present in produce—have resulted in introductions to new areas. Cargo compartments may be a different matter. Not only are they much more susceptible to invasion by night-flying insects, but the heavy-bodied moths and beetles, which make up a large proportion of the insects found in them, are known to be unaffected by the routine spray dose applied against small Diptera (Schechter et al. 1974). A more effective technique that is less prone to technical and organizational failure is needed (Dale 1980, 1982).

RECENT PEST INTRODUCTIONS

The fact that the distribution of insect pests conforms to such a large degree to the pattern of the major shipping services prior to 1960 suggests that the establishment of plant quarantine organizations in the various countries is having a significant effect. An examination of some of the cases where quarantine has failed to prevent the establishment of a new pest only serves to reinforce this view.

"Beware of Greeks Bearing Gifts"

One of the greatest threats to quarantine is generosity. Donors and recipients of gifts are apt to feel that nothing evil could accompany such a selfless gesture, and quarantine considerations are liable to be overlooked.

Brontispa longissima was introduced into American Samoa, possibly by ship, about 1974. In spite of an aircraft passenger service to nearby Western Samoa three or more times a day, this coconut pest was not found in Western Samoa until August 1980, when it appeared on a mission station where a Congress had been held a few months previously. It is believed that gifts of food (in coconut frond baskets) brought from American Samoa by participants in the Congress were the vehicle for the pest's introduction.

Plutella xylostella was found to be heavily infesting a shipment of cabbages imported by the Cook Islands in 1975 for New Zealand construction workers employed on the airport construction, a New Zealand aid project. Now that a tourist industry has grown up around the airport, Cook Island efforts to supply hotels with cabbages are being frustrated by the presence of this pest.

Panonychus citri entered the Cook Islands on citrus rootstocks provided by New Zealand scientists to improve the citrus industry in Rarotonga.

Oryctes rhinoceros entered the Tokelau Islands with soil sent from Western Samoa to enable vegetables to be grown there.

Aedes aegypti is believed to have entered Niue with taro-planting material sent as part of a hurricane relief program in 1969.

Papuana hubneri is believed to have entered Kiribati with soil imported for the mission garden.

Wars and Emergencies

Beardsley (1979) comments on the upsurge in immigrant pests during wars and immediate postwar conditions. It may be assumed that at such times quarantine receives a lower priority, and cargoes from unusual origins may be handled in unusual ways, giving new pests an opportunity to establish. In New Zealand, World War II brought a number of new insect pests whose impact was such that their occurrence could hardly have been previously overlooked. They include such significant pests as the German wasp *Vespula germanica,* the white-fringed weevil *Graphognathus leucoloma,* the green vegetable bug *Nezara viridula,* and the Australian soldierfly *Inopus rubriceps.* Such an influx in two years (1944-45) when quarantine routines were disrupted gives an indication of the value of such routines in normal years. Military aircraft are also believed to have introduced the Queensland fruit fly to Easter Island in 1973, to the Austral Islands about 1977, and to have brought *Musca sorbens* to Hawaii about 1949.

CONCLUSIONS

The distribution of crop pests in the South Pacific reveals some curious anomalies. Insects whose natural ability to travel over water is quite limited are nevertheless found to inhabit widely separated islands or even to be quite ubiquitous in their occurrence. Insects with proven ability to cover transoceanic distances may be widespread or quite limited in their distribution, and those limitations are frequently at variance with geographic or meteorological factors.

In many cases, there is evidence that human agency is involved in dispersal. Pests that are associated with the transportable portion of the host plant are generally more widespread than those associated with the rest of the plant. Those that are intimately associated with the transportable material throughout their life cycle are more widespread than those that abandon it to pupate. Moreover, islands with political or trade links often share pests that are not found in islands with which they are not linked, even though these latter islands may be geographically closer.

There is evidence that regular interisland shipping services since World War I have provided the means for dispersal of many plant pests and that various pests have been unable to cross ocean barriers where such services did not operate. Although there are exceptions, most pest dispersal seems to be associated with items carried as cargo or luggage, rather than through insects entering ships independently of host material.

In spite of the speed and frequency of air services established in the last 20 years, the organization of plant quarantine services appears to have afforded considerable protection to most of the South Pacific countries involved.

Many serious quarantine breakdowns result from disorganization of routines arising from military activity, or from well-meant but foolish actions by philanthropic persons and organizations. In general, quarantine services in the South Pacific are making intelligent use of the advantages that their geographic isolation confers on them.

REFERENCES

Beardsley, J. W. 1979. New immigrant insects in Hawaii: 1962 through 1976. *Proc. Hawaii ent. Soc.* 13:35-44.
Cumber, R. A. 1949. The green vegetable bug, *Nezara viridula*. *N.Z. Jour. Agr.* 79:563-64.
Dale, P. S. 1980. Use of residual insecticidal coatings for killing insects in aircraft. *N.Z. Ent.* 7:116-19.
————. 1982. Effectiveness of permethrin residues against insects carried in aircraft. *N.Z. Ent.* 7:310-13.
Fox, K. J. 1978. The transoceanic migration of Lepidoptera to New Zealand: A history and a hypothesis. *N.Z. Ent.* 6:368-80.
Fullaway, D. T., and N. L. H. Krauss. 1945. *Common Insects of Hawaii*. Honolulu: Tongg.
Gressitt, J. L., and S. Nakata. 1958. Trapping air-borne

insects on ships in the Pacific. *Proc. Hawaii. ent. Soc.* 16:363–65.

—————. 1959. Trapping air-borne insects on ships in the Pacific, Part II. *Proc. Hawaii. ent. Soc.* 17:150–55.

—————. 1960. Trapping air-borne insects on ships in the Pacific, Part III. *Pacific Insects* 2:239–43.

Gressitt, J. L., and C. M. Yoshimoto. 1964. Dispersal of animals in the Pacific. In *Pacific Basin Biogeography,* ed. J. L. Gressitt. Honolulu: Bishop Museum Press, 283–92.

Gressitt, J. L., J. Coastworth, and C. M. Yoshimoto. 1962. Air-borne insects trapped on "Monsoon Expedition." *Pacific Insects* 4:319–23.

Hinckley, A. D. 1969. Ecology of terrestrial arthropods on the Tokelau atolls. *Atoll Res. Bull.* 124:1–18.

Holzapfel, E. P., and B. D. Perkins. 1969. Trapping air-borne insects on ships in the Pacific, Part VII. *Pacific Insects* 11:455–76.

Johnston, C. G. 1969. *Migration and Dispersal of Insects by Flight.* London: Methuen.

Keall, J. B. 1981. *Interception of Insects, Mites and Other Animals Entering New Zealand 1973–78.* Wellington: N.Z. Min. of Agr. Fish.

Laird, M. 1951. Insects collected from aircraft arriving in New Zealand from abroad. Wellington: *Zool. Publs Vict. Univ. Coll.* No. 11.

Manson, D. C. M., and A. Ward. 1968. *Interceptions of Insects, Mites and Other Animals Entering New Zealand, 1966–72.* Wellington: N.Z. Dept Agr.

Pemberton, C. E. 1944. Insects in trans-Pacific airplanes. A review of quarantine work prior to Dec. 7, 1941. *Hawaii Planters' Rec.* 48:183–86.

Purseglove, J. W. 1968. *Tropical Crops: Dicotyledons 1.* London: Longmans.

Rainwater, H. I. 1963. Agricultural insect pests. Hitchhikers on aircraft. *Proc. Hawaii ent. Soc.* 18:303–9.

Richardson, C. A. 1979. *Interceptions of Insects, Mites and Other Animals Entering New Zealand 1966–72.* Wellington: N.Z. Min. Agr. Fish.

Schechter, M. S., W. N. Sullivan, H. F. Schoof, D. R. Maddock, C. M. Amyx, and J. E. Porter. 1974. d-phenothrin, a promising new pyrethroid for disinsecting aircraft. *J. med. Ent.* 11:231–33.

Swaine, G. 1971. *Agricultural Zoology in Fiji.* London: HMSO.

Tindale, N. B. 1981. The origin of the Lepidoptera relative to Australia. In *Ecological Biogeography of*

Australia, ed. A. Keast. The Hague: Junk, 969-75.

Willard, J. R. 1974. Horizontal and vertical dispersal of California red scale (*Aonidiella aurantii* [Mask.] Homoptera: Diaspididae) in the field. *Aust. J. Zool.* 22:531-48.

Wise, K. A. J. 1971. Trapping of air-borne insects on HMNZS Endeavour in the south-west Pacific, during the Cook Bicentenary Expedition, 1969. *Roy. Soc. N.Z. Bull.* 8:65-66.

——————. 1968. Trans-Tasman insect dispersal. Paper read at 40th ANZAAS Congr.

Yen, D. 1974. The sweet potato in Oceania, an essay in ethnobotany. *Bernice P. Bishop Mus. Bull.* 236.

Yoshimoto, C. M., and J. L. Gressitt. 1964. Dispersal studies on Aphididae, Agromyzidae and Cynipoidea. *Pacific Insects* 6:525-31.

Chapter 13

Transport and the Spread of Crop Pests in Tropical Polynesia

E. Dharmaraju

It is said that Polynesia was the last great area of our planet to be occupied by mankind.

Spreading over 12,000,000 square miles (30,720,000 km²) of the Pacific Ocean, the Polynesian triangle stretches northeast from Samoa to Hawaii; from the latter southeast 5,000 miles (8,000 km) past the Marquesas, to Easter Island, the eastward-pointing apex, which lies 2,500 miles (4,000 km) off the Chilean coast; from Easter Island southwest 5,000 miles (8,000 km) to New Zealand; and finally north again to Wallis and Futuna and Tuvalu. Within this huge Pacific pocket are numerous high islands and atolls inhabited by Polynesians (Fields and Fields 1973.)

Food crops grown in Polynesia include coconut (*Cocos nucifera*), breadfruit (*Artocarpus altilis*), yams (*Dioscorea* spp.), taro (largely *Colocasia esculenta*) and the related Araceae *Cyrtosperma chamissonis,* sweet potato (*Ipomoea batatas*), banana (*Musa* spp.), cassava (*Manihot utilissima*), water melon (*Citrullus vulgaris*), cocoa (*Theobroma cacao*), and sugarcane (*Saccharum officinarum*). *Pandanus* spp. (screwpines), which are found growing wild in Polynesia, provide delicious fruits that serve as an important item of food in some of the atolls, including Tokelau and Tuvalu.

TRANSPORT AND SPREAD OF PESTS

Table 13-1 illustrates world distribution by country of some crop pests found in Polynesia. For the purpose of this chapter only a few of the more important pests of crops will be discussed.

Rhinoceros Beetle (*Oryctes rhinoceros* [L.])

This beetle is one of the most serious pests of the coconut palm. The adults bite through the tightly packed unopened leaves in the central bud. When the damaged leaves open, triangular gashes in the form of V-shaped cuts are seen on them as though these have been cut with scissors. The consequent loss in leaf area adversely affects nut production. Heavy attacks by the beetle can also kill the palm.

In New Britain, it has been shown that the beetle *O. centaurus* is less harmful than elsewhere to coconut palms in those places where these have been interplanted with cocoa (Hoyt 1963a). It has also been demonstrated that in West Africa, burning of the jungle has a more adverse effect on the beneficial insects like predators than on the destructive beetles themselves (Hoyt 1963b).

The adult beetle lays its eggs in stumps of dead palms, sawdust, rubbish heaps, compost, and decaying vegetable matter. Eggs hatch in about two weeks. Larvae live and feed on the rotting vegetation. Larval period is about 7-8 months and pupal period about 3-3.5 weeks.

O. rhinoceros is found throughout Southeast Asia and also in the Philippines and southern China. It reached Mauritius in or shortly before 1962.

The rhinoceros beetle, which is not a native of the South Pacific, is a classic example of a pest introduced to a new area before plant health and quarantine regulations were practiced. The beetle arrived in Western Samoa during 1909 with rubber stumps packed in soil and vegetative matter from Sri Lanka.

From Samoa it spread to Keppel Island as well as the Wallis Islands. During World War II, damage to plantations and lack of crop hygiene increased the breeding sites, and military movement impeded adequate quarantine precautions. Outbreaks occurred in Palau and New Britain in 1942. Delayed by quarantine, although not prevented, it continued to spread in the Pacific to Tonga in 1951, Fiji and New Guinea in 1953, and the Tokelau Islands in 1963 (Harries 1978). It is also present in American Samoa (Stride 1977).

The larvae are known to be capable of surviving in floating logs transported by ocean currents. Wartime shipping aided its spread, and the great number of palms felled or broken in the course of military operations pro-

Table 13-1. World distribution by country of some crop pests found in Polynesia.

Pest	Distribution countries	Hosts	Ref.
Insecta			
Coconut stick insect *Graeffea crouanii*	Caroline Islands, Tuvalu, Fiji, Tonga, Vanuatu, Niue, Tokelau, Western Samoa, New Caledonia, Gambier Islands, Marquesas Islands, Society Islands, Wallis, Futuna, Australia	Coconut, Pandanus tectorius, Miscanthus japonicus, Hibiscus tiliaceus	6, 10, 15
Banana aphid *Pentalonia nigronervosa*	Widely distributed	Banana, taro, ginger	15
Pumpkin beetle *Aulacophora similis*	Malaysia, China, Australia, Solomon Islands, Vanuatu, Fiji, Tonga, New Caledonia	Cucurbits	15
Coconut scale insect *Aspidiotus destructor*	Widespread in the tropics, French Polynesia, New Caledonia, Vanuatu	Coconut, cocoa, banana, avocado, Elaeis, yam, Phoenix, citrus, ginger, guava, papaya, rubber, sugarcane, Pandanus, Artocarpus, as well as many wild plants	6, 10, 15

Table 13-1. Continued

Pest	Distribution countries	Hosts	Ref.
Insecta			
Flat moth _Agonexena argaula_	Fiji, Guam, Kiribati, Tuvalu, Western Samoa, Tonga, Wallis Islands, Futuna, Palmyra Island, Hawaii, Vanuatu, New Caledonia, Tokelau Islands, Niue	Coconut	6, 15
Banana scab moth _Nacoleia octasema_	Western Samoa, Tonga, Fiji, the Malay Archipelago, Queensland	Banana	15
Cluster caterpillar _Spodoptera litura_	Widespread over Asia, Australia, and islands of the Pacific	Taro, cocoa, head cabbage, banana, tomato	15
Coconut leaf beetle _Brontispa longissima_	Caroline Islands, Mariana Islands, Vanuatu, New Caledonia, Solomon Islands, PNG, Western Samoa, American Samoa, Tahiti, Indonesia, Mauritius, Malaysia	Coconut, _Elaeis_, _Areca_, _Caryota_, _Latania_, _Metroxylon_, _Phoenix_, _Ptychosperma_, _Roystonea_, _Washingtonia_	6, 10

Banana weevil borer Cosmopolites sordidus	Most banana areas	Banana	15
Sugarcane weevil borer Rhabdoscelus obscurus	PNG, Fiji, Western Samoa, Tahiti, Queensland, Micronesia, Taiwan, Hawaii, Indonesia	Sugarcane, Areca, coconut, Metroxylon, banana, papaya	10
Red brown weevil Diocalandra taitensis	PNG, Solomon Islands, Hawaii, Tokelau, Society Islands, Madagascar	Coconut	10
Coconut rhinoceros beetle Oryctes rhinoceros	PNG, Western Samoa, Fiji, Tokelau, Wallis Islands, Futuna, American Samoa, India, Burma, Sri Lanka, Thailand, Indonesia, Vietnam, Malay Peninsula, Mauritius	Coconut, Areca, Arenga, Borassus, Corypha, Elaeis, banana, Metroxylon, Nypa, Oncosperma, Phoenix, Pandanus, Colocasia, sugarcane	6, 10, 14, 15
Rose beetle Adoretus versutus	American Samoa, Western Samoa, Tonga, Fiji, Wallis	Cocoa, guava, rose, Bauhinia, Hibiscus tiliaceus, H. rosa, Barringtonia, ornamentals	15
Mollusca Giant African snail Achatina fulica	East Africa, French Polynesia, New Caledonia, Vanuatu, PNG, Trust Territory of the Pacific Islands, American Samoa, Western Samoa, Hawaii	Cocoa, rubber, banana, sweet potato, yams, cassava, breadfruit, citrus, bark and foliage of several fruit trees, papaya	9, 12

vided it with unprecedented opportunities for breeding (Lever 1979).

Figure 13-1 illustrates the geographic distribution of *O. rhinoceros* in Polynesia (see also Figure 12-3, Chapter 12).

Coconut Leaf Beetle (*Brontispa longissima* Gestro)

This is another serious pest of coconut palms. The beetle attacks trees of all ages. It is most feared when young palms are attacked, as their growth is severely affected. In some cases, they are killed outright (Stapley 1980).

This beetle is reddish brown or black in color. It is small, flat, and elongate, and well adapted to live within the tightly packed central shoot of the coconut palm. Eggs are laid in between the leaflets in chains of 3-4. The larval stages are yellow and are distinguished by the pincer-like termination of the body. Development takes about 5-9 weeks from egg to adult.

All stages of the insect are found within the folded leaflets. When the shoot expands and opens out, the populations move to the next unopened leaf. The adults and larvae feed on both surfaces of the closely packed tender leaflets. They make long incisions in the tissues, parallel to one another and to the veins of the leaflets. The damage results in the death of the whole of the attacked part of the leaflet.

Damage symptoms are clearly noticed when these leaflets open. Later still, the leaflets tend to shatter, especially in regions of high winds.

Severe attacks by the beetle not only reduce nut production by 50-70% but also delay the recovery of palms to normal health for a period of 1.5-2 years.

B. longissima is found in Malaysia, Indonesia (including the Moluccas), Carolines, Marianas, PNG, Solomons, Vanuatu, New Caledonia, Tahiti, American Samoa, and Western Samoa (see Figure 12-1, Chapter 12).

The arrival of the beetle in Tahiti in 1961 from New Caledonia—a distance of 4,000 km—posed a serious threat to the coconut plantations of Polynesia. By early 1973 the beetle was detected in American Samoa and by 1980 in Western Samoa.

The beetle is suspected of having been carried from Tahiti to American Samoa on the decks of oil tankers and from American Samoa to Western Samoa by interisland air and sea traffic.

The beetle can be easily transported along with items woven or made with coconut leaves (for example, baskets),

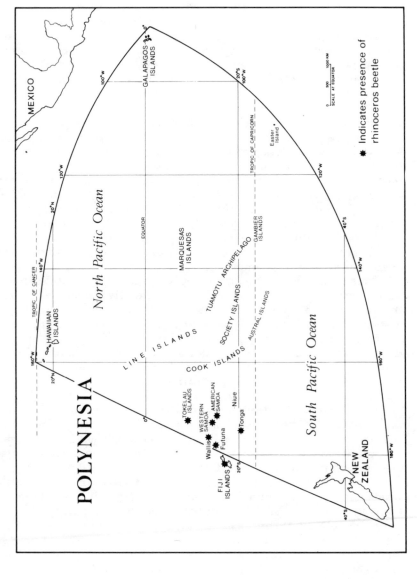

Figure 13-1. Geographical distribution of *O. rhinoceros* in Polynesia.

with seed nuts, and with seedlings. Within the islands themselves, the spread can be aided by strong winds.

The Giant African Snail (*Achatina fulica* Bowdich)

These snails are serious pests of various economic and ornamental plants. Not only are they voracious feeders, but they are also capable of extremely rapid reproduction under favorable conditions.

When first introduced into new areas, *A. fulica* attracts very little attention because its prime food source appears to be decomposing vegetation. However, once populations become significant, the snail becomes virtually omnivorous. The range of economic plant materials that it consumes shows no consistent pattern. However, the more important plants attacked (Thomsen 1980) have included cocoa (severe damage caused to seedlings), rubber, banana, sweet potato, cassava, yams, and breadfruit, as well as most shrubs and the bark and foliage of fruit trees, particularly citrus and papaya, or pawpaw, *Carica papaya*.

Besides being a serious agricultural pest, *A. fulica* is an intermediate host of the rat lung worm, which causes eosinophilic meningo-encephalitis in man.

These snails are hermaphroditic, each having both male and female sex organs. During the five-year life span, *A. fulica* lays about 6,000 eggs. These hatch in about 2 weeks. In about 5-8 months, the snails attain sexual maturity and are very active, traveling as far as 50 m during one night. When conditions are unfavorable, *A. fulica* can remain dormant for several weeks or even months, protected by a membrane that seals the opening of its shell.

A. fulica is endemic to the coastal area of continental East Africa. The species occurs from southern Ethiopia and the southern half of Somalia, through Kenya and Tanzania to northern Mozambique. The snail's ancestral homeland also probably includes certain of the small islands lying off the East African Coast, including Zanzibar and Pemba, where it is now found. Most probably, it was long ago transported by man to Madagascar. Its later introduction—usually deliberate—by man to Mauritius, Reunion, southern Asia, and the Pacific is a matter of historic record. The snail is now known from the Seychelles, Comoros, India (Andamans), Sri Lanka, Malaysia, Indonesia, Borneo, Thailand, Indochina, China, Taiwan, Japan (including the Ryukyus and Bonins), Philippines, PNG, various Micronesian islands, and Hawaii (Peterson 1957).

The snail was introduced into Miami, Florida, in 1966 by an eight-year-old boy who returned from a vacation in Hawaii with three of the snails in his pocket (Olson 1973).

It was first introduced into the Trust Territory of the Pacific Islands when a few specimens were taken to Palau in 1938. It is now established in French Polynesia, Guam, New Caledonia, and Vanuatu.

During 1977, *A. fulica* was detected in American Samoa. It is believed that the species was transported inadvertently by Japanese fishing boats operating in the region. In less than three years, as a result of the movement of goods, people, and shipping containers from American Samoa, the snail entered Western Samoa during September 1980, the first example having been detected on the wharf at Apia.

A. fulica established itself in Guam during World War II. It is not clear whether it was introduced during the Japanese occupation of Guam or after American military forces recaptured the island. It has been suggested by earlier workers that one or more accidental introductions of the snail could have taken place as a result of the numerous shipments of military equipment and war salvage materials that were moved into Guam from Saipan, Tinian, or Rota after the war.

The snail has even reached California several times, but alert plant quarantine action resulted in the invader's immediate destruction (Peterson 1957).

Adult snails attach themselves to plant material, motor vehicles, machinery, pallets, cargo containers, and metal and cement pipes. *A. fulica* is also deliberately carried from one country to another as a curiosity by tourists. Eggs may be present in plant material, especially when soil is present.

Coconut Stick Insect (*Graeffea crouanii* Le Guillou)

This stick insect is a serious pest of coconut palms in Polynesia and a large part of Melanesia, where it is responsible for defoliation and sometimes even the death of the palms (Lever 1969).

The female lays eggs that are separate and unattached. Most of these drop to the ground but some may be lodged in the leaf axils. After hatching, the nymphs climb up to the crowns of the palms, which they invade. The insects are nocturnal feeders, resting by day beneath the leaves. Generally the female is seen carrying the male on its back. The wings are vestigial in both sexes but are particularly reduced in the female. When disturbed, the insect ejects an acrid white milky fluid from the thoracic pores. The damage to coconut leaflets by both nymphs and adults takes the form of gaps cut out of the edges of the leaflets as if by scissors.

Additional food plants for *G. crouanii* include *Pandanus tectorius, Miscanthus japonicus,* and *Hibiscus tiliaceus.* It has been reported that in Vanuatu, *C. crouanii* prefers *H. tiliaceus* to the coconut palm (Lever 1969).

It has also been reported that heavy infestations are often associated with the presence of buffalo grass (*Buchloe dactyloides*) under the coconut palms (Lever 1969). It appears that the grass serves as a barrier, preventing natural enemies from reaching the eggs of the coconut stick insect that are on the ground.

Earlier workers have suggested that the eggs of *G. crouanii* can be carried by masses of vegetation floating in the sea. Within the island countries themselves, the adults and nymphs can be carried from one place to another when coconut fronds are transported by canoes and power boats. Evidence of this can be seen in the Tokelau and Tuvalu groups where the pest has spread to almost all the scattered reef islets of each atoll.

Figure 13-2 illustrates the geographic distribution of *G. crouanii.*

Sugarcane Weevil Borer
(*Rhabdoscelus obscurus* Boisduval)

This is the most destructive pest of sugarcane in Fiji (Stride 1977) and is the second major pest in Hawaii (DeBach 1974).

In addition to sugarcane, *R. obscurus* also does serious damage, of the same type as that done by *Rhynchophorus,* to coconut palms. It also damages many other cultivated plants including Areca palm (*Areca catechu*), Sago palm (*Metroxylon sagu*), banana, and papaya.

The larvae of the weevil tunnel inside the stalks of sugarcane, which eventually break and fall to the ground. Weevil-infested stalks are subsequently invaded by pathogens. The life cycle of the weevil is about 3-4 months.

R. obscurus is of South Pacific origin. It was quite possibly native to the New Guinea area, where it probably fed on *M. sagu* and related palms as well as on banana. It presumably adapted to sugarcane upon the introduction of that plant, being then spread by local people carrying sections of sugarcane for eating in their travels (DeBach 1974).

Figure 13-2. Geographical distribution of *G. crouanii* in Polynesia.

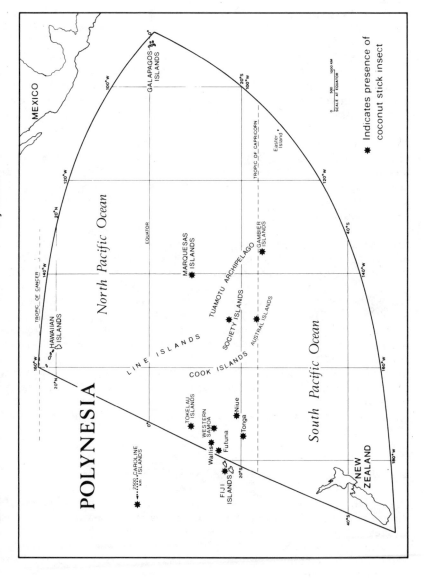

Coconut Scale Insect (*Aspidiotus destructor* Signoret)

This pest is widely distributed in the tropics wherever coconut is grown. Another important enemy of the coconut palms, it is also referred to as the Bourbon scale or the transparent scale.

A. destructor has a wide range of host plants besides coconut. These include guava (*Psidium guajava*), cocoa, banana, papaya, rubber, sugarcane, citrus, ginger, oil palm (*Elaesis* sp.), date palm (*Phoenix* sp.), breadfruit (*Artocarpus altilis*), and *Pandanus* spp.

The adults are covered by a flat, whitish, waxy scale that resembles tissue paper. The female scale is circular and the male oval. Eggs laid under the scale of the female hatch into young ones, which are very active and wander about before finally settling down with the proboscis inserted in the plant tissues. The life cycle requires about 4-5 weeks.

In severe outbreaks, the lower surfaces of the fronds are densely packed with the scale to form a continuous crust. The leaves turn yellow and sickly owing to heavy loss of sap and blocking of the stomata, and eventually die.

In recent years, *A. destructor* has *inter alia* spread from French Polynesia to New Caledonia (1961) and Vanuatu (1962) (see Figure 12-2, Chapter 12).

A. destructor can spread from one country to another through infested leaves, flower spikes, young nuts, and coconut seedlings. Infestation is severe in low lying areas of high rainfall where drainage is poor, particularly where the palms are close together and in neglected plantations.

It has been reported from Vanuatu (Lever 1969) that *A. destructor* is transported in the plumage of birds and the fur of bats.

THE NEED FOR A RIGID QUARANTINE

Pests can be spread by man, wind, water, and arthropods. Plant and animal quarantine provides the means to exclude and eradicate pests by inspection and treatment.

The appearance of *O. rhinoceros* in Mauritius by 1962 and in the Tokelau Islands by 1963; *B. longissima* in Tahiti by 1961, American Samoa by 1973 and Western Samoa by 1980; and *A. fulica* in American Samoa by 1977 and Western Samoa by 1980, afford recent examples of accidental introductions of dangerous crop pests.

The babai beetle *Papuana hubneri* (Fairmaire) is now a serious pest in Kiribati. This insect damages not only the swamp taro *Cyrtosperma chamissonis*–the principal root crop and staple food of the people–but also banana plantations. Whereas in 1971, only two villages were affected by the beetle in Tarawa, a recent survey (Dharmaraju 1982) has shown that in a period of 11 years the pest has spread to almost all the villages of Tarawa. This happened because of lack of effective quarantine action to prevent the spread of the pest.

O. rhinoceros may be carried in ships and boats from one island to another, and countries still free of the beetle should strictly regulate the visit of ships that arrive from beetle-infested ports.

The South Pacific Commission (Stride 1977) recommends that such ships should be required to be at anchor at least 2.5 miles (4 km) offshore between sunset and sunrise, and to be brightly lit during the period. The beetles fly only at night and will not leave the ship during the day, although they could then be brought ashore in cargo. They are strongly attracted by bright lights, so that those present on a lighted ship anchored at sea are likely to remain on the ship or to return to it should they fly away. Cargoes from infested countries are a hazard in the absence of effective fumigation on board ship. Some cargoes, such as timber, may be more hazardous than others because beetles may enter piles of timber in a sawmill for rest and shelter, having been attracted by the sawdust present.

A recent instance of legislation designed to exclude insect pests is to be found in the U.S. Trust Territory of the Pacific Islands (Anonymous 1979), where the introduction of coconut plants and of the nuts themselves (excluding husked nuts) is prohibited unless they have been fumigated with methyl bromide, which is lethal to all insects. Such measures need to be more widely adopted by other countries to combat the spread of pests.

Similarly, Guam's quarantine regulations strictly prohibit all parts of the coconut palm (except husked coconuts) to be imported from the following areas infested by the coconut hispid *Brontispa*: French Polynesia, New Caledonia, Vanuatu, PNG, Solomon Islands, U.S. Trust Territory of the Pacific Islands, Indonesia, Philippines, and Mauritius (Anonymous 1974).

Despite American Samoa's expenditure up to early 1983 of more than US$190,000 to control the giant African snail, this species remains a pest there.

During 1980, Western Samoa was rudely awakened to the fact that two new pests (*Brontispa longissima* and *Achatina fulica,* discussed earlier) had accidentally entered the country from nearby American Samoa. Since then the quarantine regulations have been further tightened to protect the Western Samoa's primary industries.

Although the last live snail to be recorded from Western Samoa was detected on 5 March 1981, it is too early to declare that this country is free of the pest. It will take several years of careful vigilance before such freedom can be confirmed.

The presence of *A. fulica* as well as *B. longissima* in Western Samoa has caused considerable anxiety to the neighboring island countries of Tokelau, Tonga, Niue, and Fiji.

The following are some of the steps that have been taken by the Agricultural Quarantine authorities in Western Samoa to prevent further entry of the giant African snail:

Surveillance: Cement block baits (5 cm × 5 cm × 1 cm) containing methaldehyde are placed in and around the Apia port area and in and around the stevedoring yards where shipping containers and pallets are stacked.

Movement of plants between American Samoa and Western Samoa: The movement of plants between Western and American Samoa is prohibited, except for species brought in under quarantine permits. Such plants are to be free of soil and are to be fumigated with methyl bromide at the rate of 128 g/m^3 for 24 hours (atmospheric pressure).

Shipping containers: No shipping containers from areas known to be infested by the giant African snail are permitted to leave the wharf area until they have been inspected by the Agricultural Quarantine Inspector and found to be uninfested. If traces of *A. fulica* are found on the containers, they are steam-cleaned or fumigated with methyl bromide at the rate of 128 g/m^3 for 24 hours.

Pallets: No pallets, loaded or unloaded, from areas known to be infested by the giant African snail are allowed to be taken from the wharf area until inspection has shown them to be free from *A. fulica*. If presence of the latter is suspected, the pallets must be fumigated with methyl bromide at the rate of 128 g/m^3 for 24 hours.

Cargo: No cargo, whether loose, containerized, palletized, or otherwise packed, originating from areas known to be infested with the giant African snail can be cleared for delivery until inspected by an Agricultural Quarantine Inspector and found to be free from *A. fulica*. Cargo found contaminated by the snail must be fumigated with methyl bromide at the rate of 128 g/m^3 for 24 hours.

Machinery and Motor Vehicles: All machinery and motor vehicles, whether new or secondhand, must be steam-cleaned on arrival in Western Samoa. This includes machinery and motor vehicles that have been transhipped at ports in infested areas.

Customs: The Customs Department may not clear the items listed above unless clearance is given by Agricultural Quarantine.

Agricultural Quarantine in Western Samoa has also taken the necessary steps to prevent the movement of *B. longissima* within the country by restricting the carriage of coconut materials (seedlings, leaves, baskets) from Upolu to Savaii.

CONCLUSION

With the tremendous increase in the coverage and growth of air and sea travel between the island countries, the primary industries of Polynesia are exposed to an ever-increasing risk of the introduction of exotic pests. The mere enactment of quarantine measures cannot attain its objectives unless it is supported by the means of enforcement.

The time has come for the governments of these Polynesian countries to take a more aggressive stance in educating the public about the need for strict quarantine to prevent the further movement and spread of crop pests in the region.

REFERENCES

1. Anonymous. 1959. Plant quarantine announcement: United States Trust Territory of the Pacific Islands. *FAO Plant Prot. Bull.* 7:149.

2. Anonymous. 1974. Plant quarantine announcement: Guam. *FAO Plant Prot. Bull.* 22:97.

3. DeBach, P. 1974. *Biological Control by Natural Enemies.* Cambridge: University Press, 110-13.

4. Dharmaraju, E. 1982. The babai beetle problem in Kiribati. *Alafua Agric. Bull.* 3:90-94.

5. Fields, J., and D. Fields. 1973. *South Pacific.* Wellington: A. H. & W. W. Reed Ltd.

6. Harries, H. C. 1978. *Plant Health and Quarantine in International Transfer of Genetic Resources,* CRC Press, 125-36.

7. Hoyt, C. P. 1963a. Rhinoceros beetle investiga-

tions in Papua and New Guinea. *Q. Bull. South Pacific Comm.* 13:20-21.

8. Hoyt, C. P. 1963b. Investigation of rhinoceros beetle in West Africa. *Pacific Sci.* 17:444-51.

9. Lambert, M. 1977. The giant African snail. Advisory Leaflet No. 6. Noumea: South Pacific Commission.

10. Lever, R. J. A. W. 1969. *Pests of the Coconut palm.* Rome: *FAO Agr. Studies* No. 77.

11. Olson, F. J. 1973. The screening of candidate molluscicides against the giant African snail *Achatina fulica* Bowdich (Stylommatophora: Achatinidae). Thesis submitted to the University of Hawaii for the Degree of Master of Science in Entomology, May 1973.

12. Peterson, G. D. 1957. Studies on control of the giant African snail on Guam. *Hilgardia* 26.

13. Stapley, J. H. 1980. Coconut beetle (*Brontispa*) in the Solomon Islands. *Alafua Agric. Bull.* 5,4.

14. Stride, G. 1977. Coconut palm rhinoceros beetle. Advisory Leaflet No. 4. Noumea: South Pacific Commission.

15. Swain, G. 1971. *Agricultural Zoology in Fiji.* London: HMSO.

16. Thomsen, T. E. J. 1980. Giant African snail. *Alafua Agric. Bull.* 5,2.

The Australian Redback Spider (Latrodectus hasselti): Its Introduction and Potential for Establishment and Distribution in New Zealand

Chapter **14**

L. M. Forster

INTRODUCTION*

Latrodectus Walckenaer 1805, a cosmopolitan genus of spiders, is widely known for its toxicity to humans. Australasian representatives were synonymized with *Latrodectus mactans* Fabricus by Levi (1958) who recognized only five species throughout the world. Since a great deal was then known about *L. mactans* (the black widow), little interest was henceforth shown in the biology and behavior of *Latrodectus* spiders in Australasia.

It is argued elsewhere (Forster and Kingsford 1983) that there are, as originally proposed, two endemic species of *Latrodectus* (*L. katipo* Powell 1871, and *L. atritus* Urquhart 1889) in New Zealand; and that these species are distinct from *L. hasselti* Thorell 1870 of Australia. This means that *L. hasselti* must be regarded as a prohibited species if it is intercepted at a New Zealand port by the Agriculture Quarantine Service. In practice, after 1966 the Port authorities recognized *L. hasselti* as such, so that a record of interceptions is available from that time.

Between 1966 and 1978, 16 redback spiders were located in a range of goods being brought into this country either

---

*I thank Tom Smith of Wanaka for forwarding the female redback spider found near Wanaka to the Otago Museum, and Jean Clough and Doug Sanderson of the Zoology Department, University of Otago, for the illustrations and photography.

from or via Australia. From 1978 until 1982, however, at least 20 spiders were intercepted, a four-fold increase over the preceding period (Min. Agr. Fish., personal communication). The reason for this is not known but may be due in part to the greater quantity of imports as well as to changes in the methods of packaging and storage prior to transportation.

The separate discovery of three female spiders in central Otago in 1981-82 has given rise to speculation that the redback might be established in this region. The first of these was found under a log on the foreshore at Lake Te Anau, the second in a driveway in Twizel, and the third under stones just off the road between Wanaka and Glendhu Bay. About a week after capture, the Wanaka spider laid an eggsac; the spiderlings that emerged formed the basis of the present study.

Three alternative hypotheses are proposed to account for the presence of these spiders in central Otago.

1. The three spiders were introduced on separate occasions, all missed detection at the point of entry, all escaped in central Otago from the goods in which they were transported, all found suitable shelter and sustenance, and all were ultimately found.
2. A multiple introduction of spiders occurred on a single occasion. They escaped somewhere in central Otago and have now reproduced and spread further afield.
3. A single gravid female was introduced some years ago. This female's progeny survived, reproduced, and have now spread into the localities where the present discoveries were made.

While the first explanation cannot be completely dismissed, it does not seem very probable. The remaining two hypotheses are examined in the light of findings from the present study, and some suggestions are advanced as to which of them is the most likely.

The survivorship of *L. hasselti* in central Otago is considered with respect to favorable breeding conditions and minimal subsistence temperatures, habitat and predation requirements, as well as the consequences of sexual dimorphism and the likely mechanism of dispersal. Factors that might be responsible for limiting the distribution and habits of *L. katipo* are discussed.

MATERIAL AND METHODS

A gravid female spider, *Latrodectus hasselti* (Theridiidae), was dislodged from its web beneath stones a few meters from the Wanaka-Glendhu Bay road on 26 March 1982. Several days later, it oviposited; on 16 May, 105 spiderlings emerged. Note that these were second-instar individuals—the first instar is always passed within the eggsac.

Seventy-five spiderlings were isolated in tubes as described by Forster and Kingsford (1983) and fed 3 times a week as follows: 1-2 *Drosophila* in the 2nd instar, 3-4 in the 3rd instar, 1-2 houseflies in the 4th instar and 2-4 in later instars. This diet was supplemented by an occasional slater (woodlouse, *Porcellia scaber*) from the 4th instar onwards. Apparently this schedule provided spiders with a more-than-adequate food supply since not all flies were always captured during feeding intervals. No water was provided at any stage.

Three experimental series were established:

1. Thirty spiderlings were incubated at 25°C.
2. Twenty spiderlings were subjected to a temperature regime fluctuating from 5°-15°C.
3. Twenty-five spiderlings were placed in an outdoor porch where they were subjected to variable winter conditions, which included subzero ground temperatures. Mean monthly ambient temperatures from 15 May to 31 October 1982 (supplied by the Meteorological Service, Dunedin) are shown in Table 14-1. The number of ground frosts for each month is included. Overall, the mean was <10°C for the study period.

For each series, individual records of ecdyses (molts) were kept; longevity, mean instar lengths (stadia), and standard deviations for males and females were calculated independently.

Two additional studies were undertaken:

4. Communal development: Thirty spiderlings were housed together in a clear plastic container (22 cm diameter, 21 cm height) with a corked opening to allow for the introduction of prey. A plentiful supply of *Drosophila* and, later, houseflies plus occasional slaters were provided; but because the growth rate of spiders was highly variable, *Drosophila* were offered throughout the study period. The cage was maintained in an area generally heated during the day (15°-20°C) but re-

Table 14-1. Mean monthly ambient temperatures, range and number of frosts to which 15 Series 3 spiderlings were subjected from 16 May to 31 October 1982.*

	May	June	July	Aug.	Sept.	Oct.
Mean Temp. (°C) 0.5(Max + Min)	9.9	6.9	6.1	8.5	8.9	9.9
Range (°C) (Mean max-mean min)	7.2	5.2	6.7	8.8	6.7	7.1
Number of frosts (<0°C)	5	10	14	17	13	4

*Spiderlings only occasionally caught proffered fruit flies and three died during October.

Source: Climatological data were kindly supplied by the Meteorological Service, Musselburgh Pumping Station, Dunedin.

      duced at night (10°-15°C). Individual ecdyses could not be recorded, but regular observations of events within the cage were undertaken.

5.   Intersibling reproduction: Upon maturation, six Series 1 females were mated with six Series 1 males. For this purpose, females were isolated in one-pint (half-liter) mason jars for four days to enable them to establish webs. Males were then introduced.

For present purposes, the study period was terminated on 31 October 1982.

RESULTS

The results show quite clearly that, given adequate quantities of food, the developmental rate of *Latrodectus hasselti* spiders is largely dependent on temperature. Of the first three experimental series, only those spiders reared at 25°C became mature within the observation period. Three of the fed spiderlings subjected to outdoor conditions died, but the remaining 12 were in good condition although none had molted. The ten spiderlings that were not fed all died without molting; mean survivorship was 35 ± 7.5 days. At intermediate temperatures, development was variable even among individuals of the same series and mortality was high. In the communally reared group, however, three males and five females attained maturity before the end of October; at that time only one other spider (a juvenile female) was still alive.

Series 1

In this series, two spiderlings died and 15 females and 13 males reached maturity. Sexual differences are depicted in Figure 14-1. Most male spiders, which can be recognized in the third instar by a slight, transparent swelling of the tarsal region of each palp, attained maturity in 4 molts excluding the pre-emergent molt, but one male matured after only 3 molts.

Six females became mature after 6 molts while the remaining nine took 7 molts. This is not surprising since

Figure 14-1. In *Latrodectus hasselti* spiders, the sexes are strongly dimorphic. In this photograph, a tiny male approaches the very much larger female. The male, only about one-eighth the size of his potential mate, has long slender legs and a white abdomen prominently marked with black lateral stripes and two dorsal rows of contiguous black spots. The female has long black legs and a large black globose abdomen with a conspicuous red dorsal band. (A broad red patch shaped like an hourglass is present on the ventral surface of the abdomen.)

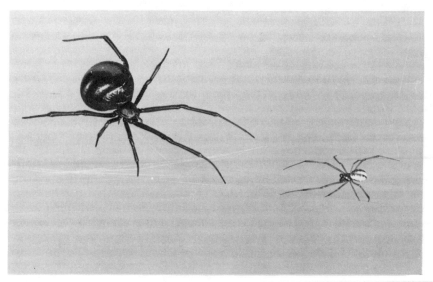

the number of molts to maturity in most other *Latrodectus* species is known to be highly variable (Kaston 1970) although Forster and Kingsford (1983) reported that the number of molts appears to be consistent for *L. katipo* and *L. atritus,* namely 3 molts for males and 5 molts for females.

Mean instar lengths (or stadia) between successive molts for males and females were calculated for each instar. In males (Figure 14-2) the 2nd stadium is greatest, being almost twice as long as succeeding stadia. (Data for the male that matured in 3 ecdyses are included since values for equivalent instars were close to the mean for the entire sample.) Mean days to maturity in males is 42 ± 5.9 while post-maturation longevity ranges from 2-4 months.

Figure 14-2. Mean instar duration (in days) for each instar in male redback (*L. hasselti*) spiders. Vertical bars represent standard deviations. The postemergence instar (second) is substantially greater than succeeding instars each of which is of about the same duration.

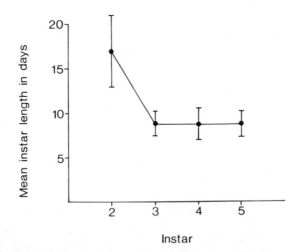

Figure 14-3 graphs values for the two groups of females, those that matured in 6 molts (mean days to maturity = 58.0 ± 6.0) and those that matured in 7 molts (mean days to maturity = 63.0 ± 4.9). In both cases, penultimate stages were of greater duration than preceding instars. A t-test for independent samples when $n_1 \neq n_2$ shows that differences in mean instar duration and time to maturity between the two groups of females are not significant (t = 0.625, df = 11, p > 0.25); and since environmental conditions and food supplies were uniform, these factors cannot be used to explain the disparity in the number of molts. Postmaturation longevity in females probably ranges from 1-2 years as reported for many *Latrodectus* females (Deevey and Deevey 1945; Kaston 1970).

Figure 14-3. Mean instar duration (in days) for each instar in two groups of female (*L. hasselti*) spiders. Vertical bars represent standard deviations. In one group (unbroken line) spiders matured in 7 molts and in the other group (broken line) spiders matured in 6 molts. Little variation was shown in the duration of equivalent instars in the two groups. In each group, however, more time was spent in the penultimate instar.

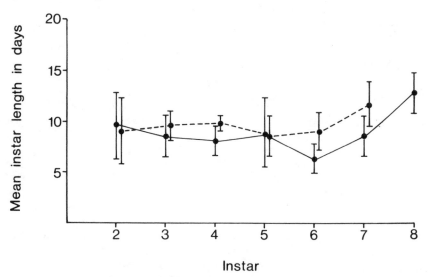

Sexual dimorphism with respect to size and appearance is well documented in *Latrodectus* species (Smithers 1944; Kaston 1970; Downes 1981), and both the juvenile characteristics and the very much smaller size of the males (see Figure 14-1) are undoubtedly a consequence of their earlier maturation. Moreover, inbreeding (endogamy) is believed to be restricted (Deevey and Deevey 1945; Downes 1981; Forster and Kingsford 1983), since this precocity and the brief life span of *Latrodectus* males (2-5 weeks in *L. katipo*, for example) mean that few survive long enough to mate with sibling females (adelphogamy) from the same eggsac, and those from earlier eggsacs have usually dispersed. Evidence presented here suggests that this may not be the case in *L. hasselti* because some of the usual controls apparently do not operate in this species.

Series 2

By comparison with the first series, development was very retarded. Mean duration for the second stadium was 29.8 ± 11.6 days (n = 20) and for the third stadium 26.1 ± 7.2 days (n = 9). One spiderling died during the second ecdysis and ten more during the third stadium. During this period, spiderlings only occasionally caught and ate fruit flies, both prey and predator being rather torpid within the lower limits of the specified temperature range. Thus, one explanation for these deaths is that spiderlings were malnourished as a consequence of their inability to catch food either through inadequate stimulation of the web by fruit flies or because they were not active enough to enmesh their prey with silk, the latter action being a necessary prerequisite to consumption.

Prior to their demise, however, spiderlings showed an abnormal thickening of the abdomen associated with a dull orange-brown discoloration, while at death they rested normally in their webs with legs extended, phenomena not consistent with death by starvation. Hence, another explanation for this mortality is that temperatures were too low for normal growth but too high to prohibit metabolic activity altogether.

Fourth instar spiders were offered houseflies but only one achieved a successful catch—the remainder were apparently too small or too weak. This spider underwent 2 more molts by 15 October and had not only grown markedly in size but had also acquired the familiar black abdominal coloration and red dorsal stripe of the redback spider. A subadult male died just after molting, but the other 7 spiders have not molted again (as of November 1982).

Series 3

The 10 spiderlings placed outside but not fed probably died of starvation (mean longevity 35.9 ± 7.2 days) rather than the cold (see Table 14-1), since twelve of the fifteen fed spiderlings survived for at least 5.5 months after eclosion. However, none of them molted during this time.

Spiderlings were very rarely seen to be eating fruit flies. Nevertheless, although quiescent, they appeared healthy. Their abdomens were generally globose and shiny as in neonatal spiderlings, in contrast to the specimens described in Series 2. It is anticipated, however, that with slowly rising temperatures, these spiderlings may become victims of the same ambivalent circumstances in which the level of predation is insufficient to sustain all facets of thermometabolism.

Communal Development

Within a short time of their installation in the cage, most spiderlings aggregated at the roof nearest the light source. When the light was transferred to the opposite side, spiderlings migrated to this area in less than 30 minutes. With successive displacements of the light on the first day, this migratory behavior was repeated but subsequently waned and eventually reversed. By the end of the second day, moreover, a substantial network of silk had been laid down throughout the cage.

Two to three days after confinement about half the spiderlings had occupied web sites in the upper regions of the cage and most of the remainder were suspended in the lower areas. The conspicuous partitioning of spiderlings into these two regions and the corresponding manifestation of individual spacing suggest that distribution patterns within the cage were nonrandom and density-dependent. Despite a superfluity of fruit flies, cannibalism occurred and after 8 days only 20 spiderlings remained. These early cannibalistic tendencies appeared to be induced primarily by competition for space and secondarily for food. Thereafter, the population remained relatively stable for 3-4 weeks, and few instances of cannibalism occurred until the later stages of development.

Spiders in the upper regions developed much more rapidly than those in the lower regions and were clearly more proficient at catching prey. Gradually the lower spiderlings vanished, but since the upper group appeared replete from eating flies, it is suspected that lower spiderlings eventually died of starvation because of their inability to compete successfully for food. After 4.5 months, the community consisted of 3 adult males, 3 subadult females, and 3 juveniles at various stages of development. A definite size gradient was evident among these spiders.

At maturity, females exhibited increased aggression towards each other. Two of the males disappeared, probably killed during or after mating (Forster, in preparation) and the second and third largest ranking females were dispatched and probably eaten by the largest. This female often patrolled the upper region of the cage, thereby restricting the four smaller spiders (1 male, 2 newly molted females and 1 juvenile) to the lower region. Spatial requirements appeared to be the paramount factor in this aggression, but in the wild such behavior could be related to the establishment of predation boundaries.

After the last male vanished, the dominant female began regular incursions into the lower region and frequently engaged in leg combat with the (now) second largest female. At that time the dominant female appeared to be gravid, and on 28 October it oviposited. This aggressiveness, which was directed solely towards the second female, became much more pronounced as it persisted with attempts to drive this spider away. At the end of the study period, however, these three adult females and 1 juvenile were still alive.

Intersibling Reproduction

Upon contact with female *L. hasselti* webs, males immediately commenced a sequence of acts similar to that described in other *Latrodectus* species (Cooke 1973). After much repetition of these acts, females were pacified and males were able to copulate with them.

Courtship and insemination were successfully accomplished in all 6 pairings and 13 eggsacs were produced within the study period. At the time of writing (November 1982), three eggsacs with a total of 317 spiderlings have hatched. From 20 spiderlings incubated at 25°C, 1 male has matured and another 7 are subadult. Within the remaining eggsacs there are visible signs of development. There seems little doubt, therefore, that when *L. hasselti* siblings mate, a high degree of fecundity is achieved.

DISCUSSION

Developmental Rates

Within the limits of the present experimental conditions, *Latrodectus hasselti* spiders achieved an optimum developmental rate when reared at 25°C. However, spiders also matured in the communal cage at temperatures fluctuating between 10°C and 20°C, although time to maturity was substantially greater. These latter conditions could be matched or improved upon in summer in many areas of New Zealand.

Evidently, growth is retarded at temperatures fluctuating between 5°C and 15°C. Hence it seems improbable that spiders could become established in the wild under such circumstances. However, these studies also suggest that *L. hasselti* spiders have the facility to withstand adverse conditions once temperatures become consistently low enough (<10°C) to restrict growth. Thus, if the Wanaka female had not produced its young in captivity, some spiderlings could well have overwintered, presuming, of course, that they had found suitable shelter and were able to capture an occasional insect.

The conclusion is that *L. hasselti* could become established in regions where existing summer parameters permit maturation, since it seems likely that spiderlings can assume a state of quiescence at other seasons if appropriately low temperatures prevail. These factors, however, are not the only requirements for their subsistence, as we shall see.

Humidity Requirements

No water was given to experimental spiders so that their fluid needs were obtained solely from prey. While this capacity to subsist on metabolically derived water has been demonstrated in some other spiders (Millot and Fontaine 1937), it has only once been reported for a *Latrodectus* species (McCrone and Levi 1964). However, there are numerous references to the generally arid environments in which these spiders live. In Palestine, for example, *Latrodectus tredecimguttatus* is found in strong dusty webs under large stones, in the corners of old buildings, or in the entrances to caves (Shulov 1940). Cooke (1973) and Levi (1959) note that in the United States, *L. mactans* webs are found in dry, shaded sites in arid and semiarid regions. In Australia, *L. hasselti* is commonly located under logs and stones, in the shaded hollows of trees, and in other sheltered and preferably dry situations (Southcott 1978; Forster personal observations). New Zealand *L. katipo* spiders, which live at the base of marram grass along sandy beaches where excess moisture drains rapidly away, have been reared successfully without access to water (Forster unpublished experiments). The implication is that most *Latrodectus* species prefer habitats of low relative humidity.

When wolf spiders (*Lycosa hilaris, Allotrochosina schauinslandi*), which have high relative humidity requirements (Forster and Forster 1973), are kept in dry tubes at 25°C, moisture from pulmocutaneous evaporation condenses on the inside of the tubes and usually within 48 hours these spiders are dead. No such condensation occurs in tubes containing *L. hasselti*. This suggests that, unlike wolf spiders, they possess ways of controlling water loss from their bodies, thus implicitly supporting the view that they are capable of living in habitats of low relative humidities.

The survival rate of adult *L. hasselti* females housed in dry cages at 25°C was 100% (N = 15), but one female kept in a container in which moisture condensed on the sides because of the presence of a damp cottonwool wick died in about 2 weeks. One explanation for this death is that the RH of the cage was too high, but more exhaustive tests are necessary to establish required RH levels with certainty.

The high success rate achieved in rearing *L. hasselti* without water, taken in conjunction with the evidence cited above, leads to the conclusion that these spiders prefer xerophytic environments and, further, that RH may be a limiting factor in their distribution.

Site selection

Suitable breeding temperatures and low relative humidity requirements clearly limit the suitability of areas in which *L. hasselti* can become established. However, differences between the ambient climate and microhabitat conditions may be considerable, hence the selection of appropriate sites within an area can greatly influence the chances of survival.

The discovery of a *L. hasselti* spider under a log and another under stones in central Otago suggests that such natural objects frequently provide warm, dry microenvironments. In addition, prey availability is a factor in the choice of suitable sites, although *Latrodectus* species are largely unspecific predators (Herms, Bailey, and McIvor 1935; D'Amour, Becker, and van Riper 1936; Kaston 1937). Furthermore, because prey blundering into their specialized webs (Szlep 1965; Court 1971) is rapidly pursued and swathed with silk, space for this predatory tactic must be available in or adjacent to the occupation site.

Recently it was reported that a nest of redback spiders and eggsacs had been discovered in an abandoned rabbit burrow in central Otago, but unfortunately the spiders were not sent in for verification. It is quite feasible, however, for such burrows, which abound in this region, to provide suitable habitats, since in various parts of the United States, black widows are often found nesting in squirrel burrows, rabbit warrens, and rat holes (Jellison and Philip 1935; Kaston 1970; Cooke 1973), where they presumably obtain protection from inclement weather. Furthermore, since the communal study suggests that a number of redbacks may coexist within specific spatial limits, it seems likely that rabbit burrows would meet many of their subsistence and habitat requirements. However, this possibility in central Otago has yet to be seriously investigated.

Dispersal

Observations of events in the community cage within the first 24-36 hours indicate that nymphal spiderlings have a strong tendency to cluster and migrate upwards towards a light source. Most probably they exhibit such a phototropism in the wild, for this behavior would liberate them from the darkened confines of the female's nest.

Araneus diadematus spiderlings, which act in this way, are usually anemotropic (they are dispersed by the wind). Aggregation and phototropism are essential preliminaries to such a dispersal mechanism (Burch 1979). It is highly likely, therefore, that *L. hasselti* spiderlings are dispersed by this method, an assumption also made by McKeown (1952). In principle, wind dispersion can carry spiderlings (and insects) for hundreds of kilometers (Bristowe 1939; Duffey 1956), but actual distance, frequency, and timing are dependent on a number of prevailing factors (Greenstone 1982). Once *L. hasselti* became established, therefore, spiderlings could spread to other areas by this means.

In unsuitable atmospheric conditions, spiderlings might revert to negatively heliotropic behavior, presumably in 1-2 days as suggested by laboratory observations. In such circumstances they probably reoccupy their original habitat or find suitable sites nearby. Density-related cannibalistic predation might then reduce the population, while simultaneously augmenting the food supply. Several spiders could thus reach maturity and interbreed.

I have not observed newly hatched *L. katipo* spiderlings aggregating or migrating phototropically, nor are there any records of this species "ballooning," as this aeronautic dispersal behavior is often called. Two factors probably account for the absence (or loss) of such a habit in this species. One is that these spiders are "linearly" distributed around the coastal regions of New Zealand, and the second concerns the fact that most of our winds are either offshore or onshore. If spiderlings were anemotropic, the majority would be blown either inland away from their preferred habitats or out to sea. Perhaps in the course of evolution such anemotropic reactions were selected against. In the one direction, the dense damp forest, which once covered the hinterlands, would have offered supposedly inhospitalbe environments to ballooning spiderlings. In the other direction, they would have faced a watery death.

Sexual Dimorphism

In all *Latrodectus* species, asynchronous sexual development results in comparatively small males that are capable of inseminating females long before their endogamic females are sexually mature. The sequential production of eggsacs with spiderlings dispersing at each emergence, in conjunction with such sexual dimorphism, can thus be assumed to favor outbreeding (Downes 1981).

Apparently *L. katipo* spiderlings do not disperse to any great extent by wind; hence, it is likely that most spiderlings develop in the same general area. This would favor endogamy despite the short life of males (2-5 weeks), but although intersibling matings were readily accomplished in the laboratory and eggsacs produced, fecundity was extremely low. Of 11 eggsacs resulting from adelphogamy, only 20 live spiderlings emerged. The subsequent mortality rate among these was much higher than previously recorded from interpopulational matings (Forster and Kingsford in review). Most eggs (several hundred) were not fertilized. In the case of those that were, the majority of spiderlings died prior to emergence. It appears that, in the absence of an adequate dispersal method in this species, endogamy has been limited by some physiological or biochemical barrier.

Anemotropic dispersal is undoubtedly the most effective barrier to adelphogamy in *L. hasselti* (Downes 1981). Males of this species have a postmaturation longevity of 2-4 months in cool temperatures (in the laboratory), whereas *L. katipo* live only 2-5 weeks under the same conditions. Perhaps because of their aeronautic habits, *L. hasselti* males need more time to locate females, although other anemotropic species (*L. mactans,* for example) are described as short-lived (2-9 weeks) (Deevey 1949). Longevity, therefore, may be partly a density-dependent characteristic. However, *L. hasselti* appears to lack the endogenous barriers to adelphogamy characteristic of

L. katipo. Moreover, longevity in males counteracts the consequences of asynchronous sexual maturation so that males can interbreed with their clone-sisters. The long-term effects of adelphogamy in this species, however, are not yet known.

CONCLUSIONS

While it is evident that temperature is a significant factor in the growth rate of *L. hasselti* spiders, only those experiments conducted under controlled conditions can be regarded as definitive. In particular, more studies are needed to determine the lowest temperature at which normal patterns of growth are possible, as well as the precise circumstances associated with delayed development. In addition, we need to know whether spiderlings can develop normally (for instance, after a sustained period of quiescence), or if other stages are able to overwinter.

Aridity is apparently important in determining the geographical distribution of *L. hasselti* spiders. This may explain why they have been able to survive in central Otago, a notoriously dry region noted for its rocky outcrops, porous soils, and rabbit burrows. Sandy beaches doubtless provide *L. katipo* with the necessary xeric conditions. Although many man-modified xerophytic environments now exist, the probable loss of anemotropic behavior in this species currently prevents its spread into these areas.

Despite the well-known cannibalistic nature of *Latrodectus* females (D'Amour, Becker, and van Riper 1936), this study shows that a degree of interindividual tolerance exists. Indeed, it seems likely that, given greater spatial dimensions, more spiders might coexist in a communal situation. A "size hierarchy" among *L. hasselti* individuals in the cage apparently resulted from competition for space and food. This in turn influenced social interactions. Since only mated females produce eggsacs (McCrone and Levi 1964; Forster unpublished observations), we know that at least one male and his clone-sister mated in the community cage. This demonstrates the feasibility of such social culturing and endogamy in the wild.

In *L. katipo,* adelphogamy is restricted by endogenous barriers probably because the loss of anemotropic behavior limits dispersal—males consequently being unlikely to come in contact with their sibling-sisters. In *L. hasselti,* there are no endogenous barriers to adelphogamy despite the fact that the postmaturation longevity of males allows them to mate with their clone-sisters. Presumably, in the wild, anemo-tropism has rendered such contraception unnecessary, as Downes (1981) also suggests. This means that if a gravid *L. katipo* was to be accidentally introduced into an alien country, its chances of becoming established would be extremely remote. In contrast, a gravid *L. hasselti* female introduced elsewhere would have a much greater chance of long-term survival provided that dispersal, in the first instance, was relatively insignificant.

The present investigations suggest that *L. hasselti* spiders could become dispersed throughout New Zealand by wind but that their survivorship would depend largely on the availability of arid habitats, as well as the suitability of summer temperatures for breeding and appropriate con-ditions for overwintering. It is unlikely that many areas will meet all three criteria. However, it appears possible that the accidental introduction of just one gravid female into central Otago two or three years ago could have led to the presence of these spiders in that area. Finally, it should not be overlooked that Closer Economic Relations* (CER) with Australia may, in fact, increase the probability of *L. hasselti* spiders entering this country.

REFERENCES

Bristowe, W. S. 1939. *The comity of spiders.* Ray Society. Vol. 1:228 pp.
Burch, T. L. 1979. The importance of communal experi-ence to survive for spiderlings of *Araneus diadematus* (Araneae: Araneidae). *J. Arachnol.* 7:1-18.
Cooke, J. A. L. 1973. Unveiling the black widow. *Nat. Hist.* 82:66-75.
Court, D. J. 1971. The behaviour and web structure of the katipo *Latrodectus katipo. Tane* 17:149-57.
D'Amour, F. E., F. E. Becker, and W. Van Riper. 1936. The black widow spider. *Quart. Rev. Biol.* 11:123-60.
Deevey, G. B. 1949. The developmental history of *Latrodectus mactans* at different rates of feeding. *Amer. Midl. Nat.* 42:189-219.
Deevey, G. B., and E. S. Deevey. 1945. A life table for the black widow. *Trans. Conn. Acad. Sci.* 36:115-31.
Downes, M. F. 1981. Sexual dimorphism in *Latrodectus*

---

*A trade agreement between Australia and New Zealand signed in 1983.

(Araneae: Theridiidae). *Aust. J. Ecol.* 6:289-90.

Duffey, E. 1956. Aerial dispersal in a known spider population. *J. Anim. Ecol.* 25:85-111.

Forster, L. M., and S. M. Kingsford. 1983. A preliminary study of development in two *Latrodectus* species (Araneae: Theridiidae). *N.Z. Ent.* 7:431-39.

Forster, R. R., and L. M. Forster. 1973. *New Zealand Spiders—an Introduction.* Auckland, London: Collins.

Greenstone, M. H. 1982. Ballooning frequency and habitat predictability in two wolf spider species (Lycosidae: *Pardosa*). *Florida Ent.* 65:83-89.

Herms, W. B., S. F. Bailey, and B. McIvor. 1935. The black widow spider. *Calif. Agr. Exp. Sta. Bull.* 591.

Jellison, W. L., and C. B. Philip. 1935. The biology of the black widow spider, *Latrodectus mactans. Science* 81:71-72.

Kaston, B. J. 1937. The black widow spider in New England. *Bull. New Engl. Mus. Nat. Hist.* No. 85.

—————. 1970. Comparative biology of American black widow spiders. *Trans. San. Diego Soc. Nat. Hist.* 16:82 pp.

Levi, H. W. 1958. Number of species of black widow spiders. *Science* 127:1055.

—————. 1959. The spider genus *Latrodectus* (Araneae: Theridiidae). *Trans. Am. Micr. Soc.* 77:7-43.

McCrone, J. D., and H. W. Levi. 1964. North American widow spiders of the *Latrodectus curacaviensis* group (Araneae: Theridiidae). *Psyche* 71:12-27.

McKeown, K. C. 1952. *Australian spiders.* Sydney: Angus and Robertson.

Millot, J., and M. Fontaine. 1937. Le teneur en eau des aranéides. *Bull. Soc. Zool. France.* 62:113-19.

Shulov, A. 1940. On the biology of two *Latrodectus* spiders in Palestine. *Proc. Linn. Soc. London.* 152:309-28.

Smithers, R. H. N. 1944. Contributions to our knowledge of the genus *Latrodectus* (Araneae) in South Africa. *Ann. S. Afr. Mus.* 36:263-312.

Southcott, R. V. 1978. *Australian Harmful Arachnids and their Allies.* South Australia: Griffen Press.

Szlep, R. 1965. The web-spinning process and web-structure of *Latrodectus tredecimguttatus, L. pallidus* and *L. revivensis. Proc. zool. Soc. Lond.* 145:75-89.

Chapter 15

Overview and Perspectives

M. Laird

INTRODUCTION

Homo sapiens being "a carrying animal, an emigrating animal" (Mason 1896), commerce in its earliest forms must have begun extending the range of undesirable insects from mankind's dawn. First and foremost among the fauna so transported must have been the ectoparasites, notably lice, carried by our otherwise initially unburdened ancestors. While human carrying abilities remained limited to what could be gripped and borne or dragged away, the nature and variety of the insects so spread about were necessarily limited. Aside from purely chance stowaways, most of the insects in question at first were probably of species associated with food and bedding. In the latter connection, Beebe's (1953) record of three cockroaches from the just-constructed "couch" of an orang-utan suggests that Blattidae and other such scavengers, as well as blood-feeders like fleas and bedbugs, must–like ectoparasites–have started along the roads to peridomesticity and cosmopolitanism in the very remote past. Opportunities for their dispersal clearly multiplied as means of carriage were devised (from the travois and sled to wheeled vehicles, and from rafts and inflated skins to canoes and sailing craft), and as domestic animals replaced people as carriers and motive power. Those opportunities were multiplied with the eventual advent of steam power and–thus Mason (1896) could refer to tenfold increase in worldwide land and sea traffic since 1850–later last century, the internal combustion engine. They took other quantum jumps during the present century, first, as larger and faster ships dominated inter-national passenger traffic and, afterwards, as these in their turn were eclipsed by aviation. Today's ever faster jet aircraft–from jumbos (with individual capacities for several hundred passengers or equivalently heavy cargoes) to supersonics–and an international shipping industry re-vamped for new modes of cargo carriage (notably con-tainerization–Piltz 1981) are presenting heightened vector, pest, and disease introduction hazards at a time when atti-tudes on the part of both officialdom and the general public have eroded the global effectiveness of disinsection, not to mention airport/port vector control. Moreover, just as containerization is presenting new opportunities for economic pests to escape detection at frontiers, more and more people still incubating vector-borne and other diseases acquired elsewhere are traveling far beyond the airport/port of arrival before developing symptoms (Goldsmid Chapter 10).

SOME HISTORICAL BACKGROUND

The beginnings of human-assisted insect dispersal by air

Had Ovid's account of how Daedalus made feathered wings (so that he and his son Icarus might escape the wrath of Minos by flying above that king's ships, deployed to pre-vent their leaving Crete) been other than legendary, we could have guessed that the pioneer airmens' own lice, or Mallophaga in their borrowed plumage, afforded the first examples of insect dispersed by air through human agency. As it is, setting aside other equally unauthenticated aerial ventures claimed from classical to renaissance times, we must search for the beginnings of our topic in early bal-looning days. An abundance of relevant literature might well repay really detailed study in this context; but even a cursory glance has been worthwhile, in moving the date of modern aircraft borne insect records back from the late 1920s (Thomas 1928) to 1803. Lowell Thomas' observation had also escaped the notice of writers on disinsection matters. Its publication preceded by a year that of Kisliuk's (1929) well-known *Graf Zeppelin* paper, and was made during a 1927 Deruluft trip in a single-engined Fokker from Königsberg, East Prussia, Germany (today's Kaliningrad, USSR) to Smolensk, USSR. He wrote: "A large insect, half the size of a locust and much like one,

seems to have been shanghaied aboard. Or is he a stowaway bumming a ride to Smolensk? He gropes along the
window edge, apparently puzzled by the transparent barrier. No doubt bewildered, too, by the tremendous vibration. Unlike poor mortals . . . he is not required to
show a passport with a Soviet visa. If the Hindus are
right, perhaps this grasshopper-aviator is Icarus himself?
Who knows?"

The 1803 data concern the second of two balloon ascents
constituting the first aeronautical ventures from which truly
scientific deductions could be drawn (Arago, in Marion
1870). This took place on 14 August of that year, when
Robertson and Lhoest rose from Hamburg in the gondola of
a hydrogen balloon to reach (over Holstein) an altitude of
ca 4,500 m at a temperature near 0°C (barometric pressure,
15 in., at-1°Réaumur). Using pigeons for the experiment,
they repeated observations made with birds a month previously on their first ascent to a rather higher altitude.
This time, "one descended in a diagonal direction, its wings
half open but not moving, with a swiftness which seemed
that of a fall." The other pigeon returned to the gondola
and clung to it. Robertson then "tried the same experiment
with butterflies, but the air was much too rarefied for
them; they attempted in vain to raise themselves by their
wings, but they did not forsake the car." These pioneer
field experiments, until now overlooked by modern entomologists, preceded by 143 years my own investigations of
the effects of low air pressure and temperature, and vibration, on mosquitoes, as related to the capacity of these
insects to survive long air voyages in the unpressurized
aircraft of the day. The results (Laird 1948) not only
demonstrated the ability of mosquitoes to survive even the
longest flights then being made, but also revealed their
reluctance to fly after the atmospheric pressure had been
rapidly reduced to that prevailing near 10,000 ft (3,050 m),
as simulated in a small decompression chamber. This confirmed original in-flight observations, including unpublished
ones made during a trip without oxygen equipment in a
Royal New Zealand Air Force Harvard trainer piloted with
élan by a wartime ace of the RNZAF—over Cook Strait we
briefly maintained an altitude of ca 17,000 ft (ca 5,200 m),
probably somewhat above that reached by Robertson and
Lhoest in their 1803 ascent of which I was ignorant until
the present literature survey.

It should be added that, as in the case of the first
orbiting vehicles, unaccompanied balloon flights preceded
"manned" ones. In the earliest of the latter, humans
deferred to lower animals for the distinction of being the

first vertebrate passengers in free-floating balloons. Then, in the presence of King Louis XVI of France (who himself had vetoed human passengers for safety considerations) the famous blue and gold Montgolfier hot-air balloon was launched from Versailles on 19 September 1783. Bearing aloft an osier cage containing either "a sheep and some pigeons," (Marion 1870) or "a *sheep,* a *rooster,* and a *duck"* (Etienne Montgolfier, as reported by Gillispie 1983), and limited in range by the fact that the iron stove from which it was inflated was purely terrestrial, it reached an altitude of 1,700 ft (520 m) and travelled for 10,200 ft (3.2 km) before running out of hot air. Its avian and mammalian* passengers, being common hosts for ectoparasitic insects (hippoboscids, lice) might perhaps have given France the honor of launching the first airborne arthropod stowaways aboard a flying machine. Alas, we shall never know. Nor shall we learn if human ectoparasites did so a few weeks afterwards—late eighteenth-century wigs, clothing, and personal hygiene having favored head and body lice, and fleas too—when following some intervening ascents in a tethered balloon (equipped with its own wire grating for a dried straw-and-wool fire to replenish the hot smoky air in flight) M. Pilatre des Roziers, now accompanied by the Marquis d'Arlandes, finally floated free over Paris. Had King Louis' initial condition that the balloon be crewed by two condemned criminals not been rescinded, the chances of lice being carried would have been higher still; and it is intriguing to consider what insects the fuel bundles might have harbored!

Domiciliary pests and transportation

Whether or not the first sailing craft were developed in Minoan Crete (it has been postulated that the Icarus legend was an allegorical reference to the invention of sailing), the evidence suggests that they plied on and from the Mediterranean. Admitting but setting aside the lack of records, Roth and Willis (1960) state that these vessels were

---

*In the same vein, a cat was aboard the U.S. nonrigid airship *America* in Wellman's unsuccessful eastbound attempt to cross the Atlantic in October 1910; while a tabby kitten stowed away on the British rigid airship *R34,* which only weeks after Alcock and Brown achieved (eastbound) trans-Atlantic flight by airplane, crossed to the United States and returned in mid-July 1919 (Collinson and McDermott 1934).

undoubtedly infested with cockroaches. This lack of records persisted until Elizabethan times, presumably because
such infestations were felt too commonplace to record.
Finally, though, a particularly heavy infestation aboard a
Spanish spice-ship captured by Sir Francis Drake was
noticed by Moffett (1634-58) in Britain's first book devoted
to entomology. Roth and Willis (1960) quote Rehm (1945)
for the information that at least 11 domiciliary species of
Blattidae have become established in other parts of the
world following shipborne dispersal from their centers of
origin. They also declare that "over 40 nondomiciliary
species have been carried by ship from the American Tropics to other parts of the world in cargoes of bananas,"
providing details for each instance. Their fascinating
summary of reports of cockroaches from vessels in general,
cites Williams (1931) for the facts that "*Blattella germanica*
was the most important cockroach pest seen on ships at New
York" and that "it was not unusual to kill 20,000 to 50,000
in the forecastle, and more than 20,000 have been taken
from a single stateroom." Of Pacific relevance is Captain
William Bligh's (1792) account of how in Tahiti (January
1789) he protected his freshly gathered breadfruit plants
(destined for the West Indies) from the depredations of
cockroaches, by ordering all the chests to be taken ashore
from HMS *Bounty* and her interior to be washed down with
boiling water to destroy these insects. Also germane to our
region is Lewis' (1836) pest-bedeviled voyage from England
to Tasmania, when hundreds of cockroaches–thought by
Roth and Willis to be *Periplaneta americana* and *Blattella
germanica*–flew about his cabin nightly. Perhaps making a
virtue of necessity, some, like Packard (1877) have put in
a good word for shipboard cockroaches, arguing their
usefulness as predators upon bedbugs. While there are
numerous earlier and later statements to the same effect,
Roth and Willis (1960) advance contrary viewpoints. In any
event, former widespread faith in this supposed virtue of
cockroaches seems to have died with the virtual disappearance of bedbugs from ships' bunks and hotel beds since
DDT and later synthetic organic pesticides became available
in powdered formulations.

Similar accounts could be presented for other now-
cosmopolitan domiciliary insects. For proper balance, too,
it should be observed that pests of other kinds than insects
also became widely dispersed by shipping long ago. Rats
and mice are obvious examples. From classical times, black
rats, or ship rats (*Rattus rattus*) and the oriental rat fleas
(*Xenopsylla cheopis*) infesting them, must have accompanied

Asian land traffic moving west—whether warrior nomads from the Huns and their predecessors to the Mongol hordes of Ghengis Khan, or the camel caravans following the silk road to the Mediterranean. With these rats and fleas and the merchants or the warriors they accompanied, came *Yersinia pestis*; the causal agent of bubonic plague, originally acquired from gerbils of this disease's endemic areas in eastern and central Asia. The earlier epidemics thus intermittently triggered in the Mediterranean area are inextricably confused with other diseases in the sketchy historical record. They radiated from eastern Mediterranean ports from Sidon (today's Saïda) in Lebanon to Alexandria in Egypt, where the ancient center of Pelusium had a particularly infamous record (Cloudsley-Thompson 1976). In particular, this meeting point of the camel caravans from the east with westward-bound shipping was central to the spread of the first of the three major plague pandemics; the Great Plague of Justinian, which reached Europe via Byzantium (Constantinople, today's Istanbul) in the middle of the sixth century A.D. In 1347 the next such pandemic—the Black Death—reached Europe, also by way of Constantinople, which presumably received shipping from the Crimea and other parts of the Russian Black Sea coast—caravans came to that region from central Asia where it is known that deaths in large numbers, including plague deaths, were already taking place among the Mongols in the late 1330s. China suffered too; as quoted by Cloudsley-Thompson (1976): "Some recorded that fleets of ships drifted about aimlessly, their entire crews dead of plague." The third pandemic arose in China in the middle of the last century. Reaching the Pacific ports of Canton (today's Guangzhou) and Hong Kong in 1894, it had spread around the world by 1922. This pandemic, still in the final stages of decline, caused outbreaks in Australia, Hawaii, and Latin America in 1899, Singapore in 1901, Thailand in 1904, and Indonesia in 1910 (Cloudsley-Thompson 1976).

European house mice (*Mus musculus*) were readily dispersed by shipping, too. According to Zárate (1556) as translated by Cohen (1981), the first were brought to Peru by a ship of the expedition despatched by the Bishop of Plasencia. Having passed through the Straits of Magellan into the Pacific, this vessel coasted northwards to Los Reyes. The rodents that it brought subsequently became extremely abundant throughout the country, their litters apparently being transported in boxes or bales of merchandise carried by land from one center to another. The Peruvian Indians dubbed the newcomer "*ococha* which means something that has come out of the sea."

SOME RECENT PEST IMPORTATIONS
BY SEA AND AIR

Rodents, snails, spiders

So might the people of Tuvalu have called the same animal
when that group's very first cargo container was winched
down to Funafuti's fine new deep-water lagoon wharf on 18
October, 1981 (Figure 15-1). As it was opened, house mice
were seen to emerge (Mr. Sam Rawlins, Agricultural Division, Tuvalu, personal communication). But "something
that has come out of the *air*" also applies at times to mice,
as well as to a host of other pests, in the modern era.
Thus Harper (1961) relates how a stowaway mouse
(*Peromyscus*) was seen descending a metal strut (it returned whence it came on finding where it was!) of a
prospector's float plane after the latter alighted at
Ashuanipi Lake, Quebec Province, Canada, in 1953. The
more startling instance reported by Dr. Takahashi in
Chapter 4—where a *Rattus rattus,* newly escaped from the
parcel in which it had reached Tokyo from South Africa,
proved to be harboring an oriental rat flea—serves as a
reminder that even though the danger of catastrophic
bubonic plague has diminished with the availability of a
vaccine and general resumption of the disease's endemic
status in wild rodent populations around the world, the
vector continues to travel about, to the extent that, for
instance, in the South Pacific, it is nowadays established in
all Australian east coast ports from Sydney northwards
(Chapter 10). As Cloudsley-Thompson (1976) expresses it,
"public health and port authorities cannot afford to relax
their vigilance. With death in the yard, one dare not leave
the door ajar."
    The giant African snail, *Achatina fulica,* has lately been
profiting from modern transportation very much along the
lines of *Mus musculus.* Like the latter, it has been finding
shipping containers a ready means of dispersal. Thus, as
Dr. Dharmaraju reports in Chapter 13, the appearance of
this pest in Western Samoa has led to legislation prohibiting
the removal from Apia's wharf of containers loaded in
A. fulica areas, until agricultural quarantine officers have
declared them uninfested. There is also a story, for which
I have yet to see confirmation, of one of these snails being
watched inching down the landing gear of an aircraft newly
arrived at Faleula Airport, near Apia, from American
Samoa. Elsewhere, a wheelbay has even provided refuge to
a child stowaway. Clearly, then, this unlikely type of
cavity must not be overlooked in the quarantine situations

Figure 15-1. Unloading part of the cargo from the *Morning Star,* Funafuti, Tuvalu. House mice emerged from the first of these containers ever to be opened on the atoll (photographed M.L., 18 October 1981).

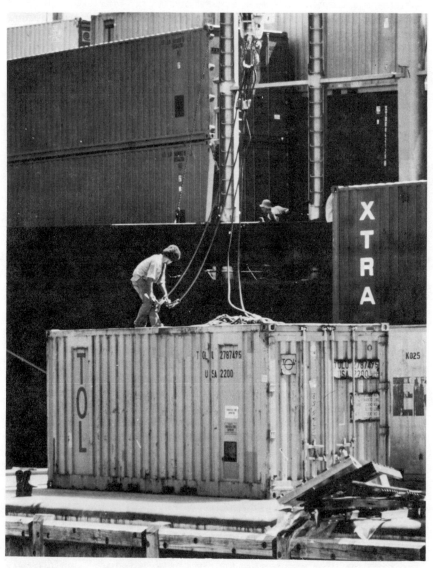

where an area is deemed at special risk to a particular pest.

Before returning to the central theme of pest insects, the Roth and Willis (1960) survey of cockroaches in banana cargoes brings back teenage memories of occasional flurries of excitement in mid-1930s Wellington when bananas and other tropical Pacific islands produce being unloaded on the waterfront yielded "a huge hairy spider" or two. As Parrott (1952) indicates, the huntsman or banana spider (*Heteropoda venatoria*) is adventive in New Zealand. With a leg-span of ca 10 cm this spider is certainly conspicuous, although harmless other than to cockroaches (it is nevertheless sobering to share a tropical Pacific bathroom with a *Heteropoda* as it slowly munches the full-sized *Periplaneta americana* clutched to its mandibles, as illustrated by Roth and Willis in their Plate 30).

The more secretive and potentially dangerous Australian redback spider, to which Chapter 14 is devoted, seems to have been aided by container shipping in gaining its first establishment in New Zealand. The discussion stimulated by Dr. Lyn Forster's presentation at Dunedin elicited the further information from Dr. Nigel Wace (personal communication) that the removal of a U.S. Coast and Geodetic Survey satellite-tracking station from Narrabri, NSW, Australia, to Tristan da Cunha in 1967-68 was responsible for an Australian redback introduction into this south Atlantic island. The freighted equipment traveled via the United States, first by air to Honolulu, Hawaii, (where while the passenger cabin was disinsected the crates remained in the hold so that even had spraying been undertaken there, arthropods imprisoned within them would have been substantially protected from the insecticide); then on to Miami, Florida, where there was a three-week stay before the station material was forwarded to Tristan by sea, being unloaded on 27 January 1968, and re-erected soon afterwards. In March of that year, while undertaking a botanical survey, Wace (1968) "was astonished to discover some specimens of the Australian red-backed spider (*Latrodectus hasseltii*)." There were no previous reports of *Latrodectus* spp. from Tristan da Cunha; subsequently, the tracking station staff killed more spiders in their equipment.

It should be added that arachnids are not commonly collected from planes (Chapter 7). Live ones were only noticed in two (0.1%) of my own ca 1,800 flights for which records were kept since 1960, one of them aboard an American Airlines Boeing 707 flight from Auckland, New Zealand, to Nadi, Fiji, in August 1972. There had been no blocks-away disinsection, so it was presumably take-off vibration that stimulated a spiderling, just as we became airborne, to let itself down from the outer edge of the overhead luggage bins into the back of a collar worn by a lady seated four rows in front of me. The seatbelt signs were on, and as it was only a tiny and distressed spider anyway, it seemed pointless to risk spoiling her flight by mentioning the matter.

Cosmopolitan domiciliary pests: cockroaches and muscoid flies

Reverting to the question of cockroach dispersal, these pests made the transition to air travel with ease. Roth and Willis (1960) summarize the earlier reports concerning aircraft, adding some previously unpublished identifications of their own and drawing attention to a 1930s problem no longer applicable in international aviation half a century later; Michel (1935) had observed that aside from the hygienic issue of the contemporary prevalence of cockroaches in airplanes, these insects were congregating in the wings to feed on the glue and dope that were then common materials of aircraft construction. While concluding that the truly domiciliary cockroaches "are likely to be pests on shipboard as they are in land-based structures," Roth and Willis (1960) felt that "all-metal aircraft would seem to provide little in the way of food or water for stowaway cockroaches." Were this indeed so, one might have expected to detect from modern records a conspicuously changed situation from the one pertaining at Darwin, NT, Australia, in 1937-38; when, at a time shortly before all-metal aircraft began to dominate aviation, cockroaches were the insects most commonly found in flight arrival searches (Chapter 7). Four decades afterwards, although dealing exclusively with all-metal aircraft from Tridents to Boeing 747s, Takahashi (Chapter 4) was not only able to report 3 families, 5 genera and 7 species of Blattidae from flights reaching Tokyo from abroad, but also he was confident that "in many cases it appeared that these cockroaches inhabited the plane. . . ."

The most dramatic example of the latter state of insanitariness to have come my way, was furnished by Dr. D. W. Roberts (1977 personal communication); who both counted "several hundred" cockroaches of all sizes crawling on the bulkhead between his seat and the kitchen of an Indian Airlines flight from Hyderabad to Bombay in November 1976, and during the first hour personally killed 100 of them. His recommendation to the airline administration that the problem be solved by regular fumigation was eminently reasonable. In this connection, Dr. A. C. Turner, Senior Overseas Medical Officer of British Airways, had shortly before written to me (1975 personal communication) that "as long as there are cockroaches, flies, rats or other pests at airports there is always the possibility they will be found on aircraft. The problem is to prevent the buildup of an infestation if the insects breed in galley areas. Any airline which ignores this will cause a problem." Dr. Turner went on to say that British Airways (Overseas Division) had thus introduced a three-monthly fumigation with the residual carbamate Ficam W on all aircraft, noting that "Boeing 747s are more liable to infestation than other types because of the galley modules which are taken off at overseas stations and replaced with others, sometimes with cockroaches present" and observing that all such modules were being so treated.

This matter of aircraft infestation with now-cosmopolitan domestic pests is germane to Dr. Turner's comments on those galley modules. The presence of module-associated colonies of insect pests is clearly distinct from more adventitious risks like the relatively less frequent carriage of free-flying pests and vectors such as malaria vectors of the genus *Anopheles*.

Such infestation with the commoner domestic pests is in fact primarily a biological indication of poor sanitation. In "bush" accomodation in the tropics, it is commonplace for cockroaches and other domiciliary pests, such as *Pheidole* ants in the South Pacific, to enter baggage—especially when left open to air, as it so frequently has to be. As often as not, a few such insects will be trapped in bags when these are closed and locked for departure. If the closure is tight, these stowaways are likely to avoid exposure to pesticides even when baggage holds are routinely disin- sected. Depending on whether or not there are customs checks, they may not escape until the traveller finally unpacks; perhaps in a hotel or at home in a country far from where the baggage invasion took place. Dale and Maddison (Chapter 12) make a related point with regard to economic pests stowing away in luggage. As even hospitals may be plagued by cockroaches at times (Roth and Willis 1960), it is no surprise that the most exemplary hotels may also be—whether the presence of these pests in bedrooms represents spill-over from infestations elsewhere in the building, or the survival of examples brought in with a previous occupant's belongings. Cabin baggage among the latter can also contain cockroaches acquired at intermediate stops. Thus in the otherwise clean but, in my experience, usually cockroach-infested washrooms of Papeete's inter- national airport, compulsory disembarkation on early morning stopovers provides (a) passengers (on long eastbound flights from Australasia to the west coast of the USA) with the chance of freshening up, and (b) resident cockroaches with travel opportunities via exploration of the open overnight bags scattered along the floor under the washbasins.

Whatever the route involved, I had *Supella supellectilium*—listed by Rehn (1945) among the originally African species that reached the New World aboard slave ships—as a fellow-guest in rooms occupied during the 1970s in such impeccable hotels as New York's Waldorf Astoria and Sydney's Wentworth. Some earlier records of this species from aircraft are summarized by Roth and Willis (1960), and a species of *Supella* is among the cockroaches lately identified from flights arriving at Tokyo (Chapter 4).

Turning to recent examples of the carriage of Blattidae by sea and land, the *Evening Telegram* (St. John's, Newfoundland) for 21 October 1977 reported Royal Canadian Mounted Police testimony that when 6.5 tons of Colombian hashish were intercepted aboard a yacht off Nova Scotia in May 1977, the resultant two truckloads of seized freight had first to be fumigated to kill the large cockroaches swarming in the contraband. An 8 January 1979 item in the same newspaper reported that in Milwaukee County, Wisconsin, cockroaches were finding urban buses "a nice spot for a banquet" because of littering. This example of a decline in public hygiene could be endlessly duplicated in a world where standards in such matters continue to fall as an inevitable outcome of increasing disrespect for authority on the one hand, and reluctance to enforce regulations on the other.

Such a state of affairs is also only too obvious as regards muscoid flies, particularly the housefly, *Musca domestica* and its diminutive relative, *Fannia canicularis*. There are innumerable records of muscoid flies from routine collections of aerosol-killed insects made aboard aircraft. Thus 295 (31.6%) of 928 aircraft reported upon by Takahashi (Chapter 4) were positive for them—955 examples in all, referable to 4 families, 8 genera, and 9 species, with *M. domestica* being the commonest of these. Throughout the past two decades I made personal observations concerning the presence of insects on aircraft and other disinsection matters, during some 1,800 flights involving landings in more than 100 countries. Being purely sight observations within the passenger section, these records are in no way comparable with properly organized collections by quarantine officers; the bulk of whose material is in the form of dead (often long-dead, Chapter 7) insects both hand-collected and sifted from vacuum-cleaner bags.

Moreover, much of the material reported upon (as in Chapters 3 and 7) is from baggage and cargo compartments. Even so, my records of live muscoid flies (*Musca domestica* being most commonly identified, with *Fannia canicularis* in second place) extend to 115 (6.8%) of 1,677 aircraft of many types from helicopters and small private planes through all the major commercial models up to the Concorde. In the last-mentioned connection, which concerned a 1978 British Airways flight from Heathrow Airport, London, to John F. Kennedy Airport, New York, a few *M. domestica* had been active during the preflight champagne and caviar festivities in the departure lounge. I had entertained hopes of logging the species once on board, but in the event no stowaway insects were to be found during the flight. However, an air hostess serving exclusively on Concordes assured me that she had been noticing houseflies during about every second supersonic flight that she made. Interestingly enough, the incidence of houseflies aboard jumbo jets appears to be substantially higher than on smaller aircraft, for which the percentage of 6.8% already given applies. My relevant figures for 102 flights in wide-bodied jets of all kinds show that 20 (19.6%) exhibited live muscoids, which were particularly evident near galleys. The specific figures for the Boeing 747 are highest of all, these flies having been observed in 12 (35.2%) of my 34 flights, bearing out an earlier published observation (Laird 1975).

Buffalo-flies, mosquitoes, and biting midges

By 1938-41, the buffalo-fly (*Lyperosia exigua*) was being intercepted aboard aircraft reaching Darwin, Australia, from the north (Chapter 7). So were the widespread mosquito vectors of disease, *Aedes aegypti* and *Culex quinquefasciatus*, and northwestern Pacific anophelines of four species including "good" malaria vectors. The buffalo-fly and the first two mosquitoes had already become established in Australia long before. For example, Tillyard (1931) believed that *Lyperosia exigua* had originally entered from the north "by way of Melville Island at the time when the first buffalos were introduced there. This was as early as 1825." Then, in 1826, Hawaii's freedom from mosquitoes (something that the earlier foreign visitors and residents had rhapsodized about in their correspondence home) ended (Bryan 1934) with the shipborne arrival of *Culex quinquefasciatus*. Hawaiians now began coming to the missionaries for help in connection with a new disease, characterized by reddish, itchy bumps on the skin, and a buzzing in the ears!

C. *quinquefasciatus* continues to be prominent among collections from ships and aircraft in the Pacific. Takahashi (Chapter 4) claims it to be the mosquito most frequently captured on flights arriving at Tokyo from abroad, and a recent establishment in the Tokelau Islands is discussed in Chapter 5. Besides its well-known public health importance, *C. quinquefasciatus* is also a major vector of avian malaria. The extension of its range in the Pacific could have serious implications for the transmission of *Plasmodium* spp. among birds, especially indigenous island species lacking immunity. Much the same applies to range extensions of biting midges of the genus *Culicoides* (Chapter 5), which includes vectors of other avian haematozoa.

In Chapter 5, Pillai and Ramalingan also consider the recent arrival of *Aedes aegypti* in Tokelau and Sabah (Malaysia), while Dale and Maddison (Chapter 12) note that this DHF vector apparently reached Niue as a result of hurricane relief activities in 1969. *A. aegypti*'s 1979 interception at San Francisco International Airport, the subject of Chapter 6, also serves as a reminder that vectors (like economic pests such as the "Medfly") absent from certain parts of a continental area can as readily be imported via the national aviation network as from abroad. Moreover, and recollecting the point made by Dale and Maddison about bewaring of Greeks bearing gifts, it must be admitted that researchers themselves sometimes bypass the proper official channels in mailing strains of exotic insects to one another, in what they consider to be the best interests of science. Such action can lead to new field acclimatizations of potentially dangerous insects long-established in laboratory colonies for research purposes. Thus during the 1960s, in the midst of intensive efforts by WHO (via the Pan American Health Organization and with strong United States Public Health Service involvement) to eradicate *Aedes aegypti* from the Americas, it proved that eggs of this vector were being blithely shipped from scientist to scientist all over North America, without the slightest regard to quarantine implications. When taxed with such behavior, scientists are sometimes defensive, Canadian-based ones, for example, rather scornfully stating that even if *A. aegypti* escaped north of the 49th parallel, conditions would be too severe for it to breed. I would question such an excuse with respect to some parts of Canada, British Columbia for example, Surtees et al. (1971) having demonstrated the survival and development of an outdoor experimental colony of *A. aegypti* in southern England.

Again, as the late Bill Sullivan reminded me to include in the book that we were planning to write in the 1970s, *Glossina* spp. have been even more widely shipped about in recent years for the establishment of laboratory colonies earmarked for research purposes; often in countries far beyond their African natural habitat and sometimes in savanna situations where it is not beyond the bounds of possibility that escaped tsetse flies (and not all of the facilities concerned are rigidly maintained in properly insect-proofed state) could establish feral populations.

Something rather alarming along these lines happened in the North Pacific just over a decade ago, when Africa's most notorious malaria vector, *Anopheles gambiae*, was imported to the island of Palawan, Philippines, by Japanese investigators planning to use the mosquito in testing antimalarial drugs following the failure of efforts to colonize indigenous anophelines in this connection (Gabriel 1972). Although it was claimed by the investigators concerned that following their experiments all remaining *Anopheles gambiae* were destroyed, this led to a great deal of adverse news-paper and other publicity in the Philippines. The incident serves as a prime example of how utterly irresponsible it is to place any possibly receptive locality at risk in such a fashion. Any tropical Pacific island with surface water must be considered at risk with respect to *Anopheles gambiae* and indeed malaria vectors in general. Similar risks inevitably arise from the deliberate importation of *any* mosquitoes, aside from such special cases as the nonbiting *Toxorhynchites* spp. sometimes imported because of the biocontrol value of their predacious larvae (even then it is, of course, essential to ensure that such importations are made in the complete absence of other larvae—those of *Aedes aegypti*—used as food for these predators in laboratory colonies or production facilities). In venturing these remarks I have particularly in mind past arguments advanced by professional entomologists for the deliberate establishment of strains of *Aedes albopictus* in eastern Polynesia, with a view to attempting the competitive displacement of *A. polynesiensis* (a vector of Bancroftian filariasis, dengue and RRV). Surely, however plausible such experiments may seem as extrapolations from the encouraging results of preliminary experiments in laboratories elsewhere, it can only be regarded as foolhardy to countenance anything of the kind; because *A. albopictus* is itself a vector, not only of dengue but also (in southeast Asia—Gould et al. 1968; Rudnick and Chan 1965) of DHF.

Thus, while some investigators have advocated the use of *A. albopictus* for competitive displacement experiments in eastern Polynesia, others have been viewing with alarm the spread of this same mosquito into the southwestern Pacific, where it was unknown east of PNG before 1978, when Elliott (1980) discovered that it had become established, possibly by shipping from PNG, in Guadalcanal and the Santa Cruz group, Solomon Islands. It had been hoped to include Susan Elliott (now Mrs. Hogge) among the participants in the Dunedin Symposium in the interests of a general discussion on the prospect raised in her paper that by persisting in its advance eastwards in the South Pacific as traffic continued to increase, *A. albopictus* might further enhance the risks of dengue and DHF outbreaks; but unfortunately she was unable to accept the invitation. Chapter 5 includes further information on this recent establishment and on the still-more recent discovery of *A. albopictus* breeding in the Caroline and Marshall Islands, where flights from Saipan or Guam may have been involved. Also, Russell et al. (Chapter 7) record interceptions of this mosquito on flights reaching Perth, Western Australia, and Darwin, NT, in 1974-79 from tropical airports to the north.

Ward (Chapter 8) documents the history of mosquito introductions into Guam, where no less than 14 of the 24 species now established seem to have arrived since the end of World War II. This is indeed the writing on the wall for other Pacific islands beginning to serve similarly as major crossroads of civil and military aviation—for five of those introduced species are anophelines. The first of them to become established was *Anopheles indefinitus,* which is not known to be a malaria vector in that area; the evidence suggests that it had been introduced several years before its discovery in 1948, as a result of wartime troop movements. Two more anophelines were recorded from Guam by Darsie and Ramos (1971). These were *Anopheles vagus* (which is not considered a vector of human disease), and *A. subpictus,* (an important malaria vector in parts of Indonesia and perhaps of some importance in parts of India). By 1975, when there had been a history of several years of intensive military air traffic between Guam and Vietnam, two further anophelines had arrived. These were *Anopheles barbirostris* (a possible vector of malaria and filariasis in Sulawesi, Indonesia) and *A. litoralis* (a known malaria vector on at least one island of the Philippines). The latter species was not recorded with certainty from Sabah, Malaysia, until 1974 (Chapter 5).

Two of the anophelines now established on Guam (*A. barbirostris,* the identification of which was queried, and *A. vagus*) had been collected aboard flights reaching Darwin from the north shortly before World War II. So had two other members of the genus, including *A. sundaicus,* which (along with more examples of *A. barbirostris* and *A. vagus* and a third member of Guam's introduced anopheline fauna, *A. subpictus*) Russell et al. (Chapter 7) also identified from their 1974-79 interceptions. Moreover, *A. vagus* and *A. subpictus,* together with a fourth species of Guam's present anopheline complex, *A. indefinitus,* are among the mosquitoes recorded from aircraft reaching Tokyo, Japan, from the south in the 1970s (Chapter 4). It should be added that *Anopheles sundaicus* is a significant malaria vector in parts of Indonesia and elsewhere in south and southeast Asia. Like the other anopheline stowaways mentioned in this paragraph, it does not occur in Australia, where potentially suitable larval habitats are present in the vicinity of Darwin (Chapter 7).

These data surely indicate that countries of the Pacific from which malaria has been eradicated or where vectors do not occur, have been at risk for a long time, and continue to be so, from anophelines clearly inadequately controlled on and around southeast Asian and Indonesian/Melanesian airports from which they receive traffic—the risk equally clearly being higher in the case of night departures as mentioned in Chapter 1. From Chapter 4 it would seem that the international airports of Manila, Taipei, and Hong Kong have been acting as major sources of mosquito pests and vectors for aircraft flying from them to other countries. Like Port Moresby, PNG, and Denpasar, Indonesia (see Chapter 7), they appear to lack effective airport insect control systems. To give but one example of the likely magnitude of the control problems involved, a survey by Basio (1973) revealed that no less than 60 species of mosquitoes were present within the Manila International Airport and its environs, 14 of them being anophelines. The latter included three of the species established in Guam since the late 1960s, *Anopheles litoralis, A. vagus,* and *A. indefinitus.* The last two are among the importations intercepted on aircraft arriving in Tokyo from the south in recent years, while *A. vagus* was collected aboard aircraft arriving in Darwin, Australia, from the north both before World War II and in the late 1970s.

In so far as is known, recent anopheline range extensions in the Pacific have been confined to the tropical northwestern sector. However, there have been numerous apprehended importations of these mosquitoes elsewhere, besides a decided increase of imported malaria in people entering or returning to Australia (Goldsmid Chapter 10). Moreover, a Great Circle line drawn from Sabah through Guam, weighted at the latter island by its five now-established anophelines, can be viewed as a dagger pointing towards Hawaii, which offers a wide range of larval habitats seemingly suited to these vectors although currently harboring only imported culicines. In its turn, Hawaii, with Honolulu's large and busy international airport, is the major aviation crossroads between North America, southeast Asia, the malaria-free tropical Pacific Islands east of Buxton's Line (170°E) and the islands, including New Zealand, south of 20° South. Three decades ago studies of larval mosquito ecology throughout this fortunate area (to this day not yet penetrated by any species of *Anopheles*) showed clearly that there is no cryptic ecological reason for such freedom from *Plasmodium* vectors and malaria. The situation simply reflects the fact that vast ocean barriers have so far disposed against anopheline introductions and establishments (Laird 1956). Of all major geographical regions, this one is certainly the most vulnerable to relevant accidents, for example, that of RRV into Fiji, the tropical crossroads for South Pacific aviation (Chapter 11).

World War II ended on a note of much anxiety in Australia (Chapters 7, 8), New Zealand (Chapter 13), and Fiji (Laird 1951), that exotic species of *Anopheles* efficient as *Plasmodium* vectors might become established after escaping from arriving aircraft. Conscientious efforts to kill insects aboard arriving aircraft were thus made from the mid-1940s onwards at the main international airports of Australia, New Zealand, and Fiji as aviation steadily expanded. These efforts fitted in well with the disinsection measures already enforced at Honolulu under the pressure of the continuing establishments of agricultural pests as summarized by Van Zwaluwenburg (1947), who held aviation chiefly to blame for the establishment of 28 exotic species of insects (including 9 agricultural pests) in Hawaii between 1944 and 1947–this despite the fact that what were probably the world's most thorough airport disinsection measures were then already enforced at Honolulu airfields receiving military as well as civil international flights.

Over the years 1957-77 there was a seven-fold increase in overseas flight arrivals at Haneda, Tokyo, from 3,711 to 25,842 (Takahashi Chapter 4); while in the past decade alone the volume of air traffic recorded by some member countries of WHO's Regional Office for the Western Pacific has increased ten-fold (Self and Smith Chapter 9). Such facts, and the recent recognition of so many new vector establishments, emphasize the present urgency of the problem. To instance just one new route of particular relevance, there are now direct flights by Air Pacific directly from Port Vila, Vanuatu (where malaria is increasing and *Anopheles farauti* abounds) to Nadi, Fiji. Even though these are daytime flights, the fact that such services now exist foreshadows the continuing development of an aviation network that will inevitably bring malarious Melanesia into more and more frequent contact with the *Anopheles*-free Pacific islands—with potentially disastrous consequences unless adequate preventive measures are adopted.

As a final note on a mosquito introduction relevant to the "Beware of Greeks Bearing Gifts" sentiment expressed by Dale and Maddison (Chapter 12), Hawaii received its fifth accidentally established mosquito species when the neotropical leaf axil-breeder *Wyeomyia mitchellii* was brought in, apparently via an illegal importation of bromeliads from Florida. By the time this new arrival was first collected (4 July 1981) in Oahu, it had already adapted to native aroids as larval habitats (Shroyer 1981).

International dispersal of crop pests

Soon after Pemberton (1941) warned that because the moth taro pest (*Prodenia*)=*Spodoptera litura* had begun to fly into aircraft at night on the islands of Midway and Canton, it might thereby be brought to Hawaii, it duly became established there (Pemberton 1944). Laird (1952) afterwards identified as this species moths reared from egg masses that had earlier been recorded from exterior surfaces of aircraft reaching New Zealand from Fiji. Like some other widely dispersing insect pests (for instance, *Chrysomya*; Chapter 3), *S. litura* is now known to be capable of windborne transoceanic trips of upwards of 2,000 km (Fox 1978). Furthermore, as suggested by Dale and Maddison (Chapter 12), it could conceivably be spread from island to island via propagative material of taro (*Colocasia esculenta, Cyrtosperma chamissonis*)—a route earlier proposed (Laird 1956) as a possible means of dispersal for certain aquatic micro-hemipterans throughout tropical Polynesia in pre-European days.

Nevertheless, regardless of the possible significance of either of these two routes—one involving purely natural agencies and the other, ancient Polynesian canoe travel—*S. litura* is continuing to be found entering New Zealand via newer means of transportation, for example, seaborne cargo containers (Keall 1981).

Chapter 12 and 13 provide other examples of establishments of economic pests that have taken place lately in the South Pacific, both of them referring to the coconut stick insect, *Graeffea crouanii*. "Devoid of obvious aids to dispersal," this pest may have been helped on its way to so many of the Polynesian islands by the fact that its eggs often become lodged at the bases of palm leaflets and may thus be worked into the region's characteristic coconut-leaf baskets (Dale and Maddison Chapter 12). Perhaps adult insects themselves, after creeping into the same baskets, have been similarly transported; for while in Apia in April 1978 I watched a fully grown *G. crouanii* slowly descending a wooden pillar into a heap of miscellaneous baggage (belonging to a group of Polynesian entertainers) piled at its base. Including many plaited-leaf baskets and trunks, also rolled mats, this baggage was awaiting transport from a city hotel to the airport, and then on to an overseas destination.

Dispersal of economic pests
by air within a continent

During the disinsection-conscious days of World War II, the Japanese beetle (*Popillia japonica*) was found at Canadian airports beyond its then North American range. One record involved the discovery of two adult beetles in planes at an airport near Montreal (Baker 1944). Another (Gardiner 1945) concerned the presence of one of these beetles in an aircraft and a second one—which had presumably escaped from an aircraft—in the airport at Hamilton, Ontario. Here is an example of an aircraft-borne pest hazard from a member-country of the Pacific Science Association, which nowadays does not concern itself with aircraft disinsection except where CPAir undertakes spraying when required to do so by countries to which that airline flies in the South Pacific. One cannot but wonder whether at times the Spruce budworm (*Choristoneura fumiferana*) may not have been helped on its way to devastating eastern Canadian coniferous forests via the network of flights serving the whole area concerned? While windborne dispersal is usually blamed for this insect's recent eastward depredations, perhaps, as in the case of *Spodoptera litura* in Polynesia, commerce may be involved too?

THE PRACTICE OF DISINSECTION

"Bug bombs"

Prewar American experience concerning "insect quarantines" in Hawaii proved enormously beneficial to South Pacific islands that became involved in military activities during World War II and that must also be regarded as virtual "faunal vacuums" from the standpoint of exotic pest establishments. The availability of American aerosol dispensers, thanks to the pioneering efforts of Dr. Bill Sullivan and consequent development by USDA (Chapter 2), certainly greatly reduced vector-borne disease transmission in the military areas by placing "bug bombs" (a substantial proportion of the 30 million then manufactured) in the hands of members of the allied armed forces. The same aerosol dispensers were widely used for aircraft disinsection on wartime flights between the various Pacific islands. Undoubtedly, this greatly reduced accidental insect dispersal of all kinds.

Attitudes to disinsection

In view of the vast benefits due to "bug bombs" and many of their lineal descendants (Figure 15-2–the black dispenser shown on the bottom shelf is an example of the original Westinghouse "bug bomb"), it is ironic that so much of what we hear nowadays about aerosols is sheer speculation concerning a postulated adverse effect on the ozone layer and, hence, heightened cancer problems. Environmentalism has, in fact, been prominent among the factors causing a falling-off in the efficacy of international disinsection. For example, the testing of improved pesticide dispensers aboard commercial aircraft–a field in which many advances were made under the personal direction of Bill Sullivan from the 1950s through much of the 1970s–is nowadays likely to be interrupted by a demand "not to squirt that thing near me" from some passenger who has never been exposed to the real and immediate danger of vector-borne disease; and whose information on the alleged threat symbolized to him or her by the word "aerosol," "chemicals," or worse still, "DDT," comes from distorted tales published by the media with a view to selling newspapers and improving radio or TV program ratings.

Such fears have unnecessarily troubled aircrew members on occasion. Thus, at the height of the environmental activism brought to bear by the media against DDT in particular, an air hostess in the cabin crew of a Boeing 747, having made an announcement that postarrival disinsection would take place on arrival at Sydney, Australia, told me in response to questioning that she was in fact personally worried about exposure to DDT (from the WHO-recommended aerosol dispenser formulation then being

Figure 15-2. Part of the aerosol dispenser collection assembled by Mr. Jens A. Jensen, developer of the vapor disinsection system (Jensen 1968), USPHS, Savannah, Georgia. By 1962 more than 290 different products from "bug bombs" (that at front center, right, is the Westinghouse World War II version) to "Christmas snow" were being sold in aerosol containers (Fulton and Sullivan 1962) (photographed M.L., 9 November 1959).

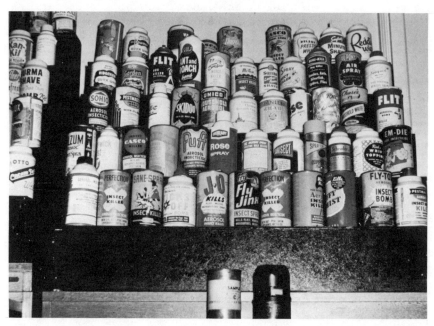

used), particularly as regards cumulative exposure among flight crew members. Apparently the recent death of a relatively young colleague had caused (altogether baseless) concern in this regard among her team. A few years afterwards, legal action was taken in the United States on behalf of The Association of Flight Attendants, and others, to try to stop the USDA's "practice of spraying airliners with insecticides such as DDT," the suit alleging "that the fumigation of the passenger and cargo compartments of planes, mostly to kill Japanese beetles and prevent them from being transported to other areas, could be injurious to the health of passengers and flight crews." (*The New York Times* 1977, datelined Washington 12 November). Had it been successful, that suit, filed by the Aviation Consumer Action Project (which was supported by Ralph Nader) could have done incalculable harm to aircraft disinsection in its broader aspects, thereby materially increasing vector establishment hazards and consequent human health problems.

Such misguided actions point to an information gap so wide that it will only be bridged by the most patient and sustained educational efforts by health and agricultural quarantine authorities. Fortunately, where relevant instruction forms part of an airline's routine training procedures, such troubles are not experienced. The necessary instruction has long been given to British Airways—formerly BOAC—cabin crew members (Laird 1960; Dr. A. C. Turner, personal communication 1975), enabling all concerned to acquire necessary expertise and a proper understanding of the rationale for disinsection, with full safety assurances respecting themselves (from the standpoint of their intermittent exposure to spraying over long periods of time) and the passengers, of all ages, for whom they are responsible.

Present requirements for aircraft disinsection on international routes

Recollecting the wide awareness of the logic of aircraft disinsection in the embattled world of 40 years ago and for the following two decades or so, it is a matter for concern that the past 20 years, which have seen such tremendous growth in international passenger transportation by air as well as fundamental changes in the movement of freight between countries by both sea and air, have also seen substantially less insistence upon such spraying than formerly. One factor in this has been worry in some of the third world countries—that stand to benefit most from the tourism has engendered much of the increase in air traffic—that the tourists in question might entertain strong objections to being sprayed with insecticide.

Thus since WHO (1961) laid the groundwork for universal standardization of aircraft disinsection, the pertinent recommendations in the IHR have been ignored by many of the recently independent states, which often have most to gain from consciencious application of those recommendations. I have the African countries particularly in mind, having over the period mentioned made 91 flights that landed in a total of 23 of the nations of Africa. During these flights, active arthropods were observed within the cabin on 25 (27.5%) occasions. Yet only once (1.1%) was disinsection ever practiced on any of the 13 types of aircraft of 23 companies concerned. That single instance of disinsection was well performed by a ground orderly following arrival in Cairo (aboard a Comet of United Arab Airlines) on 22 February 1965. However, the doors were then opened for disembarkation after only 2 minutes. This represented inadequate "holding time," the aerosol/pesticide spray requiring access to insects for at least 5 minutes to ensure proper insecticidal effect.

Taking my approximately 1,800 flights over this period as a whole, disinsection was only practiced (whether before departure, in flight, or following arrival) in 46 (2.6%) instances. Twenty-nine (63%) of these 46 disinsected flights took place in the Pacific region. The persisting awareness in that region of insect introduction hazards associated with aviation is particularly well displayed by these figures when it is appreciated that only 158 (8.8%) of those 1,800 flights took place there. Moreover, never once was on-arrival disinsection overlooked in my 10 international arrivals in New Zealand, or 6 in Australia. In the latter country, however although treatment was unfailingly well performed, a holding period of 5 minutes following spraying was only achieved once. On the other 5 flights, the commencement of disembarkation averaged 2-3 minutes after spraying ended. Much the same can be said for Fiji. Although on-arrival spraying usually took place there (and when it did was well conducted), a holding period of 5 minutes was not achieved prior to any of five disembarkations. In fact, after spraying ended, disembarkation once began immediately and otherwise after from only 1 to 2 minutes. At Auckland and Wellington, New Zealand, on the other hand, spraying was not only invariably well conducted but on nine (90%) of 10 occasions the aircraft doors were kept closed for at least 5 minutes (average 5.1 minutes) following the conclusion of spraying.

In all ca 1,800 flights "blocks away" spraying was only performed 5 times—twice at Honolulu (Hawaii) and once each at Pago Pago (American Samoa), Nadi (Fiji), and Sydney (Australia). The flights concerned were bound for Auckland (New Zealand) and Pago Pago from Honolulu, for Noumea (New Caledonia) from Sydney, for Honolulu from Pago Pago, and for Los Angeles from Nadi. "Blocks away" disinsection was advocated by WHO's Expert Committee on Insecticides in 1960 (WHO 1961) for the reasons that (a) on average more than 5 minutes had proved to elapse between the closing of aircraft doors following embarkation and actual take-off (thus allowing adequate "holding time" during which the efficacy of the pesticide spray was favored by the fact that this is a period when cabin ventilation is minimal), and (b) at the outset of an air journey passengers tend to be less impatient about any minor inconveniences associated with spraying than when eager to disembark on arrival. The actual time elapsing between the closing of the doors after embarkation and actual take-off, had proved to average 9.7 minutes on 27 flights aboard aircraft of 10 types (ranging from the war-time Dakota to Comet jets) in various parts of the world during a WHO consultantship undertaken as part of the preparation for the above WHO Expert Committee meeting (Laird 1960). In contrast, the period elapsing between touchdown on the same flights and the opening of the doors after the aircraft had halted on the tarmac outside the air terminal was always less than 5 minutes, indicating that postarrival spraying would inevitably delay disembarkation even if undertaken by cabin staff; it clearly would have caused rather longer delays if undertaken by airport per-sonnel entering planes on arrival, when at the least the delay solely ascribable to disinsection should amount to the few minutes required for actual spraying plus 5 more min-utes' holding time. Either way, it is clearly prudent to enforce such holding time (Smith and Carter Chapter 1) wherever circumstances demand on-arrival disinsection.

Despite the fact that the main disinsection recommen-dations published by WHO (1961) were repeated in sub-sequent editions of the IHR with emphasis on "blocks away" and postarrival timing, a substantial sector of world aviation (particularly the various airlines of America) continued to practice in-flight disinsection whether or not this was reinforced by "blocks away" or postarrival treatment called for by the national administrations of the countries of arrival or departure. In all my flying since the early 1960s I saw in-flight disinsection practiced 15 times, (that is, only 0.8% of ca 1,800 flights). Seven of these flights (operated by PAA, TWA, CPAir, and Qantas) concerned the Americas, and four (operated by British Airways, Swissair, and Air France) southern Asia. The remaining four took place in the Pacific (during Qantas and Air Pacific trips). One of these was one of two in-flight disinsections of my two-decade experience preceded by an announcement over the passenger address system. The flight concerned was operated by Qantas from Honolulu to Nadi, and the announcement warned passengers that they might feel momentary irritation as disinsection took place. Before two of the "blocks away" treatments and four of the postarrival ones already referred to (all 6 being in the Pacific), some preliminary information was also given to passengers.

This ranged from what I consider to be an undesirable approach to achievement of the perfect note. The first example (from a Continental DC10 flight on 26 October 1980 from Honolulu to Pago Pago) took a very negative stance. It failed to inform passengers of why disinsection is necessary and concentrated on the theme that there "is nothing in the insecticide spray to hurt humans . . . but if you have sinus problems keep your hot towel that we're handing out now, and hold it over your face during spraying." A negative announcement of this kind can only cause a degree of anxiety among the listeners, as was evident from comments heard from nearby seats. At the other extreme, a cheery announcement aboard a Qantas B747 bound from Sydney to Noumea on 19 February 1983 ran: "Disinsection is about to take place. We'll be spraying any nasty little insects that New Caledonia's quarantine wouldn't want. It's not so much the insects themselves as the fact they don't have a ticket. If you find the spray bothers you, place a handkerchief over your nose and mouth." That was received with laughter, and no complaints were heard. To my mind, a reassuring announcement of that kind goes far towards ensuring optimum public relations in the matter of disinsection. As was discussed during the 11th session of WHO's Expert Committee on Insecticides, an appropriate printed notice, perhaps associated with the safety information on the usual seat-pocket cards could prove effective too, particularly if the same combination of light approach and commonsense advice were achieved.

The optimum timing of disinsection

Reverting now to the question of precisely when disinsection should be carried out, the ideal remains as expressed by WHO (1961, 1968) and in subsequent annexes to the IHR (for example, WHO 1974); namely, that an automatic or semiautomatic built-in system be installed to inject an appropriate vapor pressure type insecticide into the cabin during flight (for a sufficiently long time to compensate for loss of active material via the air exchange system), thereby providing for an adequate holding time. In 1960, such a system was well advanced as a result of USPHS enterprise. Eight years later (Jensen 1968), it seemed as if it would be possible to install it in all pressurized commercial aircraft in the very near future. With practicality at last imminent—the World Health Assembly had in anticipation (WHO 1968) "recommended to Member States that pressurized aircraft in international flights should be equipped with the vapor disinsection system by 31 December 1970 and that, after that date, dichlorvos disinsection in flight or aerosol disinsection on the ground on arrival would be the only approved measures" (for nonpressurized aircraft the choice was to be between "blocks away" or on-arrival aerosol disinsection)—it proved that the vapor-pressure type pesticides could cause some corrosion of certain materials of aircraft construction.* During the 1970s, therefore, considerable time and effort by the late Dr. W. N. Sullivan and his group went into the developing of improved insecticidal formulations and their approval by WHO (Chapter 2) and the perfection of relevant low-pressure aerosol dispensers, notably "single shot" models discarded after one use. The question of whether in-flight disinsection with these really affords sufficient protection thus still applies, and good grounds remain for continuing to require that the choice should be between "blocks away" and on-arrival methodologies. A major problem with "blocks away" has been that some national administrators have proved quite unwilling to accept the degree of protection offered via disinsection before departure from another country, whether undertaken by ground personnel or the cabin crew.

This is a pity, because continuing flight observations have confirmed beyond any doubt that the predeparture period, besides being the best one from a psychological standpoint in terms of passengers and public relations, is the only regular segment of a flight operation during which disinsection may be effectively performed without any delay to normal aviation procedures of other kinds.

Thus, the elapsed times between the closing of the doors and the actual take-off for those of the approximately 1,800 flights already referred to, for which full data are available, breaks down as listed on page 318 (each figure is for 100 flights, except in the case of that for 1980-83 which includes 121; any postembarkation delays of longer than 30 minutes being discounted).

The overall mean interval (10.64 minutes) for the time elapsing between door-closing and take-off was remarkably close to the figure of 9.7 minutes reported by Laird (1960) from a sample of only 27 flights. Minor fluctuations evident from the list can be linked with specific explanations. For example, the lowest figure (8.86 minutes for 1960-63) reflects both the more leisurely air traffic of those years (see Table 1-1, Chapter 1) and the fact that a high percentage

---

*However, Qantas has developed an ingenious aerosol-can treatment system for the cargo holds of all its Boeing 747 aircraft, activated automatically by the pilot during take-off (Chapter 7).

Year	Mean Intervals	Range
1960-63	8.86 mins.	2.00-24.00 mins.
1963-66	10.66 mins.	1.50-27.75 mins.
1966-68	11.47 mins.	2.50-28.75 mins.
1968-69	11.00 mins.	4.00-28.25 mins.
1969-70	11.13 mins.	4.50-29.00 mins.
1970	10.75 mins.	3.50-26.00 mins.
1970-71	11.01 mins.	3.00-23.00 mins.
1971-72	10.20 mins.	4.25-24.50 mins.
1972-73	10.50 mins.	1.50-29.75 mins.
1973	9.29 mins.	2.75-26.00 mins.
1973-74	9.61 mins.	3.50-30.00 mins.
1974-75	11.88 mins.	0.25-29.50 mins.
1975-76	10.22 mins.	1.00-26.00 mins.
1976-77	10.52 mins.	1.50-28.50 mins.
1977-79	10.81 mins.	4.50-28.00 mins.
1979-80	11.78 mins.	3.50-27.00 mins.
1980-83	11.14 mins.	3.50-27.75 mins.

of flights were made aboard aircraft, such as C47s and Viscounts, having a capacity for rapid departure by comparison with today's large jets. The lowest figures in the ranges reported from 1963-66, 1972-73, 1975-76 and 1976-77 are due to departures aboard surviving such aircraft and also light aircraft, such as Cessnas; the lowest figure reported (0.25 minutes for 1974-75) is for one of several trips made aboard Bell Ranger helicopters that year. Interestingly enough, the mean for 1974-75, 11.8 minutes, is highest of all despite the inclusion of 6 helicopter take-offs, because many of the commercial flights made in that period took place aboard jumbo jets leaving busy major airports featuring traffic queues, 26 of the intervals between door-closing and take-off being above 15 minutes. It should be added that several of the means would have been rather higher had exceptional departure delays been included. Over the entire period in question, and discounting flights that were simply cancelled or for which no data were recorded, I experienced 32 take-off delays of more than 30 minutes. These were all due to exceptional circumstances, sometimes of a mechanical nature but mostly related to Canadian winter conditions.

On-arrival data for the same flights gave the following results: (each figure is for 100 flights except in the case of that for 1982-83 which includes only 48: any postlanding delays of longer than 15 minutes being discounted).

Year	Mean Interval	Range
1960-63	3.45 mins.	1.50-8.00 mins.
1963-66	3.95 mins.	1.50-8.00 mins.
1966-68	4.29 mins.	1.00-10.00 mins.
1968-69	4.62 mins.	2.25-9.00 mins.
1969-70	4.34 mins.	1.25-12.50 mins.
1970	4.44 mins.	1.75-12.00 mins.
1970-71	4.49 mins.	1.50-9.00 mins.
1971-72	4.82 mins.	1.25-15.00 mins.
1972-73	4.26 mins.	1.00-15.00 mins.
1973	4.31 mins.	1.00-12.50 mins.
1973-74	3.80 mins.	1.50-14.00 mins.
1974-75	4.55 mins.	0.00-10.00 mins.
1975-76	4.14 mins.	1.00-10.25 mins.
1976-77	4.00 mins.	1.50-12.00 mins.
1977-78	4.77 mins.	1.50-15.00 mins.
1978-80	4.62 mins.	1.50-12.50 mins.
1980-82	5.12 mins.	2.00-14.50 mins.
1982-83	4.63 mins.	1.50-14.00 mins.

The overall mean interval for the time elapsing between touch-down and the opening of the doors for disembarkation was 4.37 minutes.

Once again, there were a few abnormal delays—for example, once for 32.50 minutes through heavy snow and poor visibility and once for as long as 40 minutes when there was no ramp free at a major airport. Before walkways and loading ramps became part of major air terminal equipment, lengthy delays between landing and disembarkation were rare; thus only 2 longer than 6 minutes (8 and 8.5 minutes) were recorded for the 100 flights reported on for 1960-63, and 4 (2 of 7 minutes, 1 of 7.5 and 1 of 8) were recorded for the following 100, up to 1966. The first loading ramps then began to be introduced, and early in 1968 I experienced 10 minute and 21 minute delays while awaiting a free ramp position at O'Hare Airport, Chicago, and Dorval Airport, Montreal. By 1980-82, when the highest mean interval for landing-disembarkation (5.12 minutes) was recorded, no less than 10 (10%) of the flights in question were delayed for periods of from 9 to 45 minutes while awaiting free gate positions. This suggests that subject to continuation of the trend towards steadily increasing air traffic evident over the past two decades (see Figure 1, Chapter 1), the mean interval between touch-down and the opening of the doors may eventually increase to the point where postarrival disinsection by cabin crews would no longer mean delaying aircraft turnaround. For present purposes, however, it is obvious that the arguments against postarrival disinsection remain little changed from the situation prevailing at the beginning of the 1960s.

Smith and Carter (Chapter 1) restate the case against in-flight disinsection (although stressing the preoccupation of cabin staff with avoiding upsetting passengers, rather than considering the ineffectiveness of an aerosol spray too-early dispersed via the air exchange system); and while pointing to the relative effectiveness of on-arrival spraying, they recognize that from the standpoint of the aviation industry this still means increasing aircraft "turnaround" time. We thus necessarily get back to the timing most favored by the 11th session of WHO's Expert Committee on Insecticide, 1960 (WHO 1961), that is, "blocks away" disinsection.

At this point we must consider the factor that has caused some countries (especially in the malaria-free zone of the Pacific) to insist upon spraying by their own trained ground personnel. This is the question of whether flight crew can be relied upon to undertake the task efficiently. I personally believe that they can, especially when the training is as thorough as it has been for British Airways staff. At the same time, it must be conceded that especially since environmental activism became a political issue at the end of the 1960s, cabin crew members have often had to face levels of hostility among their passengers that would make it understandable were they not to perform disinsection as conscientiously as it must be done. There are, therefore, compelling reasons to have disinsection performed by ground personnel working under the mandate of local health or agricultural authorities. Just when the task is best carried out, though, remains to be settled. There is an additional reason beyond the common failure (for example, as in Australia and Fiji) to keep the doors closed for a full 5 minutes after spraying, why the on-arrival time is inappropriate. This is that because winged insects tend to be stimulated to flight at an aircraft's landing, there is the chance of their flying out of the door through which the ground personnel enter. This point was discussed by Laird (1948) with attention to the insect flight stimuli involved.

For example, on 22 April 1982 two houseflies were watched flying about the cabin of a De Havilland Heron of Air Tungaru, following landing at Tarawa, Kiribati, from Funafuti, Tuvalu. They continued to do so as the aircraft parked at the terminal; where, the door being opened for the entry of a local disinsection officer, one of the flies was seen to escape just as the door was closing again. This was the only such observation made in my ca 1,800 flights. However, it is considered that the implied 0.06% chance of such an eventuality, falls far short of the actual percentage probability; for in the great majority of today's commercial airliners, passenger seats are much less favorably located than mine was in that DH Heron for such an observation.

It suffices to accept that such escapes do occur intermittently, on the basis of the evidence that establishments of accidentally introduced pests and vectors continue to take place, and that escaped tropical vectors can sometimes survive long enough to transmit disease even where local circumstances preclude establishment (see Chapter 1).

One way of making it difficult for actively flying insect stowaways to escape during either the entry of airport personnel for on-arrival spraying before passenger disembarkation, or debarkation prior to on-arrival spraying as provided for in a 1979 U.S. regulation (Chapter 9), would be to have split curtaining at the doorway as suggested by Self and Smith. Whether this would be acceptable on grounds of safety and convenience is, of course, another matter. Another possibility where the aircraft is connected to the terminal building by an air bridge or walkway (lacking in many of the larger tropical airports and all of the minor ones) would be to treate them with suitable residual pesticides, as is being explored by USDA (Chapter 4).

On the whole, though, it must be concluded that pending some acceptable future procedure for automatic or semiautomatic in-flight disinsection, the "blocks away" procedure still offers the best guarantee that undesirable insects will not be accidentally exported to the airport of destination. In a discussion of this timing question at the conclusion of the Symposium, it was mentioned from the floor that the reinstitution of "blocks away" disinsection is under consideration in Australia. It was also suggested that because of past governmental lack of confidence in the ability of the cabin crew to perform this task efficiently, the best compromise solution might be for "blocks away" spraying to be conducted by quarantine personnel at the airport of departure. There was a general feeling that these matters merit the earliest possible solution at the international level.

Under what circumstances should it be mandatory to enforce vector and pest control on aircraft and ships?

The short answer to this question is wherever a particular country or region is demonstrably vulnerable to a perceived hazard from a particular pest or vector—for example, Brisbane, Queensland, Australia, to *Culicoides belkini* from Nadi, Fiji, as these places are now linked by Air Pacific (Chapter 5); and Nadi to *Anopheles farauti* from Port Vila, Vanuatu, for the same reason. However, the level of that risk reflects the opportunities for entry into aircraft or ships of the pest or vector in question, at an airport or port from which direct journeys take place to the receptive area. Thus one of the most recent reports of the north-ward advance of africanized "killer" bees from the American tropics concerns the arrival of a swarm (subsequently captured) in Baltimore aboard a containership (Morrill 1983).

In practice, there is rarely enough information available to the authorities of the country of arrival concerning the satisfactoriness of airport/port vector and pest control in the country of departure—hence, the continuing demand for on-arrival disinsection, despite the weaknesses of this approach and the delays imposed thereby. Once again there is need for action at the supranational level to pro-mote the achievement of adequate airport/port vector and pest control along international transportation routes—the present too-common neglect of these matters being some-thing for which the responsible governments must shoulder full responsibility.

CONCLUSION

Rather less than a quarter of a century ago, Roth and Willis (1960) predicted "that when man develops a suitable vehicle, cockroaches will someday accompany him into space." As they wrote, USDA research and development were already under way using restrained Madeira roaches experimental subjects in space vehicles (Sullivan et al. 1962, Chapter 2). Although this particular project had to be abandoned, other entomological investigations have since been undertaken in space. Indeed, as I conclude this chapter (20 June 1983) tonight's TV news has mentioned that the experiments currently in progress aboard the American space shuttle *Challenger* include one featuring ants. Scientifically planned experiments are one thing; but the presence of *any* uninvited living organisms on any space vehicle is quite another. Those alleged mosquito stowaways on an early Skylab trip (Chapter 2) do indeed raise the prospect that Dr. Dora Hayes suggests was in Bill Sullivan's mind (it was: he spoke of it to me in Australia in 1972), namely, that eventual permanent manned satellites might become infested with domiciliary insects. On present evidence, the exportation of such life from earth seems rather more likely than extraterrestrial importations. What better way is there to prevent such a contingency than by making real efforts to clean up our terrestrial disinsection act *now,* as a contribution towards WHO's professed goal of health for all by 2000 A.D.?

REFERENCES

Baker, M. R. 1944. Review of the Japanese beetle situation in Canada. 74th *Rep. ent. Soc. Ontario*:7-8.

Basio, R. G. 1973. The mosquito control program at the Manila International Airport and vicinity (Philippines) with comments on problems encountered on the aerial transportation of mosquitoes. In *Vector Control in Southeast Asia.* Singapore: Proc. 1st SEAMEO Workshop in Vector Control, 17-18 August 1972:78-84.

Beebe, W. 1953. *Unseen Life of New York as a Naturalist Sees It.* New York.

Bligh, W. 1792. *A Voyage to the South Sea . . . In His Majesty's Ship the "Bounty" . . .* London: Nicol.

Bryan, E. H. 1934. A review of the Hawaiian Diptera, with descriptions of new species. *Proc. Hawaii ent. Soc.* 8:399-468.

Cloudsley-Thompson, J. L. 1976. *Insects and History.* London: Weidenfeld and Nicolson.

Collinson, C., and F. McDermott. 1934. *Through Atlantic Clouds: The History of Atlantic Flight.* London: Hutchinson.

Darsie, R. F., Jr., and A. Cagampang-Ramos. 1971. Additional species of *Anopheles* on Guam. *Mosquito Systematics Newsletter* 3:28-30.

Elliott, S. A. 1980. *Aedes albopictus* in the Solomon and Santa Cruz Islands, South Pacific. *Trans. roy. Soc. trop. Med. Hyg.* 74:747-48.

Fox, K. J. 1978. The transoceanic migration of Lepidoptera to New Zealand—a history and a hypothesis. *N.Z. Ent.* 6:368-80.

Fulton, R. A., and W. N. Sullivan. 1962. Billions of bombs. In *Yearbook of Agriculture,* USDA: 358-59.

Gabriel, B. P. 1972. The *Anopheles* anxiety. Editorial, *Kulisap* (a quarterly publ. of the Philippine Assn Ent.), 4:2.

Gardiner, J. G. 1945. In *Rpt Min. Agr. Dominion of Canada, for the Year ended 31st March 1945.*

Gillispie, C. C. 1983. Aloft with the Montgolfiers. *The Sciences* 23:46-55.

Gould, D. J., T. M. Yuill, M. A. Moussa, P. Simasathien,

and L. C. Rutledge. 1968. An insular outbreak of dengue haemorrhagic fever. *Amer. J. trop. Med. Hyg.* 17:609-18.

Harper, F. 1961. In *Land and Fresh-water Mammals of the Ungava Peninsula.* Lawrence, Kansas: University of Kansas Press.

Jensen, J. A. 1968. Disinsection of aircraft used in international transportation—a description of the vapour disinsection system. WHO/VBC/68.85. Mimeographed.

Keall, J. B. 1981. *Interception of Insects, Mites and Other Animals Entering New Zealand 1973-78.* Wellington: N.Z. Min. of Agr. Fish.

Kisliuk, M. 1929. Air routes, German dirigible "Graf Zeppelin" and plant quarantines. *Ent. News* 40:196-97.

Laird, M. 1948. Reactions of mosquitoes to the aircraft environment. *Trans. roy. Soc. N.Z.* 77:93-114.

————. 1951. Insects collected from aircraft arriving in New Zealand from abroad. Wellington: *Publ. Zool. Vict. Univ. Coll.* 11.

————. 1952. Insects collected from aircraft arriving in New Zealand during 1951. *J. aviation Med.* 23:280-85.

————. 1956. *Studies of Mosquitoes and Freshwater Ecology in the South Pacific.* Roy. Soc. N.Z. Bull. 6.

————. 1960. Aircraft disinsectization and airport insect control. Ins. 11/Working Paper No. 1, WHO Expert Committee on Insecticides, Geneva. Mimeographed.

————. 1975. Insects from elsewhere. Guest editorial, *Can. J. publ. Hlth* 66:447-50.

Lewis, R. H. 1836. Notes made during a voyage from England to Van Diemen's Land, with a sketch of the entomology of the Cape of Good Hope. *Trans. ent. Soc. Lond.* 1:79-81.

Marion, F. 1870. *Wonderful Balloon Ascents; or, The Conquest of the Skies.* transl. London: Cassell.

Mason, O. T. 1896. Primitive travel and transportation. *Rep. U.S. Natl Mus. for 1894:*237-593.

Michel, C. 1935. Destruction des moustiques et autres insectes à bord des aéroplanes. *Off. Int. Hyg. publ. Bull. mens.* 27:553-57.

Moffett, T. 1634. *Insectorum sive minimorum animalium theatrum.* London: Thomas Cotes (transl., "Mouffet" *The Theatre of Insects: or, Lesser Living Creatures.* London: E. C. 1658, reprinted New York: Da Capo Press 1967)

Morrill, A. W. 1983. News and notes. *Mosquito News* 43:245.

Packard, A. S., Jr. 1877. *Half Hours With Insects.*

Boston: Estes and Lauriat.

Parrott, A. W. 1952. The banana spider (*Heteropoda venatoria* Linn.) recorded from New Zealand. *N.Z. Sci. Rev.* 10:129-30.

Pemberton, C. E. 1941. Entomology. *Rep. Comm. exp. Sta. Hawaii. Sug. Pl. Assn 1940-41*:21-27.

—————. 1944. Insects carried in transpacific airplanes. A review of quarantine work prior to December 7, 1941. *Hawaii Plant. Rec.* 48:183-86.

Piltz, H. 1981. The use of containers for stored products. *Eppo Bull.* 11:151-153.

Rehn, J. A. G. 1945. Man's uninvited fellow traveler—the cockroach. *Sci. Month.* 61:265-76.

Roth, L. M., and E. R. Willis. 1960. *The Biotic Associations of Cockroaches. Smithsonian Misc. Coll.* 141.

Rudnick, A., and Y. C. Chan. 1965. Dengue Type 2 virus in naturally infected *Aedes albopictus* mosquitoes in Singapore. *Science* 149:638-39.

Shroyer, D. A. 1981. Establishment of *Wyeomyia mitchellii* on the island of Oahu, Hawaii. *Mosquito News* 41:805-6.

Sullivan, W. N., M. S. Schechter, S. R. Dutky, J. C. Keller. 1962. Monitoring electrophysiological responses of cockroaches for space research. *J. econ. Ent.* 55:985-99.

Surtees, G., M. N. Hill., and J. Broadfoot. 1971. Survival and development of a tropical mosquito, *Aedes aegypti,* in southern England. *Bull. Wld Hlth Org.* 44:707-9.

Thomas, L. 1928. *European Skyways. The Story of a Tour of Europe by Aeroplane.* London: Heinemann.

Tillyard, R. J. 1931. The buffalo-fly in Australia. *Jour. Council Sci. Indus. Res.* Nov. 1931.

Van Zwaluwenburg, R. H. 1947. The insects of Canton Island. *Proc. Hawaii. ent. Soc.* 11:300-12.

Wace, N. M. 1968. Australian red-backed spiders on Tristan da Cunha. *Aust. J. Sci.* 31:189.

WHO. 1961. Aircraft disinsection. Eleventh Report of the Expert Committee on Insecticides. *Wld Hlth Org. techn. Rep. Ser.* 206:1-26.

—————. 1968. Twenty-first World Health Assembly. *WHO Chronicle* 22:334.

—————. 1974. International Health Regulations (1969). Second Annotated Ed. Geneva: WHO.

Williams, F. X. 1931. [Original not located: quotations secondary from Roth and Willis 1960].

Zárate, Agustín de. 1556. *Historia del descubrimiento y conquista del Peru. (Transl. of Books I to IV with additions, J. M. Cohen). The Discovery and Conquest of Peru.* 1981. London: The Folio Society.

Index

---

*Note: Page numbers in brackets refer to illustrations.

About the Editor

During World War II Professor Marshall Laird served in the Pacific campaign as Entomologist, Royal New Zealand Air Force; remaining with the RNZAF except while completing further university studies including his doctorate, until transferring to the Reserve of Air Force Officers in 1954 with the rank of Squadron Leader. His earlier research included investigations of reactions of mosquitoes to the aircraft environment, a project that took him to Japan in the spring of 1946 and led to the publication of reports in the *Transactions of the Royal Society of New Zealand* and in *Science* in 1948. Several more of his papers over the next few years also concerned aircraft disinsection, appearing in journals including *Nature,* the *Journal of the Royal Aeronautical Society,* and the *Journal of Aviation Medicine.* A move in 1954 to the Faculty of the (then) University of Malaya at Singapore led to a detailed study of airport insect control there, during which his wife, Elizabeth, assisted materially in field work. In 1959 Professor Laird traveled widely as a consultant to the World Health Organization while gathering material for the Eleventh Session of WHO's Expert Committee on Insecticides, which he chaired in Geneva in 1960. This meeting laid the foundations for the relevant section of the International Health Regulations. Subsequently, Professor Laird and the late Dr. W. N. Sullivan, Jr., maintained close contact over aircraft disinsection matters, joining forces in scientific presentations at meetings in Miami (1971, AIBS National Biological Congress, "Man and Environment II," "Symposium" World Trends in Epidemic Diseases") and Canberra (1972, 14 International Congress of Entomology). In November 1974 the former was invited to Ottawa to deliver a Banquet Address ("Jet aviation and international health") to the Tropical Medicine and International Health Division of the Canadian Public Health Association. This, and a consequent Guest Editorial in the *Canadian Journal of Public Health* ("Insects from elsewhere") furnished him with opportunities for expressing his growing concern over increasingly widespread neglect of the practice of disinsection.

Over the years his extensive travel in other connections enabled him to continue observations relating to aircraft disinsection, as summarized in Chapter 15 of this book.